THE
IMPACT
OF
FREUDIAN
PSYCHIATRY

THE
IMPACT
OF
FREUDIAN
PSYCHIATRY

Edited by Franz Alexander, M.D., and Helen Ross

FRANZ ALEXANDER, M.D.

THERESE BENEDEK, M.D.

HENRY W. BROSIN, M.D.

MARGARET W. GERARD, M.D.

MAURICE LEVINE, M.D.

JOHN W. LYONS, M.D.

LEON J. SAUL, M.D.

LOUIS B. SHAPIRO, M.D.

THOMAS S. SZASZ, M.D.

Phoenix Books

THE UNIVERSITY OF CHICAGO PRESS

CHICAGO & LONDON

First published in an expanded edition as
DYNAMIC PSYCHIATRY

THE UNIVERSITY OF CHICAGO PRESS, CHICAGO 60637
The University of Chicago Press, Ltd., London

International Standard Book Number: 0–226–01355–3

PREFACE

THIS volume offers to students of psychiatry a comprehensive view of dynamic psychiatry. The dynamic trend in psychiatry is the result of the impact of psychoanalysis, its theory, its method of investigation, and its therapy, upon the whole of psychiatry. Essentially this trend can be defined as the advancement of the study of psychiatry from a descriptive into an explanatory phase.

Through the application of the principle of psychological motivation to seemingly irrational psychopathological phenomena, it became possible to understand the deterioration of behavior as seen in neuroses and psychoses. This understanding was blocked so long as only the nature of conscious mental processes was known, since psychopathological phenomena do not follow the rational principles of conscious thought-processes. Psychopathology is characterized by regression to the primitive forms of unconscious processes similar to those which appear in dreams. The similarity between schizophrenic thought-processes and dreams was first noticed by Bleuler; the universal significance of unconscious processes and their peculiarities was first recognized by Freud and his followers.

Before Freud made known his discoveries and theories, the most that psychiatrists could do was to give a valid and detailed description of the symptomatology of psychiatric conditions, just as Cuvier and Linné did in the fields of zoölogy and botany. It was only after the principle of evolution was discovered by Darwin that their descriptive systems could be replaced by a dynamic concept and the differences between species understood.

The influence of Freud upon psychiatry was similar. In Europe, this influence was at first retarded by the feud which grew up between Freud and academic psychiatry and later by the deterioration of scientific activities, which followed the world wars. In the United States the emotional conflict between psychoanalysis and academic psychiatry was more remote and did not interfere substantially with the penetration of psychoanalytic concepts into psychiatry.

v

This penetration began about thirty years ago. The pioneers of this scientific movement were William A. White, Smith Ely Jelliffe, and Adolf Meyer. During the last three decades the assimilation of psychoanalysis by American psychiatry has gained momentum, and in recent years there has been a trend toward academic incorporation.

The impact of psychoanalytic concepts upon scientific developments is to be observed on six frontiers. (1) In clinical psychiatry proper, there have developed a psychopathology, based on dynamic concepts, and a psychotherapy, based on etiology. (2) On the border line between psychiatry and anthropology the study of personality development in different cultures has broadened the concept of basic human nature. (3) In experimental psychology another cross-fertilization has taken place, particularly in the field of clinical tests. (4) In animal psychology, particularly with the American disciples of Pavlov, another point of contact with psychoanalysis was made. (5) On medicine as a whole the influence of psychoanalytic concepts and methods is shown in a new orientation: the psychosomatic approach to physiology, general pathology, and therapy. (6) In child psychiatry perhaps the greatest influence of psychoanalysis has taken place.

The outgrowth of this sixfold scientific cross-fertilization is what may be termed "dynamic psychiatry."

This edition deals primarily with clinical and child psychiatry. For a comprehensive description of the impact on all six frontiers, the reader is referred to the original volume, *Dynamic Psychiatry*, from which these chapters have been drawn.

FRANZ ALEXANDER, M.D.
HELEN ROSS

CONTRIBUTORS

FRANZ ALEXANDER, M.D. Director, Psychiatric and Psychosomatic Research Institute, Mount Sinai Hospital, Los Angeles, California

THERESE BENEDEK, M.D. Staff Member, Institute for Psychoanalysis, Chicago, Illinois

HENRY W. BROSIN, M.D. Director, Western Psychiatric Institute and Clinics; Professor and Chairman, Department of Psychiatry, University of Pittsburgh School of Medicine, Pittsburgh, Pennsylvania

†MARGARET W. GERARD, Ph.D., M.D. Staff Member, Institute for Psychoanalysis, Chicago, Illinois

MAURICE LEVINE, M.D. Professor of Psychiatry and Director of the Department, University of Cincinnati College of Medicine, Cincinnati, Ohio

JOHN W. LYONS, M.D. University of Pennsylvania School of Medicine, Philadelphia, Pennsylvania

LEON J. SAUL, M.D. Professor of Psychiatry, Chief of Section of Preventive Psychiatry, University of Pennsylvania School of Medicine, Philadelphia, Pennsylvania

LOUIS B. SHAPIRO, M.D. Staff Member, Institute for Psychoanalysis, Chicago, Illinois

THOMAS S. SZASZ, M.D. State University of New York, Syracuse, New York

† Deceased.

TABLE OF CONTENTS

I

DEVELOPMENT OF THE FUNDAMENTAL CONCEPTS OF PSYCHOANALYSIS

Franz Alexander, M.D.

Discovery of the Dynamic Unconscious

THAT the human personality embraces more than the traditional concept of the conscious mind is a fundamental discovery of Freud. Many of the psychological functions of everyday life, such as fantasy, dreaming, and parapraxias as well as neurotic and psychotic symptoms and impulsive behavior, cannot be understood in terms of conscious motivation. They become intelligible only when unconscious motivation is reconstructed or made conscious.

The discovery of unconscious motivation had a profound influence upon psychiatric thought. It terminated a strange double standard which characterized the scientific approach to human behavior before the discoveries of Freud. Rational behavior had always been explained through conscious motivation, which could be established by introspection or by verbal communication. The moves of a chess player, for example, were explained not on a chemical or electrophysiological basis but on logical reasoning. But when the medical man was confronted with neurotic symptoms and psychotic behavior which appeared irrational and unexplainable with common-sense psychology, then he abandoned psychological causality and postulated some unknown changes in brain physiology as ultimate causes. When an adult experienced fear in high places or when crossing the street or when he had the urge to count every object in a room, this was called "psychasthenia," and certain changes in brain physiology were assumed. When a person driven by hunger killed someone in order to take away his possessions, this was considered a legitimate problem of psychology. One had only to understand the murderer's motivation to explain his deed. But if a person driven by paranoid delusions committed murder, attempts at psychological explanation were abandoned, and unknown changes in brain structure or physiology were hypothesized. The answer of Freudian psychology to this dichotomy was that both normal and pathological mental processes have their physiological side and are still largely unknown functions of the brain. Both normal and pathological mental processes can be explained, however, from psychological motivations. There is no fundamental difference between psychology and psychopathology: both follow the same basic principles. The reason that psychopathological processes appear irrational, that is to say, do not make sense, lies in the fact that they are determined by *unconscious* processes, which are more primitive than the conscious processes.

The nature of unconscious processes is revealed in dreams, in children's play, in free-floating fantasy, and in neurotic and psychotic symptoms. Unconscious processes can be understood on the basis of psychological causality only when their primitive nature is recognized. This primitive psychology is preverbal. Psychological maturation consists, to a large degree, in learning how to substitute mental processes, adjusted to reality, for wishful and preverbal thinking. Freud maintained that these primitive thought-processes and emotional reactions do not dissolve completely at maturation or become entirely transformed in well-integrated rational processes, but remain latent in the unconscious. The conscious mind defends itself against this latent influence through the mechanism of repression. Repression is responsible for the fact that personality is not a homogeneous entity.

Mental functions can be divided into two groups: rational well-integrated functions adapted to reality, and unconscious processes which make themselves noticeable directly in dreams, pathological symptoms, and errors of everyday life and indirectly through their influence on all mental processes. Their influence upon overt behavior is not obvious; but overt behavior can never be explained from conscious motivation alone. By means of a process called "rationalization," everyone covers up his unconscious motives to some degree with conscious ones, which are often of little dynamic significance. Recognition of this self-deceiving trend in man had a revolutionary influence upon contemporary thought and has gradually transformed the whole outlook of our era, just as the theories of Copernicus and Darwin influenced thinking in the past.

In the first phase of his scientific career, Freud's main concern was to demonstrate the existence of the dynamic unconscious through a study of hypnotic phenomena, hysterical symptoms, dreams, and parapraxias of everyday life. Gradually he developed techniques by which these unconscious processes could be studied by the physician and eventually brought into the consciousness of the patient. This brings us to the second phase in the development of psychoanalysis.

DEVELOPMENT OF METHODS FOR THE STUDY OF UNCONSCIOUS PROCESSES

After hypnosis was abandoned by Freud, his first significant methodological discovery was that the spontaneous, uncontrolled, so-called "free associations" offer an approach to the study of the unconscious. He considered the method of dream interpretation, which was based on free association, the most effective technique. According to Freud, the dream is the royal road to the unconscious mind. It represents the intrusion into the conscious mind of unconscious processes; it reflects in an almost pure fashion the psychology of unconscious processes and offers an unparalleled opportunity to study their peculiarities. Neurotic and psychotic symptoms are in their dynamics identical with dream processes and therefore offer a similarly suitable wedge through which the psychological laws of the unconscious mind can be explored.

The fruitfulness of the psychoanalytic technique is amply documented by the theoretical and therapeutic exploits of the first two decades of psychoanalytic history, during which Freud and his growing number of followers explored the characteristics of unconscious thought-processes. This amounted to learning a new language, the symbolic language of unconscious processes, which differs considerably from the words of conscious thinking. During these early years the fundamental dynamic processes were discovered—repression, overcompensation, substitution and displacement, projection, rationalization, sublimation, turning impulses against the self. Through the discovery of the modes of emotional expression and thought on the preverbal level, the sense of all psychopathological phenomena revealed itself. Psychological common sense was applied to psychopathology, a field where this had not been possible before. Common-sense psychology, however, had to undergo certain modifications in order to become useful in deciphering the meaning of unconscious processes. This is the essence of what is known as "psychoanalytic interpretation."

The methodological significance of the procedure of interpretation is so fundamental that we shall interpolate a brief discussion.[1]

Psychoanalytic Method of Investigation

Every science is based on the systematic development and refinement of the methods of observation and reasoning used in everyday life. Psychoanalysis, unlike earlier psychological methods, has refined the methods of common sense used to understand another person's motivations and actions.

Common sense itself is a complex faculty. It is based primarily on the fact that the observer and the observed are similar to each other. Both are human personalities. Through speech, they can convey their motivations to each other. This similarity allows identification. Knowing one's own motivations, one can easily extrapolate them to another person. This similarity between observed and observer obtains in no other science; it is characteristic of psychology alone. All psychological methods which fail to recognize and exploit this unique advantage have only a limited value for the study of human personality. So long as psychologists tried to imitate the methods of the experimental sciences and neglected to use and develop the natural faculty for understanding the mental processes of another person, psychology as a science of human personality could not develop.

Understanding another individual's mental situation through common sense alone, however, is not a reliable method. It is not sufficiently precise for scientific inquiry because of several sources of error. One of the main contributions of Freud's psychoanalysis was to improve and enlarge common-sense understanding. Four sources of error are inherent in psychological common sense:

1. Under ordinary conditions a person has no special reason to disclose his real motivations to another by verbal communication.

2. It is impossible to give a full account of one's motivations because many of them the individual himself does not know.

3. The vast extent of individual differences makes identification difficult, sometimes impossible. This is best seen if one tries to understand the mental situation of another person whose language one does not understand. The greater the difference be-

1. This methodological contribution of Freud's psychology was discussed by the author in an address given before the Harvey Society in 1930.

4

tween two minds, the greater the difficulty of mutual understanding. Difficulties in understanding the behavior of young children, savages, psychotics, and neurotics are due to just these divergences in mentality.

4. Every observer has some blind spots due to his own repressions. Either he will overlook in the other person those motivations which he tries to exclude from his own consciousness, or he will project them into the other person, discovering the mote in his fellow-man's eye while not noting the beam in his own. The obstacle which one's own repressions constitute against understanding others can be appreciated if one realizes that the uniformity and harmony of the conscious mind are guaranteed by repressions. To become an adult, it is necessary to "forget" infantile ways of thinking. The latter is to a much higher degree subject to the pleasure principle than is adult mentality, which has to adjust itself to reality. The difficulty in understanding children, savages, neurotics, and psychotics is therefore due not only to the difference between their mentality and ours but also to the repressing forces within ourselves. In order to become a rational adult, the primitive functions of the mind must be transformed into co-ordinated rational processes. The phenomenon of dreams alone shows clearly, however, that the substitution of rational functions for more primitive processes is not complete. The conscious mind has to defend itself against following the universal trend to regress to primitive forms of thought. Every night such a regression takes place during sleep. Under external stress as a result of traumatic experiences, such a regression shows itself in neurotic or psychotic symptoms or in unrestrained behavior.

By means of the psychoanalytic technique, these four sources of error, if not eliminated, have been reduced to such a degree that psychology has become a science of the personality. The disinclination of a person to give a full account of his mental state is reduced in psychoanalysis because of the therapeutic situation. The sick person, in the hope of being cured by the help of the physician, is more willing than the well person to put aside the usual restraints against revealing his most intimate feelings, as is required by the method of free association. In free association, thoughts and ideas can emerge which are usually forced out of the focus of attention. The patient's desire to be cured is an almost indispensable factor in psychological investigation, for it alone guarantees a willingness for unreserved self-revelation. As a prerequisite of the methodical study of another person's mind, this type of patient-physician relationship has not been replaced by any other human situation. It is matched only by religious confession in respect to its frankness and the desire to reveal one's self. Religious confession, however, does not utilize the confessional situation for scientific study but for giving relief to the distressed mind.

The second source of error—the inability to reveal one's self completely because of repressions—is met by the analytical technique in two ways. Through free association the conscious control of mental processes is eliminated, thus allowing a more spontaneous expression of ideas which otherwise would not appear in the stream of consciousness. Abandoning conscious control, however, does not mean that the patient is freed from his repressions. The effectiveness of the repression is diminished, since conscious control and repression work in the same direction—to keep repressed thoughts out of the conscious mind. With the elimination of the one factor, the equilibrium between the tendency of repressed mental content to appear in consciousness and the opposing force which excludes it from consciousness is changed in favor of the former. Another factor which favors the process of self-revelation lies in the emotional rapport between patient and therapist. As soon as the patient becomes convinced that he is not being judged by the therapist, that the latter wants only to understand him, frank communication becomes possible.

It is most difficult to eliminate the third source of error—the difference between observer and observed. Differences of language and culture as well as of sex and age can be bridged, however, by consistent and prolonged study in frequent and continued interviews over a long period of time. The fact that neurotic symptoms, like dreams, are manifestations of unconscious processes makes them difficult to understand by rational common sense. Painstaking study of these more primitive preverbal mental processes has resulted in a knowledge which allows their translation into verbal thought-processes used by common-sense psychology.

The last source of error—the observer's own repressions—is reduced by the training analysis which is required in every psychoanalyst's training. Through his own analysis, the physician clears up those "blind spots" which result from repression.

With these measures, psychoanalysis has developed a technique of investigation which is adapted to the special nature of psychological phenomena. By this method it has produced a theory of personality which made possible the treatment of mental disturbances on an etiological basis.

The dynamic principles established by the psychoanalytic method are valid in themselves and independent of the generalizations and speculations concerning the ultimate nature of psychological forces. The laws of optics are valid, although physicists still disagree concerning the ultimate nature of light. The dynamic principles of psychoanalysis are independent of theories concerning the ultimate nature of the instincts. Without a brief sketch of what is called the "theory of instinct," however, the history of psychoanalytic thought would not be complete. This will be presented later in the chapter.

FUNCTIONS OF THE EGO

Before the publication of *The Ego and the Id* (1923), Freud and his followers focused their attention chiefly upon the interpretation of repressed psychological content. Through a relentless study of dreams and other psychological phenomena in which the nature of unconscious processes is revealed, they developed the art of interpretation to a fine and precise instrument. In *The Ego and the Id*, Freud made the first attempt to visualize the total structure and functioning of what he called the "mental apparatus." He distinguished three structurally different parts: the id, the ego, and the superego (chap. iv). The *id* is the original power-house of the mental apparatus; it contains the inherited instinctive forces which at birth are not yet organized into a co-ordinated system. The *ego* is conceived as a product of development which consists in the adaptation of the inherited instinctive drives to one another and to the environment. The *superego*, too, is the precipitate of adaptation; it represents the incorporation of parental attitudes which are determined by the existing cultural standards. After maturation the ego becomes the dynamic center of behavior. Most important in this theory was the conception that mental functions have relationship to the total organism. The ego's function, according to Freud, is to carry out what is ordinarily considered co-ordinated rational behavior and is aimed at maintaining a constant condition (level of excitation) within the organism (stability principle). It is a homeostatic function. The homeostatic equilibrium is constantly disturbed by the life-process itself, by biological needs which arise within the organism, and by external stimuli. In satisfying biological needs and in defending the organism against excessive external stimulation, the ego performs its homeostatic task with the help of four basic faculties: (1) internal perception of instinctive needs, (2) external perception of existing conditions upon which the gratification of subjective needs depends, (3) the integrative faculty by which the ego co-ordinates instinctive urges with one another and with the requirements of the superego and adapts them to the environmental conditions, and (4) the executive faculty by which it controls voluntary behavior. Through the latter, the ego can implement the results of its integrative function, which consists fundamentally in the rational cognitive faculty.

In performing this function (homeostasis), the ego has to struggle continually against the primitive dynamic trend existing within the organism, namely, the tendency of every psychological urge to seek immediate gratification. This tendency, characteristic of the infant, is what Freud called the "pleasure-pain principle." He assumed that the gratification of every subjective need is connected with pleasure; its frustration, with pain. To relieve immediately any painful tension and to obtain immediate pleasure is the fundamental primitive motivating force within the organism.

This pleasure-pain principle, however, eventually causes more pain for the organism than pleasure, since immediate gratification often has painful consequences and may endanger survival. Under the influence of adverse experiences, the ego gradually develops the capacity to co-ordinate psychological impulses with one another and to adapt them to external conditions in a way that assures the best possible outcome in a given situation. The ego learns to postpone certain desires when satisfaction might endanger more important urges. It learns to compromise, to modify the desires, to subordinate less important to more important needs. In other words, the ego learns what is considered rational behavior. Because rational behavior appears to most adults as something natural, requiring no further explanation, its study has been neglected for many years.[2]

2. Recently, Thomas French has focused his main interest on analyzing the principles of rational behavior and describing in more detail what Freud called the "reality principle" (see *The Integration of Behavior,* Vol. 1: *Basic Postulates* [Chicago: University of Chicago Press, 1952]).

Well co-ordinated rational behavior is acquired by an arduous process of learning. Through continual groping experimentation the ego finds adequate behavior patterns, and through repetition their performance becomes routinized, automatic, and hence less energy-consuming. This tendency to accomplish the homeostatic task with a minimum expenditure of energy through repetition is the *economy principle*. Because the organism constantly changes during the process of growth and because conditions in the environment also change, it is necessary for the ego constantly to modify adaptive behavior patterns acquired earlier in the individual's life. Each change requires renewed experimentation until new adaptations are learned. Because of the economy principle, however, there is a tendency to keep old behavior patterns and to resist learning new ones. This manifestation of the economy principle can be aptly termed the "inertia principle." The phenomena of fixation, regression, and repetition compulsion are all based on the inertia principle. "Fixation" designates the tendency to retain previously successful behavior patterns. "Regression" is the tendency to return to them whenever new adjustments are required which are beyond the ego's integrative capacity. Regression is most common under experiences so traumatic that there follows a disintegration of the arduously acquired adaptive pattern into its constituent parts. These "parts" are patterns acquired earlier and gradually woven into more complex integrated behavior. "Repetition compulsion" is the propensity to repeat previously acquired patterns in accordance with the general principle of economy (inertia) instead of undertaking the energy-consuming task of finding new ways of behavior through the integrative process.

The human being does not learn everything through trial and error. "Identification" is another method of learning, a process by which the growing child takes over behavior patterns and attitudes from adults.

For the understanding of psychopathology, it is important to note that co-ordinated rational behavior can be maintained only through a constant struggle on the part of the ego, because the instinctual tendencies retain their original inclination for immediate gratification. This is the original basis of Freud's structural concept of differentiation between ego and id. He assumed that a tendency toward nonco-ordinated, isolated gratification is always present and manifests itself in all those psychological phenomena which are not rational or co-ordinated, such as dreams, free fantasy, impulsive behavior, and all that is known as "psychopathological." Whenever the ego is threatened by impulses which are not in harmony with its accepted standards or reality, a conflict and concomitant anxiety arise. To anxiety the ego reacts by defenses which are erected against these tendencies threatening from within. These defenses are partly bulwarks which favor repression, such as overcompensation or rationalization, and partly vents by which the repudiated tendencies can find an outlet, such as projection, substitution, displacement, or turning impulses directed against external objects against the self. Mental disease represents a failure of the ego to secure gratification for subjective needs in a harmonious and reality-adjusted manner and a breakdown of the defenses by which it tries to neutralize impulses that cannot be harmonized with internal standards and external reality.

Defenses of the Ego

1. *Repression.*—Whenever the ego fails in its integrative task of co-ordinating impulses with one another and with the existing environmental conditions, it adopts one or more of the defensive mechanisms it learned in earlier years. The basic mechanism consists in excluding from the consciousness the psychological content which it is unable to include harmoniously in its scope. This is called "repression" and was considered by Freud as the principal defense of the infantile ego, which has not the capacity to withstand temptation, postpone, or modify by compromise the gratification of an impulse. Whatever impulse appears in consciousness has to be converted into action immediately. Repression remains, therefore, the only effective defense. Repressed impulses, however, do not cease to exist merely by exclusion from consciousness and thereby from motor expression. To deal with the tension of these pent-up impulses the ego has to resort to further defenses, which can be classified in two groups: (*a*) further reinforcements of repression or (*b*) substitute vents by which the original impulses can find at least a partial, modified ego syntonic release and by which their pressure is decreased.

2. *Overcompensation.*—The ego may make use of an acceptable attitude to help an ego-alien attitude stay repressed. Thus pity may cover up unconscious cruelty, shyness can serve as a defense against exhibitionism, temerity against timidity, and boastful conceit against a feeling of inferiority. The conscious attitude

in these instances is the polar opposite of the repressed ego-alien tendency.

One of the most important overcompensations is that of love by hate or hate by love. This is observed when either love, such as homosexual desire, or hate directed against a benefactor becomes unacceptable to the ego. This attitude is based on the clinically important phenomenon of ambivalence—love and hatred toward the same person. A certain amount of ambivalence is universal, because the narcissistic nucleus of the personality "hates" every loved object which depletes the ego's self-love. The utilization of one component of the ambivalent conflict in order to keep the other in repression is therefore a very common phenomenon.

3. *Rationalization.*—This is a common technique by which the ego keeps certain tendencies repressed. Rationalization means the selection from coexisting motivations of those most acceptable to the ego. Emphasis upon the acceptable motivation allows the ego to keep the unacceptable repressed, since the selected motives can sufficiently explain the act in question ("I attack him because he is wrong and not because I envy him").

4. *Identification.*—Under certain conditions the mechanism of identification which plays such an important role in the healthy growth of the ego may become a defensive measure. Most common is identification with an object (a person) lost in bereavement or by separation or rejection. The ego in a way re-establishes the lost one by identifying itself with that person. Identification with a powerful enemy is another use of identification as a defense. By assuming the qualities of the opponent, anxiety is mastered.

5. *Substitution and displacement.*—Another common defensive measure consists in displacing an emotional attitude from one object to another. In this way hatred can be diverted from the person, whom to hate would cause conflict, to someone else, who may be justifiably disliked. Sometimes not the person but the act which is objectionable is replaced by another less objectionable one. This defense is characterized as "substitution." A murderous impulse may be replaced by a minor aggression or released by some impersonal destructive act, such as wood-chopping or boxing at the punch ball.

6. *Sublimation.*—The defense most important to society consists in substituting for an unacceptable tendency another one

which is appropriate for relieving the original tendency and at the same time has a socially useful aspect. Common examples are the substitution of all forms of creativity for sexual impulses or certain activities by which inanimate nature can be mastered for hostile aggressive tendencies.

7. *Projection.*—When a repressed tendency can no longer be kept out of consciousness, a radical defense may become necessary. An example is attributing a repressed tendency to another person. The ego can neither accept the subjective tendency as its own nor repress it. The only solution is then to deny its belonging to the scope of one's own personality. Through projection the ego abandons, to some degree at least, its reality-testing function by misinterpreting reality and thus returns to a primitive stage of development when external reality and internal (psychological) reality were not yet differentiated.

8. *Provocative behavior.*—In provocative behavior a person may express his original hostility against another person by inducing the other person to attack first. One's own aggressive behavior then appears as self-defense; this allows one to express one's hostility without internal conflict and at the same time keep one's motivations repressed.

9. *Turning feelings toward one's self.*—Another defense against unacceptable tendencies which threaten to break through the barrier of repression is turning them against one's self. Instead of expressing hostility or hatred against another person, the hatred is turned against the own self in the form of self-criticism and self-accusation. By the same mechanism, the feeling of love can be withdrawn from another person and turned into self-love.

10. *Isolation.*—Isolation is a technique mainly restricted to compulsive neurosis. Ego-alien tendencies which appear in consciousness are separated from the rest of the mental content and thus made innocuous. The patient may master his neurotic anxiety by carefully separating acceptable psychological content from the objectionable. This is the basis of many compulsive rituals—touching, washing, and all kinds of avoidances of trivial activities.

11. *Regression.*—Already described is the universal trend toward regression. An ego-alien tendency—for example, a sexual urge toward a tabooed person—can be replaced regressively by some pregenital, less objectionable attitude toward the same per-

son. Sexual desire may then be evaded by means of a dependent attitude, which has no obvious sexual connotation.

Regression is a universal mechanism. It is accentuated in neurosis. In fact, every neurotic symptom has a regressive connotation, inasmuch as adequate co-ordinated behavior is replaced by activities in fantasy, the content of which always shows a return to previous modes of gratification.

12. *Defense against guilt feelings.*—Defense mechanisms by which guilt feelings are prevented from becoming conscious are the most complex of all. Most phenomena qualified by the expression "masochistic" belong to this type of defense. By inflicting punishment upon one's self or provoking suffering, guilt feelings can be reduced or eliminated without the person's becoming conscious of their nature.

Like regression, these masochistic defenses have an outstanding significance in psychopathology because they are ubiquitous in neurotic processes. Regression to earlier modes of gratification—pregenital and oedipal fixations—creates of necessity either guilt feelings or feelings of inferiority or both. Owing to the deep-rooted emotional syllogism that suffering atones for guilt, guilt feelings and anxiety can be temporarily removed from consciousness through atonement by means of suffering.

13. *Defenses against inferiority feelings.*—Regression to earlier dependent states creates inferiority feelings (shame) which many patients try to repress and keep repressed by overcompensatory bravado (counterphobic behavior). This is particularly noticeable in delinquent behavior. Many wanton violations of law are motivated by deeply repressed inferiority feelings, which the delinquent denies by flaunting his independence and courage in destructive and aggressive behavior (see above, Sec. 2, "Overcompensation").

14. *Conversion.*—Ego-alien tendencies may be thoroughly repressed and find no expression on the psychological level or in co-ordinated behavior. The pent-up tension may then be relieved by changes in the field of the skeletal and laryngeal muscles or in the sense organs. These changes (paralyses, muscular contractions, spasms, convulsions, different kinds of sensory symptoms, such as anaesthesia and paresthesia or blindness and deafness) have a symbolic meaning and serve both the expression and the negation of the repressed ego-alien tendencies.

In the foregoing pages we have discussed the dynamic processes underlying the functions of the ego and its ways and means of dealing with instinctual forces. As stated before, these dynamic formulations are independent of speculations concerning the ultimate nature of the instinctual forces. Now we shall attempt to outline briefly the development of psychoanalytic views about the nature of the instincts.

THEORY OF INSTINCTS

Originally, Freud assumed the existence of two basic instincts, the instinct of self-preservation and the sex instinct. He referred to them as "ego instinct" (*Ich-triebe*) and "libido." All observed psychological forces motivating behavior were considered as derivatives of one of these basic instincts. An antagonism between the two categories was assumed because sexual strivings were those commonly found to be repressed. Neurotic symptoms could be explained as substitute expressions of repressed, and thus frustrated, sexual strivings. The ego instincts tend to preserve the integrity of the organism, which is often threatened by sexual strivings not in accord with existing social standards. Incestuous cravings of the child and hostile feelings directed against the parent of the other sex are commonly repressed tendencies.

The distinction between ego instincts and sexual libido soon led to theoretical difficulties. When the existence of infantile sexuality was recognized, the concept of libido had to be extended to include not only race preservation but also the infantile manifestations of sexuality which have nothing to do with propagation. The latter center around the vegetative functions, which are in the service of self-preservation—pleasure sensations during sucking, the excremental act, and the exercise of muscles. In fact, most biological functions are the source of pleasure sensations which resemble the later sexual gratifications. Oral, anal, urethral, and muscular eroticism are connected with nutrition, excretion, grasping, and locomotion, which ultimately become subservient to self-preservation. Moreover, the emotional content of infantile sexuality is completely self-centered. Since the main object of these erotic interests is the child's own person, Freud called this form of libido "narcissistic." As soon as it was recognized that the first object of love is the self, the distinction between self-preservation and sexuality became contradictory.

The distinction between narcissistic libido and object libido called attention to the fact that love may be directed toward the self or toward other objects. The self-centered libido, however, could no longer be distinguished from self-preservation. Essentially, all functions of self-preservation were included in libido except aggression, which was relegated to the category of ego instincts. In the form of sadism, however, the aggressive hostile impulse also assumes a libidinous connotation. This made obvious the inconsistency of the original distinction between self-preservative and sexual instincts. Hostility remained the only manifestation of the ego instinct, and even this could not be claimed as nonsexual, at least certainly not on a phenomenological basis. Jung proposed a solution to this by abandoning Freud's dualism and attributing everything to libido. The Jungian "libido" became similar to Bergson's "élan vital" or to the notions of the German vitalists.

Freud was fully aware of the theoretical difficulties of the original libido theory, but only in 1920 did he revise his theory. He then introduced a new dualistic concept of instincts: life and death. He assumed an erotic principle which is a binding force and corresponds basically to the anabolic phase of metabolism. The upbuilding tendency is a manifestation of the erotic life-instinct. This force is opposed by the death instinct, which is a disintegrating force and appears biologically in biochemical catabolism. The two tendencies, according to Freud, are always mixed in their actual psychological manifestations. The erotic instinct has a narcissistic phase when it is self-preservative. In mature organisms it attracts the sexes to each other, and it then becomes race-preservative.

It is obvious that the theory of life and death instincts was no longer an attempt to describe instinctual forces but rather a philosophical abstraction. It contained, however, a valuable nucleus in distinguishing two basic vectors in the life-process—one upbuilding (anabolic) and one disruptive (catabolic). This paved the way for the psychosomatic view of the instinctual life which developed with increasing knowledge of the integrative functions of the organism as a whole.

This psychosomatic theory of sexuality attempts to reconcile both the psychology and the physiology of all those widely diversified behavioral phenomena which have one feature in common—that they yield erotic gratification. This common feature was what induced Freud to consider physical pleasure sensations, such as thumbsucking or the excitation of the anal zone, as sexual in nature. The most convincing observation was that a child may induce an erection by thumbsucking. Further studies have shown that many other functions of the body can yield erotic pleasure, such as urination, locomotion, looking, etc. Equally significant is the fact that all intense emotions can become the psychological content of sexual excitation. The craving to be loved and to love others, which is accompanied by the desire for bodily contact, is by no means the only content of sexual desires. The sadistic impulse to hurt, the inclination to suffer pain and humiliation, curiosity about sexuality, vanity about one's own body, with the wish to expose it in order to become the center of attention—all these may be emotional sources of the sexual impulse but may be expressed also without physical sexual connotation. On the basis of such observation, Freud concluded originally that sexuality is not dependent on a special emotional quality but has a quantitative basis; it is a special form of emotional discharge. Later he abandoned this view and attributed to sexuality a specific quality.

The fact that the same emotional tension, such as love or hate, can be discharged both in a sexual and in a nonsexual manner strongly supports the view that sexuality should be considered a specific form of discharge for any psychological tension. The peculiar nature of the sexual discharge can be understood from the psychological characteristics of sexual phenomena and from their biological function. Hostile aggressive behavior against a person who threatens one's security differs in many respects from wanton cruelty carried out as a form of sexual gratification. The first type of aggressive behavior is subservient to the practical goal of defending one's own interest. In the second type inflicting pain is a goal in itself, not subordinated to the interest of the total organism.

The same difference obtains in all other forms of sexual discharge. In scoptophilia, which is an erotic phenomenon, watching, observing, and satisfying curiosity are aims in themselves and are not substitutes for another goal. Learning about something, the knowledge of which is essential for self-preservation, is the nonsexual counterpart of scoptophilia. In the latter form of curiosity, self-preservation is the main goal; watching and finding out something are subordinated to it.

The same obtains to masochism. Carrying a heavy knapsack is a form of suffering the tourist has to endure in order to be comfortable when he reaches the mountain peak. It is not a source of pleasure but a necessary evil. This is not masochism but rational well-adjusted behavior. As soon as suffering becomes an aim itself, however, it assumes the concentration of sexual gratification. This is called "masochism."

Likewise, the early erotic preoccupations of the infant, such as thumbsucking or retention of excrement, are independent of the vegetative functions to which they are related: eating and the excremental act. Thumbsucking is not subservient to the utilitarian function of eating. It is carried out entirely as a source of pleasure, without serving any physiological function in the interest of the whole organism. Psychoanalysis postulated that the exercise of voluntary muscles may yield erotic gratification which is called "muscle eroticism." In early infancy the unco-ordinated movements of the child are not yet subordinated to any utilitarian goal and probably have the sole function of erotic discharge.

The psychosomatic view of sexuality here proposed attempts to assemble all the above observations into a comprehensive picture. The outstanding feature characteristic of all those phenomena which have an erotic connotation is that they discharge an *excess of excitation*. The nature of the excitation may be love, hate, curiosity, suffering, vanity—in fact, it includes the whole gamut of human emotions. Sexuality discharges any excess excitation, regardless of its quality. The sexual discharge of impulses is not integrated with other functions in the service of self-preservation. The same impulses, if co-ordinated into utilitarian functions, lose their sexual connotation.

The biological function of mature sexuality is propagation. When the organism reaches the limit of its growth, it can no longer increase and must divide. Cell division—the prototype of propagation—can be considered as the continuation of the process of growth beyond the limits of the individual unit, the cell. Surplus organic matter which cannot be integrated in a single biological unit is expelled and becomes a new organism. In multicellular organisms the same basic process takes place in a more complex manner. Propagation, then, results from surplus generated by growth. The psychological counterpart of this process is mature love. After the maturing organism becomes saturated with narcissistic love, there is an overflow of emotion, and other persons become the objects of this love: narcissistic love gives way to object love.

The pregenital manifestations of sexuality can be understood as manifestations of excitation which is in excess of what is needed for self-preservative aims. An excess of the incorporative urge which is no longer serving the utilitarian aim of satisfying hunger appears in thumbsucking or some other oral play (oral eroticism). Likewise, the anal manifestations of sexuality are not subservient to the excremental functions but serve mainly to relieve an excess of excitation (anal eroticism).

Erotic phenomena have a playful quality—in fact, all play activities are erotic in nature. For this reason, Eros is personified as a child. Most of the infant's self-preservative needs are met by the help of adults; many of his body functions are exercised mainly for the discharge of surplus excitation and for no utilitarian goal. From birth on, only the basic vegetative functions serve the vital needs of the organism. The sense organs and the muscles are not yet co-ordinated to serve utilitarian needs. The unco-ordinated movements of the infant are not suited for grabbing or locomotion and are carried out only for pleasurable discharge of tensions, as in the form of muscle eroticism. The racing colt exuberantly uses his accumulated energies, serving no purpose. The sense organs also are used for the sake of pleasurable activity alone. The eyes see for the sake of scoptophilic pleasure, and the hands touch for the sake of experiencing pleasant tactile sensations. Gradually, with growth toward independence, the functions which originally were practiced in a playful fashion become integrated for the utilitarian goals of existence. Now the eyes are used to find the food, the extremities to approach and to grab it. Erotic play gives place gradually to self-preservative functions; yet surplus energy in excess of the needs of self-preservation may be discharged in an erotic manner also in adult life. Finally, after the organism has reached the limits of growth, surplus intake in excess over expenditure is discharged in the form of propagation or its sublimated equivalents: in productive and creative activities.

This surplus theory of sexuality receives its strongest support from physiology. In the mature organism sexual excitation is discharged primarily through the genitourinary system, the physiological function of which consists precisely in discharging body products and emotional tensions which are no longer useful for the self-preservation of the organism. Physically, it discharges either waste or germ cells, which are not integrated with the rest of the organism. Psychologically, the manifestations of sexuality consist in discharging tensions for their own sake, tensions which are not subordinated to the needs of the total organism. Sexuality, with its physiological and psychological manifestation, can be considered as a drainage system of all energies which are not needed for the preservation of individual life and are in excess of the needs of the organism. The specific organ of this kind of discharge is the genitourinary tract.

The significant role of sexuality in neurotic disturbances becomes evident in the light of this view. Whenever the ego cannot carry out its homeostatic function of finding adequate gratification for subjective needs in harmony with the total personality, tensions accumulate which are not integrated with the total needs of the organism. Such unintegrated tendencies seek expression through sexual channels. When mature expression of the genital level is inhibited, the pent-up tensions seek regressive sexual expressions, which are in conflict with the accepted ego standards. In perversion they find direct pregenital expression, whereas in neurosis the ego defends itself against these infantile sexual strivings. As a result, substitute expressions are created as vents, in the form of neurotic symptoms. The latter are expressions of regressive strivings and of the ego's defenses against these unacceptable tendencies. In this view, Freud's original formulation, that neurotic symptoms are the negatives of perversions, finds a new confirmation.

Dynamics of Ego Development

Growth and maturation are fundamental attributes of all living organisms. Lifeless machines, no matter how ingenious in performance, become old and rusty with time. Before the human organism becomes old and rusty, it passes through a cycle that is basically the same in every living being: growth until maturation characterized by the faculty of propagation, then decline until death. In the human organism this cycle consists of prenatal growth until birth, then infancy, childhood, pubescence, maturity, senescence, and death.

One of the features of this cycle specific for man is the prolonged biological helplessness of the infant. For this, there is no parallel in the animal kingdom. This comparatively long duration of dependent infancy offers a clue to many riddles of human development. The human infant, unlike most animals at birth, is not fully equipped with inherited automatic behavior patterns needed for independent existence; consequently, he must learn these functions through trial and error. The biological symbiosis between infant and mother continues for a while after birth but gradually yields to independent existence. First in nutrition, later in locomotion, and still later in his orientation to the world, the child becomes more and more independent, an achievement attained through the process of learning. In this process his identification with adults is of the greatest importance. This comparatively prolonged period of dependence, during which the infant, under parental guidance, gradually learns the ways and means of independent existence, accounts for the great variety of personalities found in the human species. The infant represents an extremely pliable yet unfinished substratum, upon which environmental influences, primarily the personalities of the parents, exert their molding impression.

Scientific recognition of the formative influence of early family life is the contribution of Freud and his followers. As a result of their studies, it was concluded that not only heredity but also the conditions of infancy determine our destiny.

It is only recently that students of personality have become impressed by the fact that personality development does not stop at a certain age, that significant changes take place in all phases of the life-curve, and particularly that the formative experience of early years do not necessarily leave irreversible effects. Many of the adverse influences of early childhood can be corrected by later experiences in life. Indeed, psychoanalytic therapy is based on this view. We try by methodical treatment procedures to bring about changes in personality structure, by undoing those unfavorable patterns established in an earlier period. All psychoanalysts conform implicitly to this view, in that they practice a therapy by which they endeavor to bring changes into personality structure. Yet many psychoanalysts are strangely inconsistent, in that they underestimate the influence of later experiences in life, to which they ascribe only a precipitating significance. While this often may be the case, profound experiences in later life, such as migration from one culture to another, continued contact with certain persons, as well as many vicissitudes of life, may produce deep changes in personality. If this were not the case, psychoanalytic therapy of adults, in itself a form of later experience, could not alter a patient's personality.

Today most psychoanalysts have reached a more balanced view, which recognizes the significance of three categories of factors in respect to the personality of the individual: heredity, early experiences within the family, and events of later life.

FACTORS INHERENT IN PERSONALITY DEVELOPMENT

Heredity supplies the ground pattern that determines not only certain basic qualities but the whole rhythm of the life-span. With certain variations, the main phases of growth are rather uniformly predetermined by hereditary factors. Dentition, myelinization of certain nerve tracts, learning to speak and walk, the maturation of the sex glands, and, finally, the degenerative changes of senescence, take place—with individual variations—at about the same age and in every individual in the same sequence. This fundamental pattern of the life-curve cannot be changed by later influences.

Each phase of biological growth is characterized by well-defined psychological attitudes. Except for oxygen supply, the newborn infant is completely dependent upon the mother biologically, and consequently seeks gratification for his needs from the mother. His security is based on being loved and cared for. Gradually the child learns to use his biological equipment independently. The eye learns to focus, the hands to grab, the legs to walk. Interest in the vegetative functions of the body and curiosity regarding its anatomy are further characteristics of the first six years. Later this curiosity is replaced by an investigative interest in the external environment. Now the phase of biological mastery of body functions is followed by a period in which the development of intellectual functions predominates, gradually allowing an independent orientation to the surrounding world (chap. iv).

The next important phase, the period of adolescence, is again determined by biological factors, the maturation of the sex glands. By now the growing organism has developed all its functions, to which finally the faculty of propagation is added. Although biologically the adolescent organism has reached the end of its growth, its psychological state can be sharply differentiated from maturity. In our culture biological growth is ahead of psychological maturation. This fact offers a clue to the understanding of most of the peculiarities of the adolescent. The salient feature of this period is the novelty of the new state of being grown-up, particularly in respect to the propagative faculties. In adolescence, the biological ability to procreate is as if foisted upon an emotionally unprepared and inexperienced organism. A full-grown body is intrusted to an inexperienced mind. The main characteristics of the adolescent—his proverbial awkwardness and insecurity—follow this discrepancy. The adolescent impresses us as not knowing what to do with himself in his newly attained state. Adolescent competitiveness can be traced back to the same basic circumstance. The adolescent feels as if he were constantly in a test situation; he must prove to himself and others that he is already a man. The only way to do this is to measure himself against others.

This competition demands a continuous practice of the adolescent's full-grown capacities. During the period of adolescence the young person gradually grows emotionally into the advanced mature status that he had reached biologically several years before. The self-confident attitude of the mature person is based on taking himself and his capacities for granted. This is in sharp contrast to the insecurity of the infant and the adolescent. As a consequence of this inner security, the mature adult's interest no longer centers around the self but can be turned outward toward the environment.

The psychological attributes of maturity, like those of other age periods, can best be understood from the biological conditions of maturity. As long as the organism grows, intake and retention of substance and energy outweigh their expenditure. Otherwise growth would not be possible. The psychological manifestation of this state of affairs is that in the immature organism the wish to receive outweighs the wish to give. When the organism reaches maturity, it can no longer add anything to its own size; growth has reached its natural limits. The body cannot organize more living matter within its own system. Therefore, individual growth stops, and propagation serves as a means of releasing surplus energy. Propagation in this light can be understood as development beyond the limits of individual growth.

As stated before, all energy that is not needed to maintain life can be considered surplus energy. This is the source of all sexual activity; it is also the source of all productive and creative work. This surplus energy shows itself in the mature person in generosity, the result of overflowing power which the individual can no longer use for further growth and which therefore can be spent in creative pursuits. The mature person is no longer primarily a receiver. He receives, but he also gives. His giving is not subordinated primarily to his expectation of return; it is giving for its own sake. Just as receiving love and help are the main sources of pleasure for the growing child, so for the mature person pleasure consists in spending energy productively for the sake of others and for purposes beyond himself. This generous, outwardly directed attitude is what in ethics is called "altruism." In the light of this view, altruism, the basis of Christian morality, has a biological foundation; it is a natural, healthy expression of the state of maturity.

It is important to emphasize that the platonic ideal of emotional maturity is never reached by most persons in its complete form; it is only approached. Individual differences are enormous and account for the existence of the leader and follower types, the latter the more numerous. Whenever life becomes difficult and presents situations beyond the individual's capacity to solve, there is a tendency to regress toward less mature attitudes, in which a person may still rely on the help of parents and teachers. In our hearts we all regret having been expelled from the Garden of Eden by eating from the tree of knowledge—a symbol of maturity. In critical life-situations, most persons become insecure and seek help even before they have exhausted all their own resources.

RELATION BETWEEN PERSONALITY DEVELOPMENT AND SOCIAL STRUCTURE

Every form of social organization requires of its members the capacity to replace self-interest to some degree with an interest in others. This is the reason why no society could be run by children or adolescents. Different forms of social organization, however, require different degrees of maturity. In all authoritarian governments, the status of the majority of the people resembles that of children more than that of independent adults. Virtue consists in obeying the existing rules and in being subordinate to the rulers, whose obligation is to take care of their subjects. In such societies people express their mature state only by taking care of their progeny. All social manifestations of individual productivity are absent. With the exception of two short periods in history, humanity has always lived under some form of authoritarian system, be it feudalism, absolute monarchy, fascism, or communism. Free societies have existed for a short period in ancient Greece and during the last three hundred years in some parts of Western civilization. These two brief periods in the history of Western civilization were undoubtedly the richest in artistic, scientific, and literary productivity. There is danger that under the paralyzing threats of global wars our present experiment with freedom may be relegated to history and free societies may be engulfed by the rising tide of authoritarianism.

Social attitudes, however, are not good or bad in themselves; they are organic parts of each culture and can be evaluated only in the framework of different social organizations. Educational attitudes and methods of child rearing do not develop in a vacuum; they are determined by the total social structure. Recent anthropological studies have shown that national charcteristics are primarily due to certain uniform paternal influences, which are determined by the total social configuration.

For example, Japanese worship of authority was the precipitate of century-long feudalism. Not only was it the reflection of the feudal ideology in the mind of the individual, but it was also an indispensable guaranty for the survival of the feudal system. Similarly, the American emphasis on individual accomplishment and depreciation of authority worship are expressions of the American social structure and at the same time the guaranties of its survival. Such attitudes, transmitted to each child by family influences, have a social function. They are adaptations of the individual to the social structure in which he lives. It is clear, then, that no educational philosophy can be foisted upon a nation which does not spring organically from that nation's cultural soil. In this perspective, the naïveté of plans much discussed in postwar years to re-educate foreign nations according to our own ideals becomes transparent. The social attitudes of a nation can be changed only by changing its whole social structure.

A self-governing, free democracy requires greater independence of its citizens than does any other social system. The question is how such emotional independence can be achieved—independence that can withstand the regressive pressure of adversity.

It is obvious from what has been said that emotional independence is achieved gradually during the process of growth. The child will assume independence if he has opportunity in each phase of development for self-expression, by which he learns to make use of the faculties that correspond to his age. He will learn to assume responsibility for his own activities if his self-control is not based on fear of external authorities but is rooted in his own conscience. This conscience develops through positive identification with adults. If the socialization of the child is achieved primarily through fear of punishment, only a grudging type of conformity will develop. Rigorous discipline, enforced by corporal and other forms of punishment, is suited to bringing up a militant aggressive youth, as exemplified by ancient Sparta, Hitler's Germany, and Soviet Russia. All the hatred generated in the punitive atmosphere of the playroom, the school, and the military barracks is channelized toward foreign societies or minority groups. It is held from expression against the internal authorities of the state by terror. This form of society, therefore, must always be a police state. It goes with the complete deterioration of internal standards of self-responsibility and independence.

The process of social adjustment in free democracies must be based on favoring the development of standards that become integral parts of the personality. In the technical language of psychoanalysis, the boundary between ego and superego disappears in such a person. This type of personality structure will develop only if the process of social adjustment is based on positive identification—on love, trust, and admiration felt by the child for those who are intrusted with his upbringing. As Freud has recognized, love is a unifying force, hatred a dividing one. If social adjustment is based on hate and fear, the internal image of the external authorities—the conscience—will remain a foreign body within the personality. Only if the child loves those whose social attitudes he incorporates during his development, only if he has confidence in them, can the image of these persons become one with the rest of the personality.

In such education the emphasis is not merely on restraining the original impulses but in directing them into socially valuable creative expression. Full expression of individuality has been the chief source of every step in social progress. The major problem of our time is to produce socially minded, co-operative adults, without sacrificing individuality.

Psychodynamic Principles of Therapy

In its main phases, psychoanalytic therapy has followed the development of theory. When the dynamic influence of unconscious tendencies was discovered, the therapy consisted in bringing repressed psychological content into consciousness. Cathartic hypnosis was such a procedure, a device by which the ego's rejection of repressed material was circumvented by the artificial hypnotic state. Freud soon realized that the mobilization of the repressed is not sufficient to cure neurotic symptoms but that the ego must undergo changes in order to become capable of integrating repressed material into its system. The therapeutic aim must therefore consist in achieving changes in the ego. With this new orientation, the center of interest shifted from the understanding of the unconscious, the knowledge of symbolism, the art of translating the archaic picture language of the unconscious into verbal thinking, to the study of the defenses of the ego. The crucial discovery concerning the ways and means by which the ego's defenses can be influenced was that of the transference phenomenon. Its therapeutic significance was only gradually recognized.

In cathartic hynosis the therapeutic factor consisted in an intensive emotional experience, in the dramatic reliving of repressed traumatic experiences of the past. Freud soon recognized that the traumatic experience in itself was not the most important pathogenic factor, but those preceding experiences which had made the patient vulnerable. What the patient felt as a trauma in itself was often a quite trivial occurrence. For example, Anna, Breuer's patient, developed her aversion to drinking water when she saw her English governess' little dog drink from a dish used by the family. When she recalled this episode in hypnotic trance, she burst out with violent hatred against the governess and abused her profanely. After this, her symptom—aversion to water—disappeared. Freud correctly concluded that this trivial event in itself could not account for the symptom. Anna must have been sensitized by previous experiences in order to react so violently. Today, with our knowledge of the typical tragedies of childhood, it is not difficult to conclude that the dog for Anna represented another child with whom she had had to share the governess' attention. Her hatred of the governess was due to her inability to share love, a quality which she must have acquired in her early development.

After Freud recognized the importance of the genetic exploration of the individual's early history for the understanding of the precipitating factors in neurosis, his therapeutic efforts became focused on the reconstruction of early emotional development. This required filling in gaps of memory caused by repressions. Free association in the emotionally permissive atmosphere of psychoanalytic interviews was an ideal device for the systematic study of the patient's past. A period followed in which the genetic reconstruction of personality development became the aim of therapy. Gradually, however, the importance of the patient's emotional experiences in the transference relationship to the analyst became more and more appreciated. The most consistent evaluation of the therapeutic significance of the transference was contained in a pamphlet published by Ferenczi and Rank in 1926, in which they expounded the thesis that not remembering but reliving the traumatic experiences in the transference is the effective therapeutic factor. Memory gaps may never be filled; yet a patient may be cured if he learns a new solution for his past emotional conflicts when these reappear in his emotional involvement with the analyst. This significant publication was unfavorably received and remained buried for more than fifteen years, until in the Chicago Institute for Psychoanalysis a systematic re-evaluation of therapeutic factors was undertaken.[3] This project required experimentation with the technique of treatment. The routine of daily interviews and the so-called "passive" attitude were abandoned, and every detail of the treatment, the frequency of interviews, interruptions, and as much as possible of the patient's life-situation were planned according to the nature of the therapeutic problem.

The significance of the therapist's attitude toward the patient has also been explored. The phenomenon of countertransference in recent years has received increasing recognition. Originally, Freud conceived the analyst's role as a neutral one. The therapist was supposed to serve merely as a screen upon which the patient projected the emotional reactions that originated in childhood in relation to his parents. In the light of precise scrutiny this postulate turned out to be a theoretical construction. The analyst's personality and his reactions, in spite of his efforts to remain impersonal, influence the course of the treatment. The patient senses these reactions, although he frequently misinterprets them according to his own emotional needs. The Chicago studies paid particular attention to the mutual emotional relationship between patient and physician; the concept of the patient's corrective emotional experience as the central factor in psychoanalytic treatment has evolved.

The essence of this theory can be summarized as follows: The

3. Franz Alexander, T. M. French, *et al.*, *Psychoanalytic Therapy* (New York: Ronald Press, 1946).

neurotic condition is the result of the ego's failure to accomplish its function, which consists in finding gratification for subjective needs in a way that maintains harmony between the various aspects of the personality and the environment. This function of mediation between conflicting or partially conflicting needs and desires and their adaptation to environmental conditions are essentially problems of integration. Every person has his own integrative capacity. French subjected the integrative function to a careful study, in which he tried to evaluate its quantitative variations. The integrative faculty varies from person to person, and in the same person it is influenced by different factors. Excessive intensity of an emotional need, for example, interferes with effective integration. Postponement of immediate gratification was recognized by Freud as one essential feature of reality-adapted behavior. Intense and urgent emotions tend to seek immediate gratification and thus interfere with effective integrative functioning. Low intensity of motivations may also decrease the integrative faculty. A person not keenly interested in what he has to accomplish will be less inclined to undertake the arduous task of appraising the whole problem and trying to solve it. Anxiety, too, depending on its intensity, may either favor or paralyze the integrative functions. Past successes and resulting hope increase integrative ability; consistent failure impairs it.

Another factor which interferes with adaptive behavior is related to the basic mechanism of repression. Repression is the characteristic defense measure of the weak ego of the child, who cannot control those desires which appear in his consciousness and which are in conflict with the requirements of the environment or with other subjective needs. He has only one way to save himself from the painful experiences he was subjected to in the past when he gave in to such impulses: he has to exclude them radically from his consciousness. This saves him from a conflict with reality and/or internal conflict but, at the same time, creates a frustration. Eventually the repressed impulse will seek outlet in symptoms. Through repression the ego is deprived of dynamic force, which it could utilize if it were able to integrate the force within its system. The highest form of integrative function requires conscious deliberation. Everything excluded from consciousness is beyond the reach of the ego's integrative functions. Neurotic symptoms are like foreign bodies and represent isolated substitute gratifications which are the source of conflict and suffering.

Psychoanalytic therapy aims at the extension of the ego's scope by making repressed tendencies conscious. For this purpose it attempts to mobilize unconscious material. In order to overcome repressions by systematic psychological maneuvers, one must know the causes of repression. As shown above, the child represses those tendencies the expression of which caused him pain, such as physical suffering, punishment, withdrawal of parental love, and resulting insecurity. The emergence of such a tendency constitutes a danger to which the ego reacts with anxiety. According to Freud, anxiety is the signal for the ego to repress such dangerous impulses. Essentially, this process is similar to conditioning. The sequence of events has three links: (1) emergence of the impulse, (2) acting upon it, and (3) painful results. Originally the anxiety was aroused by the memory of a painful experience; it reappears whenever the impulse involved emerges. In order to avoid the associated anxiety, the impulse is repressed and excluded from motor expression.

Psychoanalytic therapy in this light reveals itself as a process of reconditioning. The ego is induced to face a repressed impulse by eliminating the anxiety which induced repression. This is achieved by reproducing the original situation but changing the conditions so that they lose their anxiety-producing effect. As soon as the patient senses that the analyst's response to expression of his impulses is different from that of the parents, the intimidating effect is removed. The aim of the therapy consists, first, in reviving the interpersonal situation which led to the original repressions and, second, in supplying a new kind of experience which is suitable for undoing the effects of the parental responses. Accordingly, the analyst's response to the patient's expression should be different from the parental ones: they should perhaps be the opposite of the parental reactions. This can be achieved only if the analyst is able to reconstruct the pathogenic parental influences and respond to the patient's emotional manifestations in a manner appropriate to the counteracting and neutralizing of the disturbing influence of the parents. Essentially this is nothing but emotional reconditioning.

The objective attitude of the therapist which Freud recommended is different from anything the patient has experienced before, because complete objectivity does not exist in ordinary human relationships. The corrective influence of this objective attitude can be further enhanced if the therapist's reactions are specifically calculated to counteract the effect of parental reactions.

The practical conclusion from all this is that, in place of his spontaneous countertransference reactions, the therapist must assume an attiude toward the patient which in the light of the patient's history appears appropriate to the undoing of the pathogenic influences of the parents. In this way the emotional experiences in the therapy will have a corrective influence, resulting in the lifting of repressions. The patient will be able to face what he formerly repressed because of parental censure.

It would be an oversimplification, however, to assume that repressions are always due to intimidating parental attitudes. Permissive parental behavior may create guilt and favor repression of aggressive impulses. The therapist, therefore, cannot always assume a permissive attitude. Often a strong-hand atmosphere is needed, as in cases where parental overindulgence has caused intensive guilt feelings which lead to the repression of the guilt-provoking impulses.

The emphasis on the therapeutic importance of the emotional experience during treatment is essentially a vindication of Ferenczi's postulate, that the patient's reliving of the original conflicts in the transference situation is the primary tool of psychoanalytic therapy.

All this does not disprove, however, the value of insight. By his interpretive work, the analyst assists the patient's ego in integrating the new material liberated from repression. Making conscious what was hitherto repressed requires the reduction of anxiety. This is achieved by the corrective emotional experience and by the insight which in itself has an anxiety-reducing effect. The ego's function is mastery through insight. The integrative function is based on the appraisal of the total situation—both internal and external. Hence interpretive work increases the ego's self-confidence in dealing with newly uncovered material. Something a person understands loses its threatening quality; understanding means mastery. Properly devised attitudes and correct interpretive work together constitute psychoanalytic therapy.

Recently special attention has been given to the dependent cravings of the patient which tend to prolong the treatment. The neurotically impaired ego, to some degree, relinquishes its basic function of sustaining emotional equilibrium by its integrative and executive functions. It eliminates by repression all those impulses with which it cannot deal. Instead of using independent judgment, the ego is under the influence of incorporated parental images (superego reactions). Analytic therapy tries to substitute for this automatic regulation independent judgment appropriate to the mature state. It tries to replace parental precepts by conscious judgment which is flexibly adjusted to the ever changing situations. This is the essence of self-reliant rational behavior. In the transference situation the original parent-child relationship is re-established as the analyst replaces the incorporated image of the parents. The intra-psychic conflict between ego and superego is now converted into its original pattern through the relationship between patient and therapist. While the aim of the analytic therapy consists in replacing the automatic superego regulations with conscious control by the ego, the patient's tendency is to prolong the dependent relationship and rely on the analyst's aid instead of assuming responsibility for himself. This is essentially true for all neurotics and to a lesser extent for everyone. The trend toward dependence is deeply rooted in all human beings. It is only in degree that people differ from one another in this regard. The function of analytic therapy is to counteract this trend and induce the patient's ego to accept self-government. This entails persistent effort to counteract the dependent urge. Failure in self-government increases regression toward dependence; success encourages it. Every independent and successful accomplishment of an adaptive ego function means a step toward mental health. Yet the trend toward regression because of the inertia of the organism is ever present. It is one of the most difficult tasks of psychoanalytic therapy to dislodge the dependent relationship which gives the patient so much relief in his neurotic stress. By its very nature the analytic technique necessitates the establishment of a dependent relationship between patient and therapist, in order to allow the patient to relive and face again the old unresolved interpersonal relations with the parents. Inasmuch as it encourages dependence, the analytic technique which is devised to cure the neurosis carries in itself a factor which prolongs the neurotic condition. In order to resolve infantile reactions, one feature of which is always dependence, one must reproduce them in the transference; only then can one combat them. Much of the recent technical experimentation concerns this inherent difficulty in the analytical technique. Prolonged uninterrupted daily interviews in many cases favor the development of an intensive dependent relationship and consequently postpone recovery. To overcome this weak spot in the analytic technique is one of the crucial technical issues.

From the therapeutic studies of the Chicago Institute for Psychoanalysis, a series of technical recommendations resulted. The essence of them is that, from the beginning, the therapist must be aware of the danger inherent in the regressive tendencies of the patients. To counteract this danger, the analyst must consistently give the patient as much independence as possible. Interpretations alone cannot accomplish this. The dependent tendencies can often be counteracted by reducing the contact with the patient to that minimum which is necessary to preserve the continuity of the treatment. Properly timed reduction of the frequency of interviews, shorter and longer interruptions, are indispensable in every case. Encouraging the patient to new life-experiences outside the treatment suitable to increase self-confidence and encourage hope are also potent devices in weaning the patient from dependence on the therapist.

Our present technique of psychoanalytic treatment should by no means be considered as final and in need of no further improvements. In addition to numerous successfully treated cases, there are many failures and "interminable" analyses in which the treatment has become an emotional crutch which the patient can no longer dispense with. Not all these cases should be lightly dismissed as incurables. The long duration of many analyses should also serve as an incentive to explore further the possibilities for modifications by which the treatment procedure can be made more economical. Such advancement can come only from relentless experimentation, from the constant re-examination of the psychological processes during treatment and the re-evaluation of theoretical views, and particularly of those habits in treatment which stem neither from theory nor from controlled observations but which have been preserved merely through adherence to tradition.

II

PERSONALITY DEVELOPMENT

Therese Benedek, M.D.

THE psychoanalytic theory of personality consists of concepts concerning personality as an organization of the mental apparatus in general and of concepts concerning the processes which lead to differences specific for the particular individual.

In the infinite differentiations and integrations which make up the organization of the personality, it is useful to distinguish between the processes of maturation and those of development. "Maturation" refers to processes of growth which occur relatively independently of the environment; "development" refers to the interaction between maturational processes and environmental influences which lead to higher structuralization and to individual variations in the psychic apparatus. The development of the personality is the unfolding of an innate anlage—constitution—under the influence of the environment. Since the primary environment of the individual is created by the natural parents, who transmit to the child the patterns of the culture in which they live, genetic and environmental factors become closely interwoven, and "linked together they form"—as Freud put it—"an inseparable etiological unity."

The interaction between mother and child begins immediately at conception. We assume that the intra-uterine growth evolves through continuous gratification of basic needs, sheltered from external disturbances. However, not only the physiological processes of the mother favorable for the growth of the fetus are transmitted; more recent investigations indicate that fluctuations in the mother's physical and emotional well-being may also be registered by the fetus. Such influences, as well as the effects of obstetrical techniques, may modify the newborn child's adaptability to extra-uterine life.

Birth—the interruption of the fetal symbiosis—represents a trauma under any obstetrical condition. After a precarious passage through the birth canal, the newborn is subject to an overwhelming change in his physiology: he has to become active in securing the basic needs for living; he has to breathe, suck, and swallow. These vital functions are secured by reflexes co-ordinated during intra-uterine life. They are ready to function immediately after birth. Yet, since the network of the vegetative nervous system is not yet quite organized, the first weeks of life are characterized by vegetative instability. Irregular respiration, sneezing, yawning, regurgitation, vomiting, fitful waking, startle responses, give the impression that the newborn is not comfortable. It takes about four weeks—the "neonatal period"—for the infant to advance in maturation to a level where smoother vegetative functioning occurs.

The activity pattern of the newborn reveals marked individual differences. A stimulus intense enough to pass the threshold of a "phlegmatic infant" may activate in another infant not only a startle response but also a general excitation which provokes a crying fit. Even more significant are the differences in the activity and endurance in suckling, in the functioning of the digestive system, in the rhythm of sleeping and waking. There are other, less obvious differences in the sensory system of newborn infants: their sensitivity to sound and tone, to tactile and taste stimulations, shows marked variations.

According to Freud's hypothesis, the sleeping infant is in a condition closely resembling that of intra-uterine life. Stimuli from without and from within disturb this sleep. Hunger and pain are the sensations which most often waken the infant crying. The crying fit of the infant is a general motor discharge of excitement caused by internal need. It is characteristic of the newborn that, if the need reaches the threshold which activates crying, he continues with increasing intensity until the satisfaction of his need is made available; then he grasps at the nipple and appears to "work" with concentration until his hunger is stilled. If satisfaction fails to ensue, he may cry until his physical forces are exhausted.

The mother's genuine motherliness and her ability and desire to protect the infant reduce the frequency of disturbing stimuli and diminish the intensity of the crying fits. However, the mother's behavior toward her infant is motivated not only by her motherliness but also by the current customs of nursing care. In our civilization these customs have changed during the last thirty years, moving from one extreme to the other. Three decades ago, the nursing custom could be called "indulgent breast-feeding"; the infant was permitted to sleep close to the mother and be nursed any time the desire, not just imperative hunger, arose. As a reaction to the somatic effects of this indulgence, there followed the "strict regime" introduced by the German pediatric school (Czerny, Finkelstein). These pediatricians recommended keeping the infant isolated from the mother, and they established "feeding schedules," even at the cost of the infant's having to cry until exhaustion. It was later demonstrated that the all too routinized nursing care overlooked deprivations of various intensity and significance. Recently, a better balance between the child's needs and his gratifications has been recommended, thus allowing for individual differences rather than maintaining rigid regulations.

Normally, crying is a signal for the mother to take care of the baby. The rhythmically returning course of events is this: arising need—disturbance of sleep—crying—gratification—sleep again. As far as the newborn is concerned, this process evolves within the self, without the realization of an external environment. In this phase of extra-uterine symbiosis, the mother is part of the process of gratification. Sometimes one may observe intense sucking movements before the awakening of the infant. This phenomenon can be interpreted as repetition of the intra-uterine "practice" of the sucking reflex, which, in this early period of extra-uterine life, represents an attempt to continue the symbiosis and to preserve sleep. Naturally, the need remains unsatisfied and increases until it wakens the infant crying. The rhythmic alternation between need and gratification supplies the infant with the metabolic and emotional requirements for a smooth course of developmental events.

Feeding, especially at the mother's breast, not only satisfies hunger but also conveys to the infant the tactile and kinesthetic sensations of being protected; it preserves the security of the symbiosis. A biological communication between infant and mother is repeated with each nursing: the infant turns the head toward the mother's breast, incorporates it, retains it as part of the self, then separates himself from it, and by this, from the mother again.[1] The next step in growth is indicated when the

1. This process is supposed to represent the core (and the model) of the psychological process of identification, which is one of the basic patterns in personality development.

infant, after gratification of hunger—or after alleviation of discomfort and pain—does not fall asleep immediately but exercises "activities" already attained. He continues sucking playfully on the breast, enjoying the tactile sensations of lips and tongue, of fingers and cheeks, as they touch the breast; he learns to find his mouth in order to suck his fingers. While the infant enjoys the self-produced sensations, being awake enables him to perceive that the need originates within the self and the source of gratification—the mother—is outside.[2] We usually recognize this developmental step in the visual behavior of the infant: he follows the mother with his eyes.

The visual behavior of the infant is probably the first active manifestation of his need for communication with the environment, which, in the first place, is the mother. The infant's glance appears to greet the mother, his intent stare at her seems to grasp her and to hold onto her with his eyes before he can grasp her with his mouth. Soon after the visual co-ordination enables the infant to fix his gaze on an object, his mimical expressions become a rich means of communication. Not only the mother can interpret this body language; the trained observer also sees in it the content of the infant's primary relationship with his mother.

If the developmental process is undisturbed, the infant preserves the sense of security that all his needs are (and will be) satisfied. This sense of confident expectation from the mother is the content of the earliest affective relationship. Confidence is the intra-psychic correlate to the passive, receptive, dependent state of the infant; it plays an important role in his metabolic and psychic economy (9). Confidence sustains the mother-child unity and thus protects the infant from the intensity of external stimuli. Confidence acts as emotional shelter. It facilitates learning. The diminished instinctual tension enables the infant to give attention to the environment. The normal infant learns to understand the mother's facial expressions, just as the mother discerns in the infant's behavior the "signs and signals" of his needs as well as of his desires for activity. Through this preverbal communication, the child learns to accept the mother's reassurance in any new

2. Although a discussion of the maturation sequence is beyond the scope of this presentation, the author takes the growth processes and their observable psychologic manifestations more into consideration than is usual in psychoanalytic literature. It is in this sense that the author differs with Freud's concept that the newborn attributes all the pleasant sensations to the self and the unpleasant sensations to the environment.

step which his adjustment requires. The situation is different when the affect-position of primary confidence cannot develop. The conditions which lead to the disturbance of the primary relationship between mother and child keep the infant in a state of tension. Whether this is expressed in fitful sleep and crying fits and/or in feeding difficulties, the behavior of the infant reveals the disturbance of communication between infant and mother. Not trusting that his needs will be satisfied, his capacity for learning becomes inhibited, and in extreme cases (such as hospitalism), instead of learning, a reflex behavior develops. As the maturation proceeds, the healthy infant shows signs of recognition and a willingness to wait. The three-month-old infant recognizes the mother and the four-to-five-month-old follows attentively the preparations for his feeding.

By the time the infant turns his head toward the mother and smiles at her expectantly, the following developmental steps have been achieved: (1) differentiation between the self and the new environment, (2) perception of the mother as the "needed object" for relieving internal tensions, (3) experience of need as well as of satisfaction (pleasure of satiation within the self), (4) attention to animate and inanimate objects related to needs and gratification.

Since a psychic organization in which id is distinguished from ego emerges only gradually as a result of growth, from the point of view of personality organization the neonatal period represents an undifferentiated phase (32). The whole physiology of the newborn is in the service of survival alone. The maturation of the sensory and motor apparatus and certain emotional attitudes, such as the manifestation of the early relationship to the mother, are in the service of self-preservation and later will come under the control of the ego. The same growth processes produce a surplus of vital energies, which then become the source of pleasurable sensations and form a "reservoir of later differentiable psychic energies," which is the id (19).

With each step of the maturational processes of the motor and sensory organs, new needs for activity become manifest; it takes only a short while for the "practice" of these functions, that is, the functions themselves, to become a source of pleasure. For example, the unco-ordinated movements indicating discomfort, which one observes in the newborn when his blankets are removed, later become a push-and-pull game which reveals the infant's well-being. The pleasurable sensations come from all sources of vital energies and absorb the infant's attention immediately after the tension of the body is relieved. The relaxed infant either sleeps, or he is preoccupied with the pleasurable sensations of his body. These sensations, while originally representing only pleasurable excitation, may later become a need which demands gratification. Thus, at this stage of the development, one may differentiate between id and ego. The id generates impulses which may be supportive to, or in conflict with, the maturational and adaptive processes which form the tasks of the ego.

The libido theory was originally an anatomical concept. The organs which produce libido are the "erotogenic zones"; there the instinctual need is stimulated and is gratified. "Autoeroticism" is the gratification achieved by self-manipulation of the "zone" in which the need is perceived. The lips, the mouth, the skin, the anal mucous membrane, the penis, the clitoris, are considered erotogenic zones. In the center of the developmental organization is the erotogenic zone which is dominant at a specific age. In this sense, one speaks of "oral," "anal," and "genital" phases of development.

The first stage of libido organization is the "oral phase." The mouth is the erotogenic zone which experiences oral libido and its gratifications. The aim of oral libido is incorporation, and "the process is in the service of identification." This is, however, not an oral process exclusively. Olfactory, vestibular, and tactile sensations play a role in the feeding response of the newborn; some weeks later, auditory and visual sensations are also integrated into the feeding experience. Since all the sensory manifestations are in the service of the "receptive tendencies," these sensations as well as the feeding itself are a part of the process through which the infant evolves identification with the mother as well as a primary, affective relationship to her. The infant's capacity to adapt himself to his environment—the growth of his ego—goes hand in hand with the development of object relationship with the mother.

Not all the libidinal pleasure of the infant is autoerotic, generated by the self. The infant receives libidinal stimulation through the nursing care, through tactile, vocal, and tonal expressions of tenderness. Since the satisfaction of the physiological needs is fused with erotic, libidinous sensations generated by the mother, this continuation of gratification represents an urge strong enough to maintain object relationship. The interchange between auto-erotic and object-erotic gratifications is an important factor in successful infant care. The overstimulation of the loving mother, who does not let the waking infant be alone with his self-generated pleasures, actually frustrates the child; on the other hand, an excessive amount of autoerotic gratification at this age, similar to the extensive fantasy life of older children, turns the infant away from the object world and inhibits his efforts toward mastery of it.

Recent studies (41) of institutionalized children show that infants who did not develop object relationships or had to give them up because of neglect, withdrew from the environment and lived the life of preverbal fantasies which are expressed in the monotonous repetition of some form of autoerotic manipulation. Even if the condition is not extreme, overindulgence of the passive dependent needs can lead to an abundance of autoeroticism, since overindulgence deprives the child of the gains of his own expansiveness and inhibits his tendencies toward activity. There are many gradations between the compulsive, fixated autoeroticism of the withdrawn child and the happy, autoerotic pleasures of the well-developing infant. The former are diverted by hardly any substitute, while the latter turns his attention easily toward the mother and accepts her stimulation to external activities.

The primary process of mastery of the outer world repeats, to some degree, the process of incorporation. Grasping with the mouth is the first sign of not being afraid to incorporate (spoon, bottle, new food). Grasping with the hand and leading the object toward the mouth, putting it in the mouth and sucking on it, are the next steps in dealing with objects. (The child's own finger or toe is an external object in this respect.) The three-to-five-month-old baby grasps the bottle and holds onto it; the six-to-seven-month-old baby puts the objects which stimulate his interest into his mouth, in order to investigate them with his lips and tongue and thus to become acquainted with them. This is not a receptive, incorporative attitude alone; it is the manifestation of curiosity, through which the infant learns to recognize the objects of his surroundings. Learning is a receptive function later in life, too; what one really knows becomes a part of one's self. In infancy the receptive tendency appears manifest in oral activity—as if the baby has to be one with the object before he can learn to deal with it as a part of his external reality.

In deed, the receptive and incorporative tendencies and their psychic representation, oral libido, explain the psychodynamic processes of early infancy. The oral phase of development usually comprises the first year of life. Abraham (1) differentiated two levels within the oral phase: the *passive-receptive oral phase*, which lasts until the child becomes able to reach actively for objects; the *active-incorporative oral phase*, which is characterized by attempts at mastery through incorporation (biting is such a manifestation).

Abraham's distinction between the two levels within the oral phase has more than descriptive significance. The term "active-incorporative oral phase" indicates that the receptive tendency is charged with aggressive impulses; these are usually directed toward the mother. Mothers cannot always provide infants with the requirement of undisturbed development. "Nervous" infants respond even to slight stimulation with uncomfortable tension. Since the infant has no other means than the crying fit of discharging his tension, nervous infants often respond with a veritable "storm of excitation." It depends on the degree of maturity of the vegetative nervous system and the gastrointestinal tract whether the excitation becomes bound to definite parts of the gastrointestinal system. Since these systems are immature, colic, pylorospasm, diarrhea, or constipation may disturb the infant. Pain and tension increase the urge to gain relief and re-establish security by being close to the mother. The crying infant bites the nipple with force and suckles with greed. If the mother does not succeed in pacifying the infant, his physiological tension increases, and the need for incorporation becomes more and more charged with motor energy. This is called "hostile incorporation"; although the psychic representation of hostility can hardly exist at that age, its model is formed. While the crying fit alienates the helpless mother, who feels rejected by her child, the child feels even more "annihilated" by the sense of frustration, which leads to his exhaustion. The manifestations of hostile, aggressive, incorporative tendencies thus indicate the developing interpersonal conflict between mother and child; they also represent the origin of *ambivalence* in the infant and thereby the core of *intrapsychic conflict*.

The classical psychoanalytic theory of personality development was originally formulated by Freud and Abraham and consisted of the *libido theory*. Later, Freud developed the structural concept of the personality and defined its interacting functions as id, ego, and superego. Alexander (3, 4), considering that libido is produced by the positive balance (surplus) of the metabolic processes, defined psychic energy by the direction of its function rather than by the erotogenic zones (vector concept). These concepts are not contradictory; they complement each other.

This presentation of the developmental processes has traced the structuralization of the personality during the oral phase of the libido organization. Because of the physiology of the metabolic processes and the accompanying emotional needs, this phase can be described as the passive-receptive, dependent period of infancy. During this period, the differentiation of ego and id begins to evolve hand in hand with the development of primary object relationships. If the needs of the growing organism are not adequately met, insecurity, anxiety, and conflict develop.

Rado (39), Fenichel (18), and others pointed out that the first regulator of *self-esteem* (*Selbst-Gefühl:* a feeling of the self as a whole being) is the sense of security acquired by all the satisfactions connected with feeding; these analysts assume that the early disappointments and anxiety, which some infants experience in connection with feeding and digestion, may cause a sense of helplessness, inferiority, and worthlessness. If the positive, ego feeling is too often interrupted by its opposite, the ego development is impaired. (Fixation to the negative feelings within the self may become the core of psychosis or narcissistic neurosis.) The positive balance in the ego feeling, however, tends toward further differentiation for the sake of better adaptation.

The two principles of psychic processes—the *pleasure* and the *reality principles* (21)—are manifestations of the ego's adaptive function. The pleasure principle strives toward immediate gratification, and as such it serves the id; the reality principle tends to postpone immediate gratification in order to make later gratification secure by mastering the reality situation. Indeed, the infant learns soon to differentiate what causes pain and learns to avoid it; he learns also which of his actions bring the mother's—and other persons'—approval and expressions of love and which will bring about disapproval and withdrawal of love.

When the reality principle begins to take control of behavior, the child enters the second phase—the "anal-sadistic phase" of the development. This means that the anus becomes the leading erotogenic zone. Its double function—retention and elimination—becomes the center of interest and the source of pleasure. While the terms refer to the anal processes alone, actually urinary elimination and retention and the pleasure derived from them belong in the same developmental phase.

Toilet training is a crucial learning situation. In the authoritarian Western culture it was undertaken early. In recent years, with the increasing regard for the individual needs and expressions of the child, habit training is delayed to the second year. One assumes that compliance is easier when the child has achieved a degree of motor control. Walking is a good indicator of the change in the balance of the motor apparatus. When the child begins to walk, much of his attention is turned to this function. The increase in self-esteem which the child experiences with this achievement may easily be integrated with another achievement: sphincter control. At the same age the interpersonal relationships of the child have developed far enough so that he can understand the request of the adults and thus may "co-operate" in order to gain approval. The effectiveness of the parent's approval and disapproval as an instrument of habit training depends on several factors. One is the child's already established relationship to the parent; if this is ambivalent, the habit training becomes difficult. The other consideration is timing. There is an optimal time for habit training. This is when the stimulation of the urethral and anal passages is likely to create sensations intense enough to make the child aware of them and when the pleasurable quality of those sensations has not yet been enjoyed for too long a period. If the retentive and eliminative functions have already become an accustomed source of pleasure, the child will have difficulty in establishing control over them.

Toilet training is the ego's first conscious struggle for mastery over an id impulse. The process has several phases. It is usually the mother's task to influence the child—his ego—to exert himself against his tendency for soiling—against the id impulse. Actually, the child is offered a choice between various instinctual gratifications: the praise and love of the mother is one, and the satisfaction in soiling is the other. Thus the mother induces a conflict between rivalrous id impulses: an "instinctual conflict." With his compliance the child earns not only external approval but also internal satisfaction: a sense of mastery. When this sense of mastery becomes a goal in itself, the struggle reaches its next phase: the ego, stronger through gratification, tries to exert effort against the impulse without the help of the physical presence of the mother.

The request of the mother thus becomes incorporated, and the "sphincter morality" is gradually established. This represents a new structuralization within the self: the child becomes independent in so far as his ego can deal with the id impulse; but he also acquires the responsibility to do so—and this produces a new vulnerability. From this time on, anxiety signals danger when the id impulse is threatening to break through the controlling strength of the ego. Thus a "structural conflict" (8), i.e., a conflict between the incorporated prohibitions—primary superego—and the id impulse, is established and begins to control the behavior.

The method by which this result was achieved now pays its dividend. If the training was pursued with severity and punishment, the incorporated prohibitions appear to have such a strictly punitive quality that the child rebels against them and tries to turn the hostility back onto the mother. Defiance and hostile self-assertion during toilet training represent an attempt to externalize the conflict which has just been introduced within the self. The ambivalence—love and hate—thus expressed toward the mother creates a vicious circle: it increases not only the child's conflict with his environment but also the conflict within himself. It is more favorable for the further development of the child if at this time he is permitted and able to express his hostility toward the parent directly. If not, the defiance may be expressed by a failure in the rhythm of the sphincter functions: the child may eliminate when he should retain (lack of control: enuresis, diarrhea), or he may retain when he should eliminate (constipation). Under the confusing methods of toilet training, the excretory functions and their products become a highly appreciated value of exchange—an emotionally charged organ language—between the child and the environment.

Freud (27) described passive and active tendencies within the "anal-sadistic" libido organization. Abraham (1) attributed the passive anal-erotic tendencies to the first phase of that libido organization; he assumed that the first, the "passive-anal," phase coincides with the incorporation of and identification with the mother and with the development of ambivalence toward her. The second, the "active-anal phase," coincides, according to this theory, with the establishment of sphincter control and with the erotization of aggressive and self-assertive impulses. The child soon learns to transfer the active muscular impulses from his own body to others. The erotization of the aggressive impulses makes the term "anal-sadistic phase" appropriate for the second stage of pregenital development.

The psychic economy of the anal-sadistic phase is complex and precarious. The previously dominant passive-receptive tendencies, when the infant *was always given to*, changes to the awareness that he is also *taken from*. Retaining, of course, plays an important role not only in the physiological, but also in the emotional, metabolism. Receiving, retaining, eliminating—taking and giving—regulate the physiologic and psychic economy all through life. Actually, both physiologic and psychic economy have to remain in a positive balance in order to permit the active strivings of the organism to dominate over the passive receptive needs. If the balance of the economy is negative—this may be brought about by any serious deprivation or illness—a "regression" takes place; the active tendencies diminish or disappear, and the passive-receptive tendencies will dominate the behavior.

In the anal phase of development, when a "giving" attitude toward the environment is just at its beginning, the co-operation with the demands of the training may keep the child in a fearful tension, which repeats itself several times daily. Thus regression may occur repeatedly. This is the reason that infants, formerly happy and secure, sometimes become tense and negativistic and suffer from crying fits during a long-extended training period. After sphincter control is safely established, the conflict tension diminishes, and the child becomes free for the next step in his development. The greatest part of the infant's experiences, even those of the toilet-training period, occur mainly on the level of physiology and thus remain unconscious. But the experiences are not "organically" forgotten. The conditionings, during the oral as well as during the anal phase of development, and their psychic derivatives form a complex reaction pattern of somatic and psychic functioning.

It is in another area of maturation that the child learns to speak. This occurs usually during the second and third years of life. This complex process is considered to be the result of the progressing maturation of the speech apparatus and of intellectual accomplishments and is, therefore, not usually discussed in connection with the psychodynamic aspects of personality development. While the psychology of speech is beyond the scope of this presentation, we include some of its aspects which indicate the role of speech development in the structuralization of the mental apparatus.

When the infant coos and babbles in his crib, he uses his lips and tongue, also his vocal cords, not for communication, but for autoerotic pleasure. If his mother (or someone else whom he knows) enters his visual field and interest, the baby turns to his "dependable" means of communication: he smiles, he stretches his arms, grasps with his hands; he certainly makes his wishes understandable. When he is older and has already learned that movements of the lips and the tone accompanying them have importance for the mother, he babbles and coos back to her, trying to imitate her, though he is unable to co-ordinate the movements necessary for articulation. It has often been pointed out that the prevalence of oral gratification and the surplus excitation of the lips can be held responsible for the fact that, in every language, the word which means mother and the nursing person (and nursing implements) are formed by lip sounds: *ma—mom—mama; pa—ta—fa; ba—baba;* etc. These are the sounds which are first formed and are usually first noticed by the environment. But infants often repeat "unknowingly" some other sounds even earlier, sounds which accompany affects. Some infants inhale deeply when they are surprised or pleasantly amazed, and one can hear a definite syllable, like *hee, he, hei;* or they utter guttural tones, forming syllables when they are angry, like *ghroo, ghra,* or a combination of lip and hissing tones, such as *huppe, hppe.* Whether the infant "gets the idea" of speech by the experience that certain tones and sounds are forming the same way in his own mouth when he has certain feelings, one does not know. These affective utterances usually disappear after the child has learned to articulate in speech.

Each child learns to speak in his own way and at greatly varied times. Some children can speak one- to two-syllable words at nine months. Generally, children at first acquire a vocabulary which they use in single one- or two-syllable words, accompanied by gesturing. Some children, earlier than others but usually before the end of the second year, learn to speak a sequence of two to three words and then rudimentary sentences. In the third year they usually speak short sentences correctly and begin to speak of themselves in the first person.

Speech, phylogenetically the most recent acquirement, is abandoned quickly if the child is under the influence of affects. Not only in distress does the child cry rather than tell about his situation, but other emotions are also expressed by gesture rather than by word. The child jumps around with joy but does not say "I am glad," or he hides his face or himself altogether if embarrassed. Children in early years actually communicate by speech only when they are calm and their attention is directed. Under emotional influence, they revert to mimical expression. To this, we may add the body language of the urethral and anal functions to conclude that the language of emotions is primarily a body language; the verbal language, on the contrary, brings to the ego a means of communication beyond the purely physiological and emotional patterns of reaction.

The child learns to know many objects of his surroundings and to isolate them as functional units before he learns the word which designates the object itself. Since he hears the words, the names of things, he accumulates in his mind many word symbols before he can articulate enough to speak the words; and even more highly integrated must be the speech and the mental apparatus in order to express not only concrete things and needs but perceptions and feelings which are not directly connected with needs. Thus, when the child is able to speak the word "mama," he not only knows the mother as a person, different from others, but he has accumulated psychic experiences of identification with her, love, anger, and fear, and he also has stored in his mind symbols related to those experiences. These experiences, however, and the related symbols do not ever need to reach the level of verbalization. They form the content of the unconscious as the mental representation of physiological processes and/or as word and symbol representation of memory traces. The communication between these occurs through primary processes. In infancy and early childhood before the ego defenses interfere with the free flow of psychophysiologic energy, the demarcation between psychic and somatic processes is not so well defined as it is later in life. Therefore, only careful analysis of individual cases may reveal how much of the preverbal emotional processes occur purely on the level of physiology and how much reaches psychic elaboration which can be called "preverbal fantasy," how often and under what conditions they combine or change from one to another. All this needs to be investigated. Since the ego's control is not yet well developed, the child easily reverts to preverbal expressions. It is not words, therefore, but the child's activities, movements, and games, as well as his physiological regressions, which reveal the emotional processes which form his personality.

To take inventory of the psychosexual personality of the child as he is about to outgrow the age of toilet training, we shall review the various new differentiations within the psychic apparatus.

Since the prohibitions are introjected, the child has to protect himself not only against the fear of the parent but against the anxiety produced by the structural conflict. The primary super-ego manifests itself in the defense measures of the ego. The child at this age level is capable of loathing and shame. Loathing and shame are highly charged affects which used to be considered as reaction formation of the ego against the instinctual impulse; but they can also be defined as ego defenses, since they protect the ego by making the id impulse undesirable. While shame and loathing appear to be the manifestations of a strict superego, there are also simpler defense reactions. Small children expose naïvely their impulse to undo the harm which is already done (soiling) or to deny the blame. Undoing and denial are two typical ego defenses (19). If the child's fear of the parent is too great and the ambivalence conflict too intense, the developing ego defenses have a more serious character. Expression of the hostility against the parents or against a sibling and/or discharge of hostility against animals or turning the hostility toward the self are outcomes of the anal-sadistic tendencies. Both the aggression directed toward objects and the aggression turned toward the self play a significant role in the fixation of the conflict constellation of the anal phase. The sadistic, as well as the masochistic, tendencies and the structural conflicts which they imply create the disposition for compulsion neurosis as well as for paranoid reaction formations.

Normally, the simple ego defenses, together with the positive identification with the mother-teacher, enable the child to withstand the pressure for immediate gratification of his instinctual needs. While he postpones the gratification, the suspense presents a new stimulation. Now the child is ready for substitute gratification of the diminished instinctual tensions. Masturbation may begin through the suspense stimulation of the urethral and anal zone; the stimulation may extend to the genitals, and thus genital masturbation may channelize the urethral and anal excitation. The child at this age, however, is able also to divert his attention from direct, masturbatory gratification and can enjoy substitute gratifications in play with toys, with children and adults. The fantasy gratifications of this age level are complex and serve not only the gratification of the instinctual need but also the need of the ego for mastery. Hand in hand with the expansion of the ego, the interpersonal relationships of the child become manifold. He becomes aware of other people in his orbit besides the mother in the second half of his first year. In the second year these individuals begin to play distinct roles in his life. Innumerable identifications with the father bring him closer to the center of the child's psychosexual development. At the same time, the child explores the significance of siblings and responds to them day by day, to each one in a specific way. He may envy and hate one and admire another; he may feel that one is a source of security and reassurance or that he is a cause for competition, hostility, and ensuing guilt. The interpersonal relationships of the two-to-three-year-old are not based on the need for security alone; they are motivated by many other needs of the growing personality.

During the oral phase of development, there is hardly any difference in the emotional dynamics of the children of the two sexes. In the second year, during the anal phase, when self-assertion begins to play a role, marked differences are observed between boys and girls. The emotional security which results from the undisturbed relationship with the mother affects boys and girls differently. It gives the boy permission for self-assertion and courage that he may free himself from dependence on his mother and may start a development in which identification with his father becomes the leading motive. The girl's development takes a different course: the sense of security with her mother supplies her with the most effective impulses for identification with her mother. As long as the girl's identification with the mother is undisturbed, she learns from her easily. For example, it is well known to mothers that the toilet training of girls is usually achieved more easily than that of boys. Girls probably learn from the mother willingly and by identification, while boys learn from her only if and after their need for self-assertion has been satisfied.

Several behavior manifestations appear decidedly "masculine" or "feminine" even in two-year-old children. For the psychosexual integration, especially significant are the expressions of the child's interest in his body. During the anal phase the child learns a great deal about his body; he experiences some of its capacities and limitations. The ego gratification gained from good performance is abundantly enjoyed, but this pleasure is checked by disappointment and anger when the child fails to satisfy his ambitions. These reactions to failure are stronger in boys than in girls in general, and they become more obvious if the child compares himself with others. The roots of competitive behavior originate in the struggles for achievement of sphincter control. Jones (37) assumed that the competition in urinary behavior—the control and the power of the urine stream—is the model for all competitive behavior among men. Actually, it demonstrates the psychodynamics of competition in general: (1) the admiration for the successful competitor and the desire to be like him (identification); (2) anger toward the self because one is not like him and because the sense of frustration is not relieved; and (3) the projection of anger on the competitor who thus becomes responsible for one's failure.[3] During the anal and oedipal period the boy usually compares himself with his father; the effects of the comparison may contribute to passive reactions toward the father and to inferiority feelings. If the reactions of the child are too hostile to the father, the resulting fear may add to the developing castration complex. (Urinary competition with individuals of the same age is characteristic of the latency period.) The significance of urinary competition implies that the anus as an erotogenic zone is receding and that the penis is becoming the leading erotogenic zone: the boy enters the phallic phase of development. (The girl's responses to the experiences of her body at this age will be discussed later.)

The "phallic phase" is the third pregenital phase of development. In recent psychoanalytic literature it is more often referred to as the "oedipal phase," since the oedipus complex dominates its psychodynamic constellation. The term "phallic phase" originates in the concept that children of both sexes, at a certain age level, assume the existence of the same male genital in all persons. The term "oedipal phase" indicates that the child has arrived at that developmental level when his erotically colored demands are intensified and directed for gratification toward the parent of the opposite sex, i.e., the parent of the opposite sex becomes the object of the child's libido. Oedipus Rex (Sophocles) suffered blindness and exile as punishment for his unknowingly committed incest with his mother, Jocasta. The incestuous "crime" and the "punishment" for it represent the content of the oedipus complex. Several authors have attempted to be precise by intro-

3. "Projection of anger" sounds too severe a reaction in regard to the failure of the child. Yet we know how easily a child accepts the idea that a chair, a table, etc., is responsible for his hurting himself; he is relieved when he can "punish" it for its "misbehavior."

ducing the term "Electra complex" to define the conflict of the girl, caused by the heterosexual tendency directed toward her father. However, this seems to be cumbersome, and its use has not become general.

Boys begin to concentrate upon the genitals for gratification—in general—earlier than girls do. Boys' earlier awareness of the organ which produces pleasure is motivated by the anatomical differences in the sexual organs. The anatomy of the boy permits him to gratify his partial instincts freely. He can look at his penis and exhibit it; he can play with it while he urinates, and he may have sensations of fleeting erections. To this one may add the social evaluation of the male sex, the parents' pride in having a boy, and the pleasure of many fathers in stimulating sexual comparison in their sons and thus activating sexual preoccupation. The first manifestation of the awakening heterosexual interest is an intensified sexual curiosity which is normally directed toward the mother. She is the first object of her son's dependent love, and when he reaches another phase in his sexual maturation he holds onto the original object of his love. In this sense the male oedipus complex is simple.

The girls' development is more complex and somewhat slower. When the stimulation of the anal phase recedes, the sexual energy does not find an object for outlet through the body of the girl as easily as through the body of the boy. Thus, instead of concentrating on the genitals, the little girl's interest in and love for her body remains diffuse and is expressed mostly in pleasurable sensations of the skin and of motor co-ordination. The little girl's preoccupation with the mirror is not imitative; she is curious about her body, and she can look at it and enjoy its reflection. The diffuse narcissistic libido much later becomes directed toward the genital region.

There was, and still is, much discussion in psychoanalytic literature concerning the primary sexual development in woman. Freud's thesis (28) is that the genitals of the girl, except for the clitoris, remain undiscovered and without sensations until puberty; he assumed, therefore, that the first genital (i.e., phallic) response of the girl is curiosity regarding the genitals of the other sex, which she compares with her own. According to this concept, the first genital affect of the girl originates in the realization that she has no penis; the next may be the discovery of the clitoris as a substitute; the comparison results in a sense of inferiority which motivates the intense, biologically determined wish to have a penis. "Penis envy" is the center of the "female castration complex." Karen Horney (34) was the first in the ranks of the psychoanalysts who attacked this concept and pointed out that penis envy can be explained by the instinctually and socially preferred situation of the boy rather than by a biological inferiority of the girl.

The girl's oedipal development is not easy to explain. Her dependent needs satisfied by her mother, what motivates her in turning to her father for libidinal gratification? What mobilizes her heterosexual tendency? According to Freud's hypothesis, the penis envy mobilizes the tendency to incorporate the penis, to hold onto it, to possess it. This concept attributes a primary ambivalent motivation to the heterosexual tendency of the woman.

It seems that in the normal course of the maturational process, the feminine sexual anlage directs the libido toward the male sex. This threatens the girl with an instinctual conflict; her desire for her father's love represents a threat of losing the gratification of her dependent needs by the mother. This accounts for the prolongation of the pre-oedipal phase in the girl. Since she feels guilty because of her oedipal desires, any emotional upheaval in the little girl may be decided in favor of her dependent needs. The trial-and-error sort of fluctuation between heterosexual impulse and dependent needs has a significant role in the further development of sexuality.[4] When a regression to greater dependence occurs, the concurrent, diffuse erotization of the body may sustain the pregenital autoerotic behavior, or the libido may be steered to the genitals, stimulating masturbation and probably new conflicts. Through such repetitive processes, the girl finally develops the oedipus complex. This represents two conflicting instinctual tendencies: (1) the wish to be in the mother's place and to be loved by the father and (2) the wish to be the child and be loved by the mother. The first—the competition with the mother—carries with it the fear of punishment, the fear of losing the mother's love. This may be accepted by the girl as a stop signal, and she may turn back in her development to remain infantile but safe in her dependence. The other outcome of the oedipus complex may be that the girl, to be safe with the mother, strives for identification with the father or with a brother. Such an identification would make her safe against her heterosexual

4. This is usually repeated during adolescence, on another level of maturation.

wishes and would make her lovable to the mother as—she assumes—the father and/or brother are. Such a result of the oedipus complex intensifies the penis envy and, at the same time, fixates the development on an infantile level. The post-oedipal development of the girl continues in one of these two qualitatively different directions. The quantitative differences in the fixations account for the individual differences, namely, that the same process may lead to pathology in character formation in some individuals and to normal character development in others. Differentiation of these two main types is justified not only on the basis of the emotionally significant material but also on the basis of corresponding body-build and the evolving hormonal functions. Yet it would be a mistake to assume that these types are sharply delineated and definitely fixed. "Developmental processes" mean the struggle to overcome the factor which may interfere with an integration of the personality in which all factors are balanced.

The boy's oedipal development is more direct, less hesitating, than that of the girl. Yet the oedipus complex holds the crucial conflict of the male child also. The boy who was encouraged and stimulated to grow through identification with his father feels, at this step in his development, the urge to compete with his father and to take his place with the mother. Although his phallic tendencies cannot be consummated, the boy's sense of guilt for his sexual striving becomes concentrated upon the penis. He expects retaliation to be directed toward the organ from which he receives pleasure. The fear of castration—mutilation—develops, in varying intensity, even if a threat of physical punishment was never uttered. The castration fear impels the repression of the sexual tendencies toward the mother and sets in motion the most significant structuralization of the personality.

Castration fear changes the boy's relationship to his father; it brings out the mutual ambivalence. Even if the father has not been punitive and his attitudes have not intensified the son's hostility, the internal conflict alone is sufficient to bring out the guilty feelings of the boy. He hates and fears the rival father, whom he loves and appreciates as his protector outside the conflict area. Under the pressure of guilty feelings, the boy will tend to intensify his dependence on the father; he will try to please him, and, by identifying with him in other than sexual matters, he tends to idealize his father. As the child imagines that the parents do not exercise sexuality, which they forbid, he introjects an asexual image of the parent, and thus the sexual prohibition becomes internalized. By the strength of the internalized prohibition, the boy attains the capacity to respond to the moral code of the environment, not out of fear of retaliation, but because the parents' prohibition has become a part of his own personality: in this way, the superego is established. This is such an important structuralization within the ego that Freud (21) attributed to it the quality of an inner psychic institution which controls and regulates instinctual impulses. It would be a mistake, however, to assume that the superego is a topically defined entity, functioning from above, mastering the id impulses and policing the ego. The superego represents the sum of those differentiations within the ego which develop through internalization of prohibitive influences. We have discussed one of its earlier manifestations in the adaptation to sphincter control. While the repression of the oedipus complex is a thrust for the stabilization of the superego, it does not represent its final organization. It takes many years through the process of mastery of castration fear and resolution of the oedipus complex before the mature superego becomes an integrated part of the personality.

What are the sexual manifestations of the third pregenital organization, the oedipal phase? Infantile sexuality is essentially autoerotic and is expressed in diffuse manifestations of partial instincts. The oedipal phase represents the first or primary concentration of erotic strivings upon the genitals. Yet the manifestations of this infantile genital organization naturally remain autoerotic, albeit the instinctual need has an "object" outside the self, in the parent of the opposite sex. But the father and/or the mother have "normally" a nonaccepting attitude toward the erotic impulses of the child. The rejection (nonacceptance) of the heterosexual parent, on the one hand, and the fear of the parent of the same sex, on the other, keep the oedipal tendencies of the child in check; the genital tendencies may turn toward substitute objects and are often acted out with siblings and playmates; they also supply the libidinal excitation for genital and substitute masturbation.

Besides the direct manifestation of sexual impulses, there are psychosexual activities, characteristic of this period, which reveal not only the sexual tendencies but also the ego's defenses against them. They indicate the psychodynamic processes by which the oedipus complex is finally repressed and resolved.

1. *Sexual curiosity*.[5]—The desire to gain knowledge about the sexual apparatus and its functioning is an attempt at mastery by intellectualization. In the guise of objective inquiry, the child is allowed partial gratification; in talking about it, the child expresses his sexual tension and conveys it in a limited measure to the parent toward whom it is directed. Since the answers, whether they are objectively informative or evasive, cannot lead to gratification, the child's questioning may become a compulsive preoccupation. Factual information may coexist in the child's mind with sexual theories of his own creation.

2. *Infantile sexual theories*.—Such theories are characteristic attempts at solving the riddle of one or the other aspects of the propagative functions. Usually a child has a "theory" for only one phase of sexual functioning. For example, one child is more preoccupied with the idea that impregnation occurs through the mouth; another with the theory that birth occurs through the anus; etc. Although aware of the genitals and able to perceive sensations from them, the child cannot imagine their functions or accept them emotionally. In his own "sexual theory," the child admits that the body of the adult actively participates in the act of procreation, but he attributes the process to organs the functions of which he has experienced and, in some sense, understands. In his sexual theories the child seems to charge the organs —gastrointestinal tract, mouth, anus—with new libidinal interest at a time when he is about to overcome the libidinal organization centering around them. This fluctuation between the libidinal charges actually helps to *deny* the significance of the genitals.

3. *Denial*.—Denial is an ego defense which represents a step toward the repression of an ego-alien impulse. The child, convinced that "that cannot be which should not be" in his effort to desexualize the parents, tries to believe: "My parents would not do that." And even later, when the child knows about the "facts of life," he may still cling to the idea with a slight modification and often believes that the parents have had intercourse only as many times as they have conceived children. Such denial of the parents' sexuality is the result of the incorporated taboo of sexuality. Measured by such an idealized image of the parent, his own

5. Freud (25, 29) considered sexual curiosity to be the root of all intellectual curiosity, since its instinctual energy can be transferred to other areas of knowledge: if sexual curiosity is inhibited by fear and its energy repressed, intellectual curiosity may also become inhibited.

sexual impulses appear unacceptable to the child; thus they cause guilty feelings and fear of punishment.

The repression of the knowledge about the parents' sexuality is caused not only by the anxiety implicit in the oedipal conflict but even more, or probably primarily, by the discomforting tension which the unintelligible sexual excitation activates in the child. The auditory and visual perception of the parents' sexual intercourse represents the "primal scene."[6] The concomitant sexual excitement of the child and the anxiety aroused by it may represent a trauma of pathological intensity. Its affective charge may be reactivated again and again until it has been slowly mastered through fantasies, through symptom formations, and, finally, through the developmental processes which were set in motion by the oedipal conflict. While it is easy to understand the significance of the primal scene for those who have witnessed it, it is interesting that the psychic elaboration of the parents' sexuality also plays a role in the fantasy life of those children who have never been exposed to this experience. This indicates that, if sexual impulses mobilize the ego's struggle against them, the child draws into the area of sexuality previous experiences of nongenital nature. He may elaborate all sorts of prohibitions as sexual prohibitions, all kinds of tenderness as sexual seductiveness, and all gentleness between the parents as "primal scene." Thus he may sustain fantasies which are necessary for the intra-psychic "working-through" of the oedipal conflict. We may assume, however, that the repression of the sexual impulses and with it the desexualization and idealization of the parents evolve more smoothly if the child is not exposed to overwhelming sexual stimuli. If the child is unable to repress the affects caused by witnessing the primal scene, he is impelled to rationalize his anxiety caused by sexual tension. This leads usually to the following process.

4. *A sadistic concept of sexuality.*—The anxiety-producing idea that sexual intercourse is an extremely brutal activity which endangers the life of a parent (usually the mother) changes the meaning of sexuality. Instead of love, the child attributes to it aggressive tendencies of threatening intensity. This necessarily intensifies the fear of his own sexual impulses. The increased conflict tension often leads to massive inhibition of the sexual

6. Freud referred to this also as "primal fantasy" (24).

impulses, or it may seek solution in identification with the opposite sex.

5. *The identification with the opposite sex.*—Such identification is a defense against intense castration fear and/or wish. The loss of the penis is not inconceivable to the little boy. He is "prepared" for it by previous experiences which he might have interpreted as a loss of a part of his body. Thus impressions, like the loss of the nipple from the mouth, the loss of the feces from the anus, might reinforce the fear of losing the penis (2). The fleeting tumescence of his penis, which comes and goes beyond his control, may be frightening. When the boy discovers the female genital region (his mother's or some little girl's), the danger of losing his penis may be corroborated; he realizes that there are human beings not so endowed. To the boy who, by anlage or by experience (or both), has developed intense castration fear, this discovery may be a traumatic experience. To him the female genitals appear as a devouring organ, which may incorporate his penis and keep it. To avoid this catastrophe, the identification with the dangerous individual appears to be the efficient defense. Through the identification with the mother, the boy develops a "negative oedipus complex": instead of identifying himself with the father in order to have heterosexual feelings toward the mother, he offers himself, so to speak, as a passive love object to the father and wants to replace the mother. Thus the negative oedipus complex diminishes not only the fear of the vagina but the boy's fear of the strong father (who would punish him for his sexual feelings toward the mother). During such a negative oedipal phase, the boy may hate the mother, whom he considers an intruder between him and the father, but he may also regress and intensify his passive dependent attachment to the mother, or he may try to avoid the father, especially if the father is not sympathetic toward the son's passive tendencies. Escape into femininity is not a socially acceptable solution. Soon the passive tendencies are in conflict with the need for self-assertion and masculinity. After new attempts at identification with the father, the normal positive oedipus complex may finally be achieved.

The retarding effect of the identification with the male sex on the girl's oedipal development has been pointed out before (see p. 81). Referring to this, however, we usually do not speak of a negative oedipus complex. When the girl recoils from her heterosexual tendencies and turns to the mother for love, she repeats the pattern of her dependence on the mother. Yet, if the girl's fear of the feminine sexual function becomes intensified by the sadistic concept of sexuality, the resulting "female castration complex" may interfere with the further oedipal and sexual development: the fear of the male (father's penis) impels the intensification of the girl's incorporative tendencies, the goal of which is, in this instance, the *identification with the aggressor*. The little girl's fascination with the penis and the ensuing active curiosity are manifestations of her heterosexual tendency, but its goal is the possession of the penis. Some girls, obsessed by this need, become very aggressive toward little boys in the oedipal age; other girls, more passively, try to imitate the boy's behavior. In all these instances, penis envy, as a defense against the female sexual tendencies, dominates the outcome of the oedipal conflict.

The various phases of the oedipus complex may occur not only in time sequence but also side by side in the same individual. The active heterosexual tendency and the fear of its punishment, as well as traces of identification with the opposite sex, are present in every individual. The psychodynamic significance of these factors and their interaction depend upon the tendency to bisexuality.

Bisexuality is a primary quality of the biological anlage. Its manifestations may be discerned in the variations of the child's tendencies for identification. But it takes the struggle of the oedipal phase to reveal the quantitative differences between masculine and feminine tendencies; between readiness to take the risks of heterosexual development or recoil from it because of the strength of the opposing tendencies. In the *Studies on Hysteria* Freud (15) developed the concept that the unresolved bisexual component of the oedipus complex is responsible for the fixation of libido which tends toward discharge in *conversion hysteria*. Hysteria is generally considered as a neurosis referable to the oedipal conflict, since the psychic energy maintaining its symptoms originates in the unresolved conflicts of that developmental phase.

Since the structuralization of the personality progresses, the conflicts of the oedipal period can be more clearly differentiated than those of the anal period as: (1) instinctual conflicts, arising between the various instinctual tendencies; (2) structural conflicts, arising between the instinctual tendencies and the already introjected prohibitions: superego. The ego—as an organ of adaptation—seems now to have developed far enough to undertake the function of mediation between (1) instinctual needs and their prohibitions (superego), (2) instinctual needs and external reality, and (3) internal (structural) conflict and reality. At this stage of development, the ego can best safeguard its functioning by repressing the sexual tendencies. Freed from the tensions and disturbances caused by immature sexual impulses, the personality is prepared for the next developmental phase: *the latency period*.

In our culture the beginning of the school age (six years) usually, or ideally, coincides with the emerging latency period. The desexualization of the child's interest enables him to comply with environmental requirements and thus to expand in mental and social growth. The latency period is considered, generally, as the age of character formation.

The early psychoanalytic concepts considered character traits as transformations of and reaction formations to the originally libido-charged, instinctual tendencies. Abraham (1), with a brilliant comprehension of psychic connections, ascribed specific character traits to the transformation of specific libido organizations. Thus he described oral, anal, and genital sources of character trends. According to our present concepts, character trends represent well-defined structuralizations within the ego. The previous discussion of developmental processes, such as learning of sphincter control, desexualization and idealization of the parents in establishing the superego, may serve as examples of the differentiation of psychic energies through which the integration of character trends within the personality may take place.

The primary biological tendencies of giving and taking, of retaining and eliminating, appear as habits of the ego function during the latency period. The continuation of the oral receptive pleasure is manifest in the desire to receive material as well as spiritual gifts. The need to receive may express the normal degree of dependence, or it may increase to insatiable demandingness. Some children at this age show a willingness to give and to share, while others are unable to separate themselves from possessions; others again seem always to be afraid of losing something. The tendencies for aggressive incorporation appear in manifestations of envy, jealousy, and maliciousness. The intensity of these emotions may lead to stealing. Stealing at this age does not necessarily indicate a lasting trend toward delinquency. It is considered rather the "acting-out" of an emotional tension resulting from the child's struggle with several concomitant frustrations. After the child has renounced gratification of sexual impulses, he may experience intensification of the receptive-incorporative tendencies. This may cause, for example, an irresistible desire for sweets or to own things which do not belong to him; it may also increase the child's desire to resist the authority of prohibitions set up by adults. Thus stealing, while it satisfies the child's incorporative urge, also expresses his need for self-assertion. Children resort to stealing usually when they feel helplessly abandoned to several inconsistent prohibitions. Stealing is an emergency reaction of the ego; it indicates how narrow the margin is between what we expect as normal and what we call abnormal behavior at this age. The reason for this is in the "brittleness" of the newly formed superego reactions. At first, the internalized prohibition tends to be overrigid and strict. If the frustrations are not relieved or if they are too severe, inhibiting several areas of the personality, the superego may yield, and "acting-out" or other regressions occur.

Even more complex are the character trends related to the anal retentive and eliminative tendencies.[7] The latency period is the age in which the child's attitude toward orderliness appears "characteristic." Some children cannot be taught orderliness; they lose their possessions, scatter them, forget about them. Other children are meticulous. Some children who were orderly before become rebelliously disorderly and unclean during "latency." The dynamics of this reaction is similar to stealing. Restriction in one or many areas of the personality may demand regressive behavior in another area, especially if this area was highly charged in the previous developmental phase. For example, children who were toilet trained early may become quite unclean as far as their general habits are concerned.

The retentive tendency may become manifest in the *passion for collecting* and in the desire to systematize the collection. The cherished objects may change often, since renouncing interest in previously valued objects, discarding them, or forgetting about them have their developmental significance, too. Since the objects have symbolic value, toying with them represents substitution for and/or stimulation of sexual fantasies. It is well known that the difference in the emotional makeup of boys and girls is

7. This enumeration of "character trends" is incomplete and serves only as examples of the organizational processes within the ego.

revealed in the objects they collect. Every age has its characteristic fad. Young boys usually collect stones, pieces of string, keys, mechanical tidbits—objects which represent masculine occupation. Some years later they change to stamps, to work models, to bugs and butterflies, etc. Little girls usually collect boxes, ribbons, and beads, all sorts of materials useful for dolls. When somewhat older, they collect pictures and picture cards, cutouts, and things to "trade with." If boys show interest in the objects usually cherished by girls, or vice versa, this fact is considered a sign of bisexuality. However, the interest may take definite turns. The developmental changes in the psychodynamic tendencies are responsible for the lability of emotional value (object cathexis) represented by the collected material. For some children, possession in itself remains significant even after the collective urge has diminished; for others, the possessions become a means for developing interpersonal relationships. Some children feel the need to "overpay" for friendship; they give away what they value (whether it belongs to them or to someone else) in order to gain prestige and love; others, again, develop skilful acquisitiveness by turning their interest from valued objects to objective values. None of these characteristic attitudes, although they are referable to the primary biological tendencies, can be considered simply as sublimation of, or reaction formation to, any one tendency alone. Any new attainment has to fit into the already established patterns of functioning, in order to safeguard the positive balance within the systems of the personality necessary for undisturbed development. If this cannot be achieved, the arising conflict tension motivates new attempts for solution.

Fantasy is an intra-psychic safety valve which yields relief from tension and at the same time provides intermediary steps in development. Fantasy is a form of primitive thinking which, in contradiction to logical and realistic thinking, permits the wishes and desires—the psychic representations of the instinctual needs—to appear attainable or even fulfilled. The fantasies most crucial for the personality development have been discussed in relation to the oedipus complex. The biological urge which motivates those fantasies is the impulse to grow and become like the parent. But the struggle for the repression of the oedipal fantasies and the "threat" which they imply indicate that identification with the parent in order to be safe must be achieved by small steps. Characteristic of the latency period are fantasies which, either through imagination alone or through games, repeat and channelize the developmental conflicts, paving the way for their resolution. The universal inclination of girls to play with dolls is an example. These games give the girl opportunity to express (1) dependence on the mother: "I love my doll as I want to be loved by Mother"; (2) hostile conflict with the mother: "I treat my doll badly, I hate her, as my mother hates me and treats me badly"; (3) conflict within the self: "I hate my doll because she is like me, a girl," or "I love my doll because she is like me, a girl," or "I love my doll because she is what I can be"; etc. There are innumerable variations of fantasy games played by boys and girls which prepare them for mastering situations and for satisfying their ambitions.

Since it affords autistic gratification, fantasy tends to make the child independent of the environment (in the area of the needs gratified by the imagination). Fantasy yields pleasure and brings consolation for pain. Since it reduces action to endopsychic function, it diminishes the conflict with the environment and thus serves as protection against fear. If the child feels unable to cope with a situation, the protective use of the fantasy may grow out of hand; the rampant imagination may bind an unduly great part of the child's psychic energies and thus interfere with his adjustment to reality. Not all fantasy yields protection. Some fantasies create conflicts with the superego and produce anxiety. One fantasy may even counteract the psychodynamic effect of another. Fantasies may absorb the psychic energy of conflicting tendencies and thus become the focus of developmental disturbance.

The concept of "latency period" implies that, after the psychodynamic tendencies of the oedipus complex have been repressed, the child becomes free from sexual impulses and, protected by his ego defenses, lives in a quasi-asexual environment. He has repressed his need to expose and express erotic tendencies and with it his wish to hear, to see, and to know about sexuality altogether. Yet observations reveal that sexual impulses can easily be stimulated in the child by external as well as by internal experiences, even if an asexual period has been achieved. In a great percentage of children, a complete latency period does not develop at all. Even if the content of the oedipus complex is repressed, the pregenital sexual tendencies, fixated by infantile eroticism, persist and stimulate sexual activities of various extent and significance. Whereas desexualized pregenital tendencies can be integrated in the ego as character trends and mitigated libidinous tendencies can be dealt with in ego-permissible fantasies, sexual impulses of greater intensity cannot be mastered in any way but by discharging them in sexual activity. Sexual behavior and its accompanying fantasies—disturbances of the latency period —often determine the ways and practices by which the individual will attain sexual gratification throughout his life.

The concept of latency period as a biologically determined phase of human development has provoked criticism and has caused a great deal of controversy. Objections are based mainly on anthropological data. Children of many primitive societies do not develop a latency period because the moral code of their environment does not imply sexual prohibitions like those of the Western cultures. Incest is taboo in primitive civilizations, as well as in ours, but the structure of the family organization in most primitive cultures permits a dispersion of the child's psychosexual energies among many persons, without provoking such exclusively significant focus as the father and mother are in the patriarchal family of Western civilization (38). However, individuals of the primitive cultures described in this connection do not develop such differentiation of the psychic apparatus which our superego represents.[8] Superego is the "intra-psychic institution" by which, in our civilization, the family achieves its cultural function and "carries the cultural demands from generation to generation." This educational process is the result of a continuous two-way communication between the child and his parents.

In discussing the developmental processes from early infancy thus far, we have referred repeatedly to the processes of introjection and identification; they represent basic adaptive responses of the child to the parents. We have not mentioned, however, the parents as individuals, as persons with specific wishes and ambitions, with problems of their own personality and experience. Yet the parents in their everyday living express in a way perceivable to the child their expectations and gratifications, the hopes, fears, and frustrations related to their parenthood. Parental behavior is rooted in the personality development of each of the parents; it is modified by the parents' relationship to each other,

8. In comparison with the individualistic superego in our culture, the superego in primitive societies is collective.

and it unfolds toward the child in innumerable manifestations of love, care, tenderness, as well as of impatience, anger, and punitiveness. Through countless processes of mutual identifications and projections, the relationship between the parents and the child forms an intrinsic psychodynamic unity—*the family triangle*: father-mother-child. The culmination of the complex interactions within the family triangle is reached in the superego.

Freud arrived at his concept of the superego and its function for the individual as well as for society by studying individuals reared in patriarchal families. The psychodynamic processes within the family triangle appear to have been simple in the traditional patriarchal family as compared with "individualistic" families. In the patriarchal family, the role of the parents was well defined: the father, strong, infallible, the threatening representative of the moral code; the mother, the main (or only) source of tenderness, herself abiding by the authority of the husband. The parents, supported in their function by religious and secular authority, pursuing their educational goal with unwavering but simple principles, were well suited for idealization and for becoming the core of a strict and prohibitive superego. But even in the patriarchal family the child introjects not only the aims and wishes of his parents but also their inconsistencies and shortcomings.

In our present individualistic civilization the dynamic forces of the family triangle tend to become more involved. The parents, eager to maintain and to emphasize their own individuality in relationship to each other, are inclined to minimize the differences in the role of the father and that of the mother in regard to the child. In the attempt to convey to the child the meaning of his own individuality, they often diminish the distance between themselves and the child. Thus modern individualistic parents renounce, often too early and too much, their rights and responsibilities for guiding the child. By leaving him to his own "decisions," they confuse the child about his powers and his limitations. The ambiguities of such parent-child relationship become even more apparent if the sexual education is too permissive or seductive. Thus, while the child is not compelled to repress his impulses, he is exposed to several internal conflicts without being able to resolve them after a pattern set by the parents. Such parents often interfere with the goal which they are anxious to achieve. Instead of furthering the individualization of the child, they do not afford the conditions in which a stable superego can be established. Too many children incorporate the doubts and conflicts of their parents in such a way that in specific areas of their personalities they do not learn to distinguish right from wrong. Thus a deformed character develops.[9]

Compulsion neurosis is a condition caused by the strictness of the superego. It develops when rebellion and hostility toward authority has to be repressed early and under the pressure of great fear. Indeed, the authoritarian regime of the traditional patriarchal family is conducive to the development of compulsion neurosis. It should not be overlooked, however, that personality development is motivated by too many factors to be pressed into relatively simple equations. It happens often that in families where the father is lenient and "understanding" the children may develop compulsion neurosis. Their superego responds to an unconscious guilt in proportion to the lenience of the father and sets up a rigid internal regulation of behavior.

Generally, the superego is strict and rigid during the latency period as a protection against ego-alien impulses which the father did not sufficiently control. Therefore, children in these years often suffer from compulsive neurotic symptoms. Many of the games are but compulsive activities or magic ceremonies that serve the purpose of overcoming superego demands. If the family triangle is responsible for the development of a superego which encompasses many conflicting tendencies, the intra-psychic struggle may lead to depressive or to delinquent personalities. In the former "autoplastic solution," the punishment is doled out to the self before it can become guilty in action; in the latter "alloplastic solution," the ego—too weak to stand the internal pressure of the conflicts—"acts them out" to invite the punishment of the environment.

The next developmental phase is introduced by the physiological maturation of the sexual apparatus. From the first manifestations of the secondary sex characteristics until the completion of functional maturity, several years pass. The term "puberty" indicates the time of physiological maturation; the term "adolescence" refers to the complex interaction between the physiological and psychological processes involved in the developmen-

9. Several studies of the development of delinquency demonstrate such disturbances in the ego development (Szurek, 42; Johnson, 36; Bettelheim and Sylvester, 14; Eınch, 17.

tal task of this period. *Adolescence* can be considered as a new chance for the reorganization of the personality. The disquieting manifestations of adolescence cannot be attributed alone to the physiologic upheaval of puberty. Since no developmental phase is entirely overcome and since each new developmental achievement, or its failure, possesses the characteristics derived from the earlier history of the personality, it is to be expected that puberty will bring to the fore the conflicts which were latent. Adolescence, indeed, puts the ego to a hard task; the ego, using the newly upsurging psychosexual energy (which is at the same time a source of uneasiness), must master the old conflicts and integrate them into the functions of the adult personality. It is no wonder that this process, strongly overdetermined by sociological and cultural factors, is circuitous and takes a longer time for reaching its goal than does the physiologic maturation itself.

The early signs of physiologic maturation are noticeable in many instances—in boys and girls alike—as early as the age of nine, but, on the average, the physiologic changes of puberty take place gradually between the ages of ten to fourteen. The psychology of the *prepubertal period* is largely that of the latency period, which, once established, only slowly gives way under the influences of the physiologic growth. Helene Deutsch in her study, *The Psychology of Women* (16), discusses the manifestations of the girl's "last defense" against the oncoming sexual maturation. Shyness and shame because of the growth of the breasts may trouble some girls; others may be concerned about expected menstruation. Normally, these emotions are reactions to the libidinous feelings caused by the physiologic processes and may soon give place to *positive narcissism:* a normal libidinal cathexis of the body. If, however, the *bisexual* tendency is dominant, the onset of feminization of the body may activate anger and hostility toward the self, which may be expressed in various indirect manifestations of self-destructive tendencies, for example, in overeating. In these instances, we may speak of "negative narcissism."

The boys' reaction to physiologic changes of prepuberty are normally free from denial and shyness. Since the center of his body narcissism is the penis, the boy accepts the growth of his genitals and the other signs of the beginning sexual maturation with a sense of gratification and pride. Thus the male puberty is characterized by a more or less free expression of autoeroticism.

Yet (and this is the perplexing problem of male adolescence in our culture) boys go through a complex developmental process which leads from the *early genital phase* to the *final genital phase*. The latter implies, as Abraham (1) stated, that the boy has "attained a point in his object relation where he no longer has an ambivalent attitude toward the genital organ of his heterosexual object, but he recognizes it as a part of that object whom he loves as an entire person."

Not only the male but the female also has to overcome the remnants of the castration complex in order to become able to reconcile with love the existence and function of her own sexual organ and that of the heterosexual love object. In the case of male development, the oedipal phase ended with the desexualization of the mother and the depreciation of sexuality. The rejection and loathing of the female sexual organ is an integrating part of sexual repression; the result of it is the fear of the "castrating" female sexual organ. At puberty, the arising sexual needs again mobilize the earlier castration fear with increased intensity. Psychodynamically similar are the effects of the female castration complex. At the time of puberty, the fear of the (envied) male organ is mobilized again. This recharges the defenses against the male and causes the flight from the feminine sexual role. As the sexual maturation proceeds, the libido tension finally succeeds in overcoming the fear of being hurt, and by this the sexual act becomes possible.

The hormonal function of the maturing sexual apparatus together with other processes of growth produces "surplus energy" (3, 6), which charges the body with a sense of well-being. "Primary narcissism" is the libidinal energy which originates in the positive metabolic balance. The primary narcissistic libido is channelized in activities which satisfy the ego's sexual needs as well as the needs for mastery in nonsexual areas. Through the accomplishments of ego-syntonic and ego-elating activities, the ego becomes charged with a sense of the value of its functioning. "Secondary narcissism" is the term for the libidinal charge of the ego which, originating in the satisfaction with one's self, serves as a defense against disappointments in one's self. The adolescent struggle for intra-psychic equilibrium may be described in terms of exchange between primary and secondary narcissism.

Adolescents, boys and girls alike, when they perceive sexual impulses after the latency period, attempt to master them by repeating the effort which was successful at the oedipal phase: namely, repression. As the struggle against sexuality proceeds, all the available resources of sublimation are mobilized, and expansion of interests and achievements is generated. The fascination for abstract problems, the tendency to project one's subjective problems into the realm of the absolute or into the culturally significant, and other feats of creative imagination can be considered—from one point of view—as ego defenses of the adolescent. Since they afford ego gratification on a high level, they reassure the youth of his individual merit at a time when internal turmoil threatens his equilibrium.

For the repression of the primary narcissism and its sexual manifestations, the youth is rewarded by the augmentation of his secondary narcissism. Yet the ego, even though its power is enhanced by secondary narcissism, cannot withstand for long the pressure of the instinctual impulses; the defenses yield and the instinctual tension is released. Since the span between the ego's aspirations and the sexual impulses is great, however, the sexual gratification is soon followed by remorse. This again reactivates the ascetic attitude and its gratifications, but only to fail and to yield again to the instinctual demands. Thus develops the "polarization of affects" which Anna Freud (19) finds characteristic of adolescence. It is obvious that the effect of the vicious circle between asceticism and indulgence may drive the adolescent farther away from adjustment to reality.

The normal adolescent, however, can hardly enjoy his isolation. His need to withdraw is disturbed by the internal stimulation of the sexual need, as well as by his need to conform with external reality. He is too aware that insecurity is the root of his need for isolation. Hence the shyness, awkwardness, and hypersensitivity lest others will notice what he wants to hide; hence the rebellious pride that he displays in defending his new values, which he has acquired to satisfy a new ego ideal and which he appraises as different from the old one, formed after the father and/or the mother. Thus old, hidden ambivalence conflicts become buoyant and are easily provoked into some sort of discharge by incidents which would seem insignificant at any other time. The defiant, often exasperating, behavior of the adolescent may be considered as a symptom, and, in some instances, it may actually reach a pathological, asocial degree; yet generally it is a manifestation of the resolutions of the original conflict with the parents. Through many repetitions of the rebellious, hostile behavior, the adolescent "fights it out," the boy more with the father, the girl with the mother. The emotional upheavals brought about by such hostile episodes reach deep into the unconscious and lead finally to a shift in the structure of the superego. In "The Passing of the Oedipus Complex" (26) Freud formulated one of his fundamental concepts. There he points out the dynamics of the processes by which, through many repetitions, the ambivalence conflict embodied in the superego finally reaches its resolution. Its aggressive (destructive) energy discharged, the superego loses its rigidity; it becomes more pliable than before, since it is independent of the past (parents).

In interaction with such structural changes in the personality the sexual drive reaches its integration step by step. Usually this process involves the overcoming of the auto- and homoerotic tendencies. Conflicts between these and the heterosexual impulses and between them and the inhibiting factors of the personality motivate the inferiority feelings and induce the moodiness which seems to justify the assumption that adolescents suffer from narcissistic neurosis. Through tribulations and depressions, the adolescent boy relives his early unconscious identification with his mother. The conscious manifestation of this is his conviction that he "understands" women—usually one woman whom he does not need to fear and may therefore begin to love. This phase of adolescence is governed by different dynamics in the girl's development. The bisexuality of the girl is already intensified in prepuberty and may persist with various oscillations for a long time. As the sexual maturation proceeds, the emotional manifestations of the feminine, passive-receptive tendencies diminish the effect of masculine identification and prepare the girl to find a heterosexual love object.

The resolution of the adolescent conflict does not mean merely that the adolescent has achieved the capacity for genital gratification—the male, sexual potency; the female, sexual receptiveness. Heterosexual love is not a function of sexual physiology alone. It is an achievement of the total personality which, through the *adolescent process*, reaches a new level of integration.

No doubt there are many adolescents who do not achieve maturation through the sequence described here. There are many who seem to reach the goal by passing through all phases in a relatively short time; some experience one or more phases only in dreams and fantasies; others may pass through one of the stages quickly and then may be caught in another for a long delay and struggle. In many instances the process seems to repeat itself, for regression may occur after disappointments of any kind. Therefore, many of the experts are inclined to speak of this torturous process as the "normal psychopathology" of adolescence.

The most significant difference from the process described above is presented by those individuals who do not develop a latency period. In their adolescence they do not need to "discover" the genitals of the other sex, since they "knew" of their existence all the time; they do not "learn" to accept the genitals as part of the beloved person because they reverse the process of "falling in love." Instead of expanding the love to include the genitals of the beloved, they transfer their more or less persevering ambivalent interest in the genitals to include the person whom they "love." The reason for this attitude lies in the denial of the castration fear which is a characteristic outcome of the oedipal conflict of these individuals. Since they have not succeeded in repressing the fear of the castrating effect of the female genitals (respectively for girls, the fear of the damaging effect of the male organ), through the sexual practices of a latency period, they try to prove their lack of fear. The sexual curiosity and activity of the latency period is then more a demonstration of lack of fear than a manifestation of emotional need. The adolescent process can only rarely overcome such "habit-forming" fixations; thus sexuality usually remains in these cases, even after physiological maturation, an act of self-assertion and overcompensation. This explains the cynical attitude of such individuals toward the sexual object who is sought out in order to repeat compulsively a fixated sexual pattern. Such persons avoid the painful experiences of adolescent suspense and delay of gratification, but for this "convenience" they pay with a limitation of personality development. The heterosexual affect repressed, there is no drive to set in motion the process through which a new equilibrium of the personality can be achieved. This accounts for the puerile behavior which remains characteristic of such individuals for a lifetime. Measured by the requirement of our culture, these individuals do not achieve the developmental goal.

"Sexual maturity" means that the individual learns to find gratification for his instinctual needs in the framework of his conscience. This includes not only the organization of the ego for acceptance of the sexual drive but also the adjustment of sexual gratification to the requirements of external, sociological realities. This brings about the motivation for further development. As in the earlier phases of development, each new achievement serves as an urge for the next one, so in adolescence the sexual maturation itself supplies the motivation for the next phase, which is achieved in marriage and through parenthood. In simpler societies this goal can be achieved with more safety and probably in shorter time than in ours. Here the individual himself is responsible for the choice of his love object, and sexual activities outside marriage are considered to be against society rather than a part of it; yet, since the economic basis of marriage is difficult to achieve, this often forces the man to postpone marriage. Thus the two aspects of development—sexual and social—often oppose each other and delay or even arrest maturation. In primitive societies and even in the majority of societies with strict patriarchal organization where the society takes care of and assumes the responsibility for the sexual activities of the adolescent, his place in the community is determined by the social order. Thus the co-ordination of the sexual and social aspects of maturation evolves in sequence and reaches its goal—although without that degree of individuation required by our culture—with fewer remissions and with less delay.

The maturation of the sexual function and the development of the personality are, indeed, intricately interwoven. The integration of the *sexual drive* from its pregenital sources to the *genital primacy* and to functional maturity is the axis around which the organization of the personality takes place. From the point of view of personality development, the process of interaction is the same in both sexes. Men and women alike reach their psychosexual maturity through the reconciliation of the sexual drive with the superego and through the adjustment of sexuality to all other functions of the personality. Regarding the integration of the sexual drive from the point of view of its goal—procreation—the difference between the sexes is obvious. *The sexual drive is organized differently in man and in woman, in order to serve specific functions in procreation.*

The woman's life, more markedly than the man's, is divided into periods defined by her reproductive function. "Menarche," the first menstruation, definitely indicates her puberty. Menstruation is frequently considered a traumatic event in the girl's life, since it represents an offense against the integrity of the body. Yet the anticipation of menstruation, as well as the conscious response to it, are influenced by cultural factors. In our present civilization, education and hygiene prepare the girl for menstruation in a sympathetic way and diminish her manifest rebellion against it. But the bleeding and discomfort, which often may increase to the point of pain, may stir up her latent anxiety. These sensations impel her to realize that women have to adapt themselves to sexuality, not only to its pleasurable function, but also to its discomfort.

The female sexual functions are under highly complicated hormonal controls which result in the cyclic functioning of the ovaries. The ovary has the dual function of forming the female sex cells—the ova—and of producing two kinds of hormones: (1) the estrogen, produced by the ripening follicle, and (2) the progestin, which prepares the uterus for the nidation of the fertilized ovum. From menarche to menopause, in cyclic intervals, the woman prepares for conception which, if it fails to occur, is followed by menstruation, after which the new cycle promptly begins.

The periodicity of the gonadal functions and their influence upon the behavior related to reproduction are well established in mammals. In the human the direct manifestations of the sexual drive are modified by the developmental processes which establish patterns of sexual expression and conditions for its gratification. In spite of this—in a series of investigations in which the state of the ovarian function was determined by vaginal smears and the course of affect-manifestations was followed by psychoanalytic observations, it was found that the emotional manifestations of the sexual drive, like the reproductive function itself, are under hormonal influence and, therefore, in correlation with the gonadal cycle—an emotional cycle evolves (13). The term "sexual cycle" includes both the hormonal and the emotional aspects of the process.

To summarize: the sexual cycle begins with the ripening of the follicle. The estrogen secreted by the follicle mobilizes the manifestations of active, heterosexual tendencies; these are expressed by conscious or by disguised heterosexual desires and by increased alertness in all kinds of extroverted activities. Parallel with the increasing estrogen production, the heterosexual need increases[10] and reaches its height at the time of *ovulation*. About the time of ovulation, the hormonal state is that of maximum estrogen and of incipient progestin production. The emotional state of the woman accords with the biological readiness for conception; her body flooded with libidinous feelings, she is receptive to her sexual partner. After ovulation, the direction of the sexual drive appears to change; the libido is turned toward her person, especially toward its gratifying, pleasurable care. In correlation with the increasing progestin production, the passive-receptive and retentive tendencies motivate the emotions which are expressed in wishes and desires concerning pregnancy and the love and care for a child—or in the defenses against pregnancy and in conflicts about childbearing and child care. If conception does not occur, the hormone production declines, and the woman's emotional reactions reveal her inner perception of the "moderate degree of ovarian deficiency" (35) which the premenstrual-menstrual phase represents. Her behavior often changes; the woman feels and acts less composed; she is more irritable and aggressive, or more dependent and moody than she was at the height of the same cycle. Generally, the woman reaches the most complete psychosexual integration of which she is capable at the height of the hormonal cycle. In correlation with the decline of the hormone production, the psychosexual integration regresses from the genital level to the pregenital, anal-sadistic and/or the oral-dependent level. The analysis of the sexual cycle reveals that, corresponding to the gonadal cycle, the emotional cycle represents a condensed repetition of the processes of the psychosexual integration of the woman's personality development.

The study of the sexual cycle permits significant conclusions in regard to the basic organization of the female sexual drive and its psychic representations. Helene Deutsch in her extensive study, *Psychology of Women* (16), on the basis of general psychoanalytic observation, came to the conclusion that a deep passivity and a specific tendency toward introversion are char-

10. In evaluating the intensity of the heterosexual need, one has to consider the changes in affects occurring with gratification or from frustration; in the same way, one has to consider the variety and affect-content of the defenses in order to use them as indicators for the hormone production.

acteristic qualities of the female psyche. The study of the sexual cycle confirms this assumption, since it demonstrates that these propensities of the female psyche are repeated in cylic intervals in correspondence with the dominance of the specifically female gonadal hormone, progestin, the function of which is to prepare for and help maintain pregnancy. On this basis, we assume that the emotional manifestations of the specific passive-receptive and narcissistic retentive tendencies represent the psychodynamic correlates of the biological need for motherhood.

The psychology of pregnancy belongs to the scope of this presentation only as it indicates the role which childbearing plays in the evolution of the woman's personality. The psychodynamic processes accompanying pregnancy can easily be understood in the light of the progestin phase of the sexual cycle. As the woman, through the monthly repetition of the physiologic processes, prepares somatically for pregnancy, so does the corresponding emotional state prepare her for that introversion of psychic energies which motivates the emotional attitudes during pregnancy. The enhanced hormonal and general metabolic processes necessary to maintain normal pregnancy intensify the receptive tendencies of the woman. Whether they are expressed orally in overeating and/or in a general increase of the receptive dependent needs, they are manifestations of the biological process of growth which they serve. The "surplus energy" produced by the active metabolic balance replenishes the reservoir of primary narcissistic libido which is concentrated on the self, on the pregnancy and its content, the child-to-be. Thus the psychic energy which supplies the placid, vegetative calmness and well-being of the pregnant woman becomes the source of her motherliness. Her general behavior during pregnancy may appear withdrawn and regressive in comparison with her usual level of ego integration; yet the condition which seems to indicate regression of the ego actually represents a growth of the integrative span of the personality on a biological level: motherhood encompasses the child in the psychodynamic processes of the woman.

The trauma of birth interrupts the symbiosis of pregnancy, leaving the mother with a varying degree of physiological and emotional readiness for the complex, emotionally charged functions of motherhood. After parturition, the organism of the mother is preparing for the next function of motherhood—lactation. The hormonal control, related to the production of prolactin, stimulates milk secretion and, with it, usually suppresses the gonadal production. Thus it induces an emotional attitude which is similar to the progestin phase of the sexual cycle. The trend toward motherliness in now, as then, expressed, actively or passively, by receptive tendencies. During lactation, both the active (giving) and the passive receptive tendencies gain in intensity; they become the axis around which the activities of motherliness center. The mother's desire to nurse the baby, to be in close bodily contact with it, represents the continuation of the symbiosis, not only for the infant, but for the mother as well (12). While the infant incorporates the breast, the mother feels united with her baby. The identification with the baby permits the mother to enjoy her "regression" and to repeat and satisfy her own receptive, dependent needs. The emotional experience of lactation and of the sundry activities of nursing care, through the processes of mutual identification, lead step by step to the integration of motherliness.

Motherhood, through the libidinally charged processes of pregnancy and motherliness, sets in motion a reorganization in the mother's personality. To be a good mother and love the child —to be able to respond to the child's needs in the most constructive manner—is the ego ideal of every normal mother; if she fails, she feels punished by the child as much as, or even more than, she ever felt punished by her parents. Thus the child, through his unceasing needs, becomes a strict superego of the conscientious mother. As the child becomes older, the mother's identification with him becomes more complex. While the mother consciously strives to make the child's needs and goals a part of her own ego aspirations, unconsciously she may project onto him her own expectations, hopes, and frustrations. One mother may burden the child with the hope that he will satisfy her aspirations; another may reject the child because of her own frustrations, assuming that her child, being like herself, cannot or will not be able to undo her own failures. Thus the mother, reliving with her child, and with each child in an individually significant way, those emotional experiences which determined her own development, is a conveyor of the past and a participant in the future at the same time.

Motherhood, indeed, plays a significant role in the woman's personality. Physiologically, it completes maturation; psychologically, it channelizes motherliness. The specific qualities of motherliness originate in the primarily introverted narcissistic tendencies; their sublimated expression becomes a part of the woman's personality even if physiological motherhood does not replenish its primary sources. Sympathy, responsiveness, the desire to care for others, and other sublimated manifestations of motherliness develop in every woman through similar, if not such intensive, processes of empathy and identification which govern the mother's feeling toward her children. Thus motherliness, in its sublimated manifestations, widens the span of the personality.

The organization of the sexual drive in the male is simpler than in the female. The propagative function of the male, under the control of one group of gonadal hormones—androgens—is discharged in a single act. There seems to be a coincidence between gonadal hormone production and the urgency of the sexual impulses. However, there is no regularly returning cycle of recessions and reintegrations of the psychosexual pattern directly comparable with the sexual cycle in women. Men are not prepared for parenthood by cyclical repetitions of emotional expressions originating in the reproductive need. Yet there are emotional, originally instinctual, trends which, together with cultural trends, complement those which find expression in motherhood.

Under conditions which impede the reproductive function, such as sterility of either of the marital partners, or enforced separation, such as occurs during war, man's instinct for survival in his offspring becomes accessible to study. If man's survival is threatened—directly, as in war, or symbolically in the many ways which may destroy his self-esteem—his anxiety activates dependent needs. But, in the process of growing up, man's dependent needs have fused with the aspirations of his virility. In gratifying his sexual need, man reassures himself of his virility, especially in the hope that he may create a representation of himself in his child. The analysis of such cases reveals that the instinct of propagation is but a special form of the instinct of self-preservation in adults. The psychology of fatherhood can best be understood as the manifestation of two tendencies of man's biological urge for growth. One is the urge to conquer his own dependent needs through heterosexual love and the other is to fulfil his desire to become like his father or even to surpass him. These ambitions take many turns during his development, until they triumph when he himself becomes a father: his self survives as once his father did, in his child. In man, as well as in woman, the instinctual need for parenthood originates in the narcissistic reservoir of "surplus energy." When this is discharged in the germ cells, it surpasses the boundaries of the self and creates a continuation of the self.

Since the father's biological function is completed in one act, the psychodynamic processes of fatherhood are strongly influenced by cultural requirements. In societies where the organization of the family affords the development of a family triangle, the adaptation to fatherhood is psychodynamically similar to that of motherhood. The father, like the mother, tends to identify himself with his child; he, too, repeats unconsciously through identifications and projections the steps of his own aspirations and hopes, in order to achieve completion through the child. While fatherhood channelizes man's narcissism, it also puts harsh requirements upon him and acts as would a severe and relentless superego. The responsibilities to which the father is pledged by our society become the axis around which the organization of his further development takes place.

The mother normally achieves identification with her infant through libidinally charged processes which permit her to become a child with her child again. This is not so for the father. He is impelled to renounce and repress his receptive dependent needs when they arise—as they may—in identification with his offspring. He has to become the provider. Alexander (5) has discussed the psychodynamics of this complex developmental task which requires that the man, who once needed a mother for the gratification of his dependent needs, should become the father-provider for his wife and children. Although men are prepared by previous identifications with their own fathers for the task which is taken for granted in our culture, they may often fail, or they may pay for fulfilment with various types of mental or psychosomatic suffering. Overcompensation of their dependent needs in demanding, domineering, or even despotic behavior is one, regression to direct gratification of oral needs in overeating and alcoholism is another, expression of the repressed passive-dependent needs. More complex and more disguised psychosomatic symptoms may ensue if the father overdraws his libidinal resources in the effort of being a provider.

Against the restrictions and renunciations of id gratifications on the other side of the ledger, adult man has his gratifications in and through his work. From childhood, achievement, in whatever form and level it occurs, is absorbed in the personality, enlarging its span. Mastery, through its affective gratifications of secondary narcissism, delineates the psychodynamic role which work plays in the emotional household of men in our civilization. In youth the instinctual needs are more compelling; in adulthood, especially after the father has incorporated the gratifications and restrictions which his family represents, work and its satisfactions gain emphasis in the psychodynamic processes. Fortunate is the man whose primary emotional gratifications keep balance with the spending of psychic and physical energies in work. Even the gratifications of secondary narcissism may become a steady drain upon the psychic resources, leaving but little libido for primary emotional gratification. Such a process may lead to rigidity of the ego and finally exhaust the adaptive capacity of the individual. Since work, through sublimation as well as by its material gratification, plays an integrative part in the expansion of man's personality, the renunciation of work often represents a trauma; it necessitates a readjustment of the total emotional economy. If the individual can look back upon a successful career and can give up work by his own decision, the adjustment may be smooth, although it is not always so. If, on account of social and economic circumstances or because of age and disability, the man is compelled to give up work, his ego may collapse. New attempts at success or his sense of guilt because of his failure may exhaust his psychic resources. The mental health of the adult male is best guaranteed by a smoothly functioning interchange between primary libidinal gratifications (provided by his interpersonal relationships within his family and community) and the satisfactions of his secondary narcissism, which he achieves by work.

The decline of the reproductive period in man and woman approaches slowly. Normally, it evolves as a process of maturation through continuous adaptation to the internal and external requirements of living. The term "climacterium" is often applied to the period of abating reproductive function in both sexes. Climacterium, however, according to the different organization of the reproductive function, is a dynamically different process in man and woman.

The woman experiences fluctuations in gonadal hormones

from puberty on; her organism adapts itself to the psychosomatic reactions which accompany the monthly hormonal decline. Thus, when the gonadal stimulation definitely subsides, the healthy woman's emotional economy is not severely harmed by the loss of hormonal stimulation. The integration of the personality once established, the woman appears independent of gonadal stimulation for maintaining the sublimations of the reproductive period.

Many women suffer from neurotic, psychotic, or psychosomatic manifestations which, because they occur about or after the menopause, are usually attributed to the stresses of climacterium. The psychoanalytic study of such cases reveals that the symptoms, which appear aggravated during this period, have already existed before. Even if they were not manifest, they have been pre-formed under the influence of the precarious balance of the personality. Those women who were unable to adapt to the premenstrual hormone decline and suffered from premenstrual depressions and/or dysmenorrhea usually suffer again from the vegetative discomforts of the climacterium. The study of the personality structure and life-experience of women who manifest severe emotional disturbances at climacterium reveals that in these cases (1) the bisexual component played a dominant and obviously disturbing role; (2) the psychic economy was dominated by the strivings of secondary narcissism rather than by primary emotional gratification of motherliness.

Climacterium is different for those women whose psychic economy has not been exhausted by previous neurotic conflicts. When menopause indicates the cessation of the propagative functions, these women often respond to the desexualization of their emotional needs with an influx of extroverted energy; their still flexible personalities seek and find new aims for psychic energy. As in early childhood, when repression of the sexual impulses led to superego formation and socialization, so in climacterium the cessation of the reproductive function releases a new impetus for socialization and learning. The manifold interests and productivities of women after the climacterium, as well as their improvement in general physical and emotional health, serve as evidence that woman's climacterium may be regarded in a psychological sense as a "developmental phase" (10).

In man the reproductive period lasts longer than in woman; his procreative capacity is expected to last as long as orgastic potency remains. Both the sexual urge and the reproductive capacity may be rekindled, even if they appear to be extinguished. Thus man has no definitely marked cessation of his reproductive capacities, which would justify the concept of a "male climacterium" on the basis of hormonal physiology alone. Such a concept, however, has a broader biosociological implication.

Men in our society respond sensitively to the signs of aging, and they may relate any functional decline to it, for aging is considered a menace, which they watchfully expect and detect in the oscillations of sexual potency, in work or sport achievements, in general health. Aging is a source of insecurity for the modern man. In patriarchal society the social significance of old age was different. Whatever the oscillations of his sexual potency were, man did not need to feel threatened, since marriages were stable and, socially, the man's prestige increased rather than decreased with age. In our culture, men are not protected by such tradition. They feel compelled to compensate for their lessening capacity by increasing competitive productivity. While this may enhance man's self-reliance, it may increase his intrapsychic tension: success and mastery dominate his activity at the cost of primary emotional gratification. Slowly or suddenly, as, for example, in a traumatic failure in sexual potency, the aging man's psychosexual economy becomes similar to that of the adolescent. Just as in adolescence, sexual potency and mastery in achievement have acted as opponents, now again the insecurity in regard to sexual potency enhances the narcissistic significance of each sexual act and every other activity as well. Thus the "polarization of affects" may be repeated. Any failure may appear as an irreparable damage to the personality and may activate the ever latent castration fear; this mobilizes the specific conflicts of the individual, and these, in turn, may determine the specific symptoms which, occurring at this age, make the assumption of "male climacterium" justifiable. However, "male climacterium" is motivated mainly by the multiple psychosomatic effects of man's struggle in a competitive society. If the adaptive task which men have to meet is not motivated by factors other than that of the physiology of the declining sexual function, "climacterium" does not develop, for man's aging is a continuous, not a pathological, process.

Chronological age has a different significance for the individual as well as for his community, depending upon many cultural factors. It is common knowledge that, in spite of its stresses and discomforts, civilization has extended man's life-expectancy. Even more significant is it that modern man can look forward to a much longer period of productive enjoyment in life than the average man ever could before.

The psychodynamic process of growing old is characterized by a change in the vector of the psychic and somatic processes. The giving, expansive attitudes, needed for the functions of the reproductive period, slowly become outweighed by the retentive, self-centered tendencies characteristic of old age. Since the redistribution of the vital resources induces an introversion (retention) of psychic energy, both men and women obtain manifold gratifications of a narcissistic nature. Whether the aged individual applies what he has learned in a lifetime and surveys his world in broad philosophical concepts or just cares for the grandchildren, the pleasure which "warms his heart" is the gratification of being able to think, to do, to feel, to be aware of the self in special activity and achievement. There is no doubt about the enhanced narcissism of the old, which, since it cannot draw on the resources of newly produced surplus energy, enlarges the gains of their available resources by identification with the young and by rekindling the memories of past achievement and gratification.

In the obviously self-centered phase of senescence, the receptive dependent needs dominate the aged individual's relationship to his environment, often causing great irritation in the younger generation, who complain about the egotism of the old. The gratification of the dependent needs, however, serves more than the mere maintenance of life. In old people as in children, the gratifications of the dependent needs are taken for manifestations of love; being loved increases the sense of security and enhances the value of the personality. The senescent individual, aware of the failing of his own capacities, becomes hypersensitive in regard to the fulfilment of his dependent needs, which are often expressed as a need for prestige and recognition. While the old person is dissatisfied with himself, he demands from those who love him the impossible, namely, that they shall make him unaware of his weakness. Thus the regression within the personality structure of the senescent often manifests itself in a paranoid conflict with the environment.

As the exhaustion of the vital energies proceeds, the restriction of the emotional household becomes more and more manifest. Expenditure has been limited long before; at that late stage, also, the receptive needs diminish because abundance can no longer be enjoyed. When life has no more strength than to maintain itself at a low metabolic rate, mental functioning is reduced to a minimum, and one can no longer speak of the structuralization of the personality.

In this chapter, we have discussed the processes through which biological and cultural forces become organized and form the personality. "Personality" is the capacity of the total organism to function as a whole—a unique, discernible self, distinguished from other members of the species and from other members of the same social group. In the most general psychodynamic terms, one may define personality as the product of the various ways of dealing with psychic tensions which, in turn, produce recognizable trends and predictable behavior. Personality is a continuous function, resulting from infinite interactions between the individual and his society. "Emotional maturity" is a term often used to describe a personality which has fully developed its potentiality for reconciling internal, instinctual needs with the external requirements of society. "Emotional maturity" in this sense does not mean a consciously applied philosophy; it indicates rather an unconsciously functioning psychic economy which operates with a positive balance. This implies that the organization of the personality allows for an easy mobilization of psychic energies whenever a new adaptive task requires it. Thus emotional maturity is a relative concept. It can be evaluated only in reference to the question: "Mature—for what?"

The key to the understanding of all pathological processes is the evaluation of the adaptive task in respect to the total psychic economy. Preventive psychiatry has as its purpose the diminution of the gap between the requirements of the adaptive task and the individual's capacity to master it. This aim, however, is beyond the scope of any single discipline. When all cultural and economic forces of a society bend their efforts together in behalf of the individual, then we may secure that stability and security which will reduce the risks involved in the complete individuation of the personality.

BIBLIOGRAPHY

1. ABRAHAM, K. *Selected Papers* (London: Hogarth Press, 1927).
2. ALEXANDER, F. "Concerning the Genesis of the Castration Complex," *Psychoanalyt. Rev.*, 22:49, 1935.
3. ALEXANDER, F. *Fundamentals of Psychoanalysis* (New York: W. W. Norton & Co., Inc., 1948).
4. ALEXANDER, F. "The Logic of Emotions and Its Dynamic Background," *Internat. J. Psycho-Analysis*, 16:406, 1935.
5. ALEXANDER, F. "A Note on Falstaff," *Psychoanalyt. Quart.*, 2:592, 1933.
6. ALEXANDER, F. *Our Age of Unreason* (rev. ed.; Philadelphia: J. B. Lippincott Co., 1951).
7. ALEXANDER, F. *Psychosomatic Medicine* (New York: W. W. Norton & Co., Inc., 1950).
8. ALEXANDER, F. "The Relation of Structural and Instinctual Conflicts," *Psychoanalyt. Quart.*, 2:181, 1933.
9. BENEDEK, THERESE. "Adaptation to Reality in Early Infancy," *Psychoanalyt. Quart.*, 7:200, 1938.
10. BENEDEK, THERESE. "Climacterium: A Developmental Phase," *Psychoanalyt. Quart.*, 19:1, 1950.
11. BENEDEK, THERESE. *Insight and Personality Adjustment* (New York: Ronald Press Co., 1946).
12. BENEDEK, THERESE. "The Psychosomatic Implications of the Primary Unit: Mother-Child," *Am. J. Orthopsychiat.*, 19:642, 1949.
13. BENEDEK, THERESE, and RUBENSTEIN, B. B. *Psychosexual Functions in Women* (New York: Ronald Press Co., 1952).
14. BETTELHEIM, B., and SYLVESTER, E. "Delinquency and Morality," in *The Psychoanalytic Study of the Child*, Vol. 5 (New York: International Universities Press, 1950).
15. BREUER, J., and FREUD, S. *Studies in Hysteria* (New York: Nervous and Mental Disease Publishing Co., 1936).
16. DEUTSCH, H. *The Psychology of Women*, Vols. 1 and 2 (New York: Grune & Stratton, 1944–45).
17. EMCH, MINNA. "On 'the Need To Know' as Related to Identification and Acting Out," *Internat. J. Psycho-Analysis*, 25:14, 1944.
18. FENICHEL, O. "Frühe Entwicklungsstadien des Ichs," *Imago*, 23:243, 1937.
19. FREUD, A. *The Ego and the Mechanisms of Defence* (London: Hogarth Press, 1937).
20. FREUD, S. *Collected Papers*, Vols. 1–5 (London: Hogarth Press, 1924–50).
21. FREUD, S. *The Ego and the Id* (London: Hogarth Press, 1927).
22. FREUD, S. "Female Sexuality," *Internat. J. Psycho-Analysis*, 13:281, 1932.
23. FREUD, S. "Formulations Regarding the Two Principles in Mental Functioning," in *Collected Papers*, 4 (London: Hogarth Press, 1925), 13.

24. FREUD, S. *A General Introduction to Psychoanalysis* (New York: Boni & Liveright, 1920).

25. FREUD, S. *Leonardo da Vinci: A Study in Psychosexuality* (New York: Random House, 1947).

26. FREUD, S. "The Passing of the Oedipus Complex," in *Collected Papers*, Vol. 2 (London: Hogarth Press, 1924).

27. FREUD, S. "The Predisposition to 'Obsessional Neurosis,' " in *Collected Papers*, 2 (London: Hogarth Press, 1924), 122.

28. FREUD, S. "The Psychology of Women," in *New Introductory Lectures on Psycho-Analysis* (New York: W. W. Norton & Co., 1933).

29. FREUD, S. *Three Contributions to the Theory of Sex* (New York: Nervous and Mental Disease Publishing Co., 1930).

30. GESELL, A., *et al. The First Five Years of Life* (New York: Harper & Bros., 1940).

31. HARTMANN, H., and KRIS, E. "The Genetic Approach in Psychoanalysis," in *The Psychoanalytic Study of the Child*, 1 (New York: International Universities Press, 1945), 11–30.

32. HARTMANN, H.; KRIS, E.; and LOEWENSTEIN, R. M. "Comments on the Formation of Psychic Structure," in *The Psychoanalytic Study of the Child*, 2 (New York: International Universities Press, 1947), 11–37.

33. HARTNIK, JENO. "The Various Developments Undergone by Narcissism in Men and Women," *Internat. J. Psycho-Analysis*, 5:66, 1924.

34. HORNEY, K. "On the Genesis of the Castration Complex in Women," *Internat. J. Psycho-Analysis*, 5:59, 1924.

35. HOSKINS, R. G. *Endocrinology* (New York: W. W. Norton & Co., 1941).

36. JOHNSON, A. M. "Sanctions for Superego Lacunae of Adolescents," in *Searchlights on Delinquency* (New York: International Universities Press, 1949), p. 225.

37. JONES, E. "Urethralerotik und Ehrgeiz," *Internat. Ztsch. f. Psychoanal.*, 3:156, 1915.

38. MEAD, M. *From the South Seas* (New York: Wm. Morrow & Co., 1939).

39. RADO, S. "The Problem of Melancholia," *Internat. J. Psycho-Analysis*, 9:4:20, 1928.

40. REICH, W. *Character-Analysis* (3d enl. ed.; New York: Orgone Institute Press, 1949).

41. SPITZ, R. "Hospitalism: An Inquiry into the Genesis of Psychiatric Conditions in Early Childhood," in *The Psychoanalytic Study of the Child*, 1 (New York: International Universities Press, 1945), 53–74.

42. SZUREK, S. "Notes on the Genesis of Psychopathic Personality Trends," *Psychiatry*, 5:1, 1942.

III

NEUROSES, BEHAVIOR DISORDERS, AND PERVERSIONS

Franz Alexander, M.D., and Louis B. Shapiro, M.D.

Neurosis Defined

FREUD defined neurotic symptoms as substitute gratifications in fantasy for co-ordinated action, adequate to satisfy impelling subjective needs. Because fantasy gratification can never completely relieve the pressure of unsatisfied needs, neurosis is always connected with frustration. Neurosis is, then, an inadequate, unsuccessful attempt to restore the emotional equilibrium disturbed by the presence of unsatisfied or poorly satisfied subjective urges.

The adequate satisfaction of subjective needs is the function of the ego. Every neurosis can be understood in final analysis as a disturbance of ego functions. In this respect, neurosis can be compared with any other disease. Disease is a result of inadequate functioning of an organ system. In the case of neurosis, the failing organ is the co-ordinating center; it fails in its biological task of gratifying subjective needs in harmonious co-ordination with one another and in congruity with existing external conditions upon which the gratification of the subjective needs depends.

Any or all of the four fundamental functions of the ego may be disturbed: (1) internal perception of subjective needs, (2) correct external appraisal of the environmental situation, (3) integration of the data of internal and external perception with each other, and (4) the executive function based on the ego's control over voluntary behavior (see chap. iii). In most neuroses all four functions are to some degree disturbed. For example, in hysteria, the internal perception is primarily disturbed by repression, whereas in behavior disorders chiefly the executive function of the ego is impaired.

As discussed before (chap. iv), the ego acquires its functional efficiency during postnatal development by a gradual learning process. The first requirement for integrated and goal-directed behavior is an adequate capacity for controlling one's impulses, a capacity which is only gradually acquired. The child's capacity for conscious control—renunciation or postponement of impulses —is weak; and, in order to maintain the integrity of the ego, he can only resort to the process of excluding from consciousness all impulses that the ego cannot control and harmonize, those impulses which would otherwise give rise to anxiety, guilt, and shame. This process is called "repression." Repressed impulses represent quantities of energy which have either to be held constantly in check or to be drained off in some other manner not threatening to the ego. Many of the psychodynamic phenomena in the field of psychopathology (chap. i) are auxiliary methods which support repression or represent substitutive vents for repressed psychological forces.

Repression is essentially denial. In a sense the ego denies the existence of an internal impulse or an external event that might lead to a painful consequence. Ideas—the carriers of instinctual strivings—must become conscious in order to gain motor expression. In repression the ego excludes from consciousness any pain-producing idea or impulse by refusing it entrance to its domain. Repressed impulses are therefore not permitted any modification through the learning process. The more the infantile ego has to make use of the drastic measure of repression, the less it can fulfil its function of gratification of the subjective needs by modifying them and adapting them to one another and to external conditions. Excessive repression has a twofold result: (1) the ego's supply of energy will be impoverished, since the dynamic forces over which the ego rules are excluded from its territory; (2) a great deal of the ego's energy will have to be utilized for defense against the pressure of repressed tendencies. Having once repressed an objectionable impulse, the ego's task is not finished. Energy is constantly required to maintain the repression. This may be manifested clinically in the neurotic's complaint of fatigue and lack of energy adequate to meet the daily problems of living. In many cases the ego's task of dealing with a dangerous or unpleasant impulse by repression proves to be unsuccessful, and the ego is therefore forced to take recourse to auxiliary defenses.

Although neurotic symptoms represent inadequate gratification, still they contain a component of gratification which they both seek and deny. This is the basis of the "neurotic conflict." This conflict, which exists in the mind and yet is unknown to the person, is a struggle between two sides of the total personality. It can be demonstrated when one attempts to cure a patient of his symptoms. When the therapist applies the analytic technique of unraveling the symptom, the patient unknowingly and unwittingly opposes this effort with strong resistance. This becomes apparent when the therapist is about to make conscious to the patient some unconscious material related to the symptom and at the same time particularly painful to the patient. It becomes obvious that the patient prefers to retain his unwelcome symptom rather than to become conscious of the particularly painful association. The symptom is a substitute for the latter, which remains in the unconscious. This struggle of the patient to obtain relief from his symptoms and yet to avoid making conscious the unconscious processes underlying his symptoms is the core of every neurosis. All symptoms can be understood as results of the conflict between repressed and repressing forces.

Neurotic disturbances can be classified according to the type of defenses which the ego employs or according to the nature of the repressed impulses. In the actual clinical classification of neuroses, as a rule, a combination of both criteria is utilized. Freud suggested that there may be an intimate connection between special forms of defense and a particular neurosis, as, for example, between repression and hysteria. He also called attention to the relation between aggressive and sadistic impulses and reaction formations in the ego, such as overcleanliness, exaggerated scrupulousness, meticulousness, and defensive techniques employed in obsessional neurosis. Helene Deutsch (2) has noted that possibly each defense mechanism arises at first to master some special instinctual impulse during infantile development. Anna Freud (3) has suggested that repression is used against sexual impulses, while other mechanisms are employed against aggressive impulses.

The fact that repression is generally the chief technique used by the ego in hysteria is probably due to the attitude in our culture toward sexual impulses. Adults often behave as though sex were nonexistent. In hysteria we see the same attitude adopted; that is, the unacceptable impulse is viewed as if it simply did not exist. In other words, the cultural attitude toward the instinctual impulses supplies the tool that the ego uses in dealing with sexual impulses. Aggressive impulses, on the other hand, although acknowledged as existing, are stamped by our culture as bad, and the ego is called upon to exercise various techniques, such as "overcompensation" or "undoing," to counteract this force. This explains the presence of overcompensatory techniques in those neurotic pictures characterized by aggressive instinctual drives, as, for example, in obsessive-compulsive neurosis.

Neurotic disturbances can be divided into two large categories —chronic and acute. Emotions of excessive intensity, such as anxiety, rage, and frustration, may temporarily impair both the integrative and the executive functions of the ego. Anxiety, if excessive, may have a paralyzing influence. The same is true for rage. An enraged person is likely to concentrate on one single aim—that of vengeance—and leave out of consideration everything else. In all excessive emotional states the primary objective of the organism is to find immediate relief from the tension. This urgency interferes with a comprehensive handling of all external and internal factors.

Common examples of acute neuroses are the so-called "traumatic neuroses" (see chap. vi). In the traumatic situation the ego is incapable of carrying out its co-ordinating and adaptive functions. This failure may precipitate not only a regressive evasion of the traumatic situation but also a strong regressive movement toward a more dependent, helpless state of infancy. Loss of consciousness, of the faculty of locomotion or of speech, or of the co-ordinated use of the extremities may be the result. Acute conditions may easily develop into chronic neurotic states, and therefore it is important that acute conditions should be treated early. In the early phases supportive measures frequently suffice to prevent the development of chronic neurotic states as a result of an acute neurosis. The emotional support may serve as encouragement for the ego to make new attempts to regain its mastery, which was only temporarily disturbed under the influence of the excessive stimulation of the trauma.

The chronic failures of the ego functions usually can be traced back to disturbed interpersonal relationships in childhood. Sometimes traumatic interpersonal relationships are of later origin. Accordingly, there is a continuum between acute, subacute, and chronic states. In the development of a chronic neurosis the following phases in general can be distinguished:

1. Circumstances that precipitate the actual situation with which the patient cannot cope.

2. Failure in solution of the actual problem after some unsuccessful attempts.

3. Replacement of realistic adaptive measures by regressive fantasies or behavior.

4. Reactivation of the old conflicts which in the past induced the ego to give up the old adaptive patterns in the course of maturation.

5. Efforts of the ego to resolve the infantile conflict revived through the evasion of the actual life-situation. As has been said, the differentiation between the several forms of neurosis is based to a great extent on the type of defensive measure employed to resolve the anxiety, guilt, and inferiority feelings resulting from the reactivated original neurotic conflict.

6. Secondary results of the chronic neurotic state. The symptoms, which are the ego's attempt to resolve the conflict, absorb the patient's energy and make him even less effective in dealing with the real problems of his life. This secondary conflict necessitates further regression and produces new symptoms which, in turn, decrease the ego's efficiency by absorbing more energy. This is the neurotic vicious circle which results as the end-effect of the chronic neurotic state.

TYPES OF NEUROTIC CONDITIONS

In the following discussion the main criterion used for classification of the several forms of neurosis is the differentiation of defenses used by the ego to resolve the neurotic conflict. Only secondary consideration is given to the nature of the ego-alien impulses against which the ego has to defend itself. According to the authors, classification based on "instinct-qualities" is much less reliable. In fact, the validity of some customary generalizations concerning the nature of ego-alien impulses and the degree of regression postulated in the different conditions is questioned by the authors.

HYSTERICAL CONDITIONS

Three clinically well-defined conditions belong in this group: (a) anxiety neurosis, (b) phobia, and (c) conversion hysteria. Although these three neurotic states outwardly appear as quite different, the one common feature which justifies classifying them together is that the principal defense employed in all three is repression. In anxiety neurosis, repression is not supported by any other defense mechanism; in the phobias, repression is supported by displacement; and in conversion hysteria, the symbolic use of body innervations serves as a substitute expression of ego-alien tendencies. The validity of the statement common in psychoanalytic literature that in hysteria the repressed impulses are mainly of genital-sexual nature is not fully convincing. The presence of pregenital tendencies, particularly oral and sadistic, are commonly observed both in anxiety and in conversion hysterias. The argument that these pregenital impulses are regressive retreats from genital impulses is true in all forms of neurosis. There may be a preponderance of genital-sexual impulses in this group, but this generalization still requires further confirmation.

a) *Anxiety neurosis.*—Some form of anxiety is a well-nigh universal concomitant in all forms of neurosis, and it is also a common reaction in healthy individuals. Anxiety is the ego's reaction to the internal danger represented by the pressure of impulses, the gratification of which would involve the person in conflict with external or internal standards. In anxiety neurosis, anxiety is the central symptom, a constant or regularly recurring condition which has a paralyzing effect upon behavior. It appears without conscious motivation—it is "free-floating," without being firmly attached to any ideational content.

Free-floating anxiety, as a rule, is a reaction to repressed hostile impulses and represents a fear of retaliation. The hostile impulses are mostly aroused by sexual competitive drives, no matter how deeply these drives may be repressed. The unconscious content of anxiety in man, accordingly, is castration fear or masochistic homosexual fantasies; in women it is typical masochistic fantasies resulting both from guilt toward the mother and from hostile (castrative) fantasies toward the man.

Free-floating anxiety, seldom a chronic state, is the introduction to the development of some other more stable neurotic condition. Since neurotic mechanisms serve to allay anxiety aroused by the central conflict, anxiety neurosis can be considered as an initial phase, which exists before the ego forms adequate defenses against the anxiety. Nevertheless, free-floating anxiety may persist occasionally for a long period of time or may flare up periodically under conditions which mobilize the patient's conflict. The central mechanism is repression without any of the auxiliary defenses which are utilized in other neuroses to circumvent anxiety. Accordingly, anxiety neurosis can be considered the simplest form of neurosis, and the other neurotic conditions can be understood as different methods by which the central core of neurosis —neurotic anxiety—is handled by the ego.

The following case illustrates the dynamics and clinical picture seen in anxiety neurosis. It particularly high-lights the etiology and demonstrates how the anxiety neurosis can be the initial phase of a breakdown in ego functioning and then lead into the development of a clinical picture characterized by phobic and depressive features as the ego's defenses become operative.

A 34-year-old married white woman, following a serious quarrel with her mother-in-law, developed an acute attack of anxiety. Her free-floating anxiety, obviously a reaction to repressed hostile impulses, became manifest in tachycardia, palpitation, loss of appetite, and weakness and tremulousness of both upper and lower extremities. The anxiety soon became attached to the idea that she had heart trouble and that she was going to die. This phobia persisted for several months and finally led to hospitalization and cardiac study. After six weeks she returned home to her husband and three children, relieved of the thought that she had heart trouble. However, the unconscious hostility toward her mother-in-law and marriage now became displaced by obsessive thoughts that her husband and children would die or that he would divorce her. By the time she was referred to the psychiatrist, she was deeply depressed and full of remorse and self-accusations.

b) Phobias.—In the phobias, in place of generalized anxiety as seen in anxiety neurosis, the fear is focused on certain highly specific situations, such as being in the dark, in crowds, in inclosed places (claustrophobia), in wide-open spaces (agoraphobia), or high places (acrophobia). It is not our purpose to give an exhaustive description of the great variety of specific forms which phobic anxiety may take. In all instances the patient reverts to some early childhood fears, which are common and normal in infancy, such as fear of strange people, of darkness, of falling, of being alone in a crowded street. The etiological question is to establish the cause of the regressive reactivation of childhood fears.

The phobic fear reveals itself as a substitute for an actual fear of the problems of life which the patient cannot meet. The most common among these problems which the patient tries to evade are those connected with mature sexuality, the responsibilities of marriage, having children, and occupational tasks requiring independent decisions, competition, and all those complex interpersonal relations which are a part of adult existence.

A common example is the street phobia of women, who displace their anxiety because of prostitution fantasies (street-walking) to the fear of crowded streets. In acrophobia, the fear of ambition, responsibility, and leadership is symbolized by being "high up"; and the wish to accept a more humble position—in men, often a female position—is frequently replaced by the fear of falling.

Phobic anxiety has a tendency to spread, making the patient avoid more and more of the trivial situations of everyday life. In severe cases the patient retires completely from independent activity and indulges in a vegetative existence within the four walls of his home. This end-phase demonstrates clearly the unconscious trend toward infantile dependence—an escape from all the risks and efforts of adult existence.

The following case illustrates the clinical picture of a phobia:

A 31-year-old single white woman, in addition to vague complaints of chronic indigestion, suffered from a street phobia. This became particularly manifest when she was about to cross a street. She usually waited until others came along and then surreptitiously joined them as they went to the other side of the street. Her fear was that she would fall or faint. The street phobia in this woman was not only a displacement of her anxiety of unconscious prostitution fantasies but also a fear of her intense ambition and masculine strivings. Her feminine sexual strivings, repressed by her masculine protest, found discharge in the rich prostitution fantasy that led to one part of her street phobia. Her masculine protest led to a professional life, bringing her into a competitive relationship with men. However, strong unconscious trends toward infantile dependence became activated whenever she made important advances in her professional career and moved into positions calling for greater responsibility and leadership. Following such an advancement in position, her fear of falling became so acute that she felt giddy and dizzy even when walking on the sidewalk along the buildings. Her gastrointestinal distress also became more acute. In short, her unconscious infantile longings to be nursed and cared for became so intensified that the fear of ambition and the wish for a more humble position was replaced by the fear of falling.

A second example of a phobia is the case of a young lawyer who had a morbid fear that he would someday contract rabies. Not only was he fearful of being bitten by a dog, but he was afraid even to be near or touch anyone who owned, petted, or had been near a dog (example of the tendency of phobic anxiety to spread). As a youth he was exposed to the frequent quarrels of his parents, and often heard his mother refer to his father as a "baser Hund" ("mad-dog"). In fantasy the young lawyer often pictured himself as the rescuer of his mother and the avenging destroyer of his father. It is clear that his fear of rabies is a displacement and reaction to both his hostile wishes as well as his passive submissive trends toward his father.

The phobic anxiety in the latter case is similar to that of "little Hans" and the "Wolf man" from Freud's clinical studies (4, 6). In little Hans the fear of the falling, kicking horse was a displacement of the fear of the father who little Hans wished would fall over dead, while the Wolf man's fear of being bitten was a reaction to his unconscious passive feminine strivings toward his father.

c) Conversion hysteria.—The underlying mechanisms in conversion hysteria are essentially the same as in the common expressive innervations of the body, such as weeping, laughter, and blushing. Conversion symptoms express and relieve emotional tension through bodily changes, which have no other function but to relieve emotional tension. The differences between normal bodily expression and hysterical conversion symptoms is that the latter are individual uncommon innervations and the underlying emotional content is completely repressed into the unconscious. On the other hand, the normal channels of emotional expression may also be utilized for the drainage of unconscious ego-alien impulses, in which cases we deal with hysterical uncontrollable weeping or laughter. These patients are unable to say why they are laughing or weeping. A woman patient reported repeated instances of uncontrollable laughter at funerals and condolence visits. In her case unconscious malicious pleasure about the tragedy which befell persons against whom she had ambivalent feelings was the unconscious motivating force.

The forms which conversion symptoms may take are extremely variegated and are determined by the traumatic experiences of the individual. Contracture and paralysis of the limbs are the most common conversion symptoms in the field of the voluntary muscles. The contracture or paralysis has a symbolic meaning, which, at the same time, expresses both the gratification and the denial of the unconscious content. A contracted leg may symbolize the castrated male organ and thus express both the unconscious castrative wish as well as the punishment for it. In the great hysterical attack described in the older textbooks of psychiatry, several details of sexual intercourse are represented, such as the rhythmic movements, episthotonus, forced respiration, etc. What is missing is the experience of sexual gratification.

Hysterical conversion symptoms may appear not only in the voluntary muscles but in all sensory systems, producing an immense variety of paresthesias, anesthesias, pain, blindness, deafness, etc. The unconscious meaning is the denial of some ego-alien gratification connected with the affected sense organ.

The functions of some smooth muscles under the control of the autonomic nervous system may be the seat of hysterical conversion. The most common example is hysterical vomiting, the unconscious meaning of which is the rejection of some oral fantasy (fellatio, oral impregnation, biting, etc.). Such symptoms are not contradictory to the statement that conversion hysteria is restricted to the field of the sensorium and voluntary movements, because swallowing is a part of a complete co-ordinated physiological function, the first phase of which is the voluntary act of eating.

The excretory functions, also, are controlled by a combination of voluntary and automatic innervations. Accordingly, a combination of hysterical conversion mechanisms with those of vegetative neurosis is a common occurrence in the gastrointestinal tract.

It is a widely held view that hysterical conversion symptoms are utilized primarily for the expression of genital impulses, in contrast to depressions and compulsive obsessional states, in which pregenital (oral and anal) impulses are prevalent. The detailed study of conversion symptoms, however, seems to indicate that all kinds of instinctual tensions may find expression in conversion symptoms.

The prevalence of genital impulses holds more true in what is often called the "hysterical personality." These patients are inclined to go through the motions of feeling without actually experiencing the very emotions to which they often give an extremely dramatic expression. The feelings which the hysterical patients so desperately try to capture and which they are unable to experience are, as a rule, those characteristic of mature sexuality. This emotional shallowness is particularly frequent in connection with the sexual act itself and is the basis of the widespread phenomenon: sexual frigidity. Many frigid women go through the external motions of sexual gratification without being capable of experiencing it. Play-acting in place of actual experience, however, usually spreads out to all interpersonal relationships.

In connection with conversion hysteria, a phenomenon described very early by Freud deserves special mention. The patient identifies himself with another person but restricts the identification to assuming the sufferings of the chosen person. He imitates the disease symptoms (such as coughing or pains and aches of all kinds) of the one whom he both loves and hates. In the identification the patient gives unconscious gratification to his wish to be in the other person's position—for example, to have the same lover—and at the same time he gratifies the need for punishment by sharing the suffering of the envied person.

The following case is an illustration of conversion hysteria:

A woman of 32 developed a hysterical paralysis of her right arm and hand after her husband lost his job and developed a gradually increasing degree of impotency. The frustration she experienced as a result of his inadequacies led to the generation of strong unconscious hostile impulses. These, as well as substitutive sexual expressions, were repressed, but found expression in her conversion symptom of paresis. This occurred through the process of displacement and symbolization.

A dream reported during the second week of analysis reveals her unconscious hostile castrative impulse toward her husband as well as the masturbatory strivings. She dreamed that she returned home with a bag of groceries. She put her hand into the bag and took out an onion. She looked at it and said: "It has gone to seed, it is rotten." The hand, which is innervated by the hostile as well as the masturbatory impulse, is punitively immobilized. The onion that has gone to seed is an obvious reference to her husband's atrophied testicle.

In this case the conversion symptom has a symbolic meaning which, at the same time, expresses both the gratification and the denial of the unconscious impulses. The hand paralyzed is a symbol of punishment and gratification for the hostile castrative wish against the husband's genitals, as well as punishment and gratification for the infantile masturbatory impulses.

OBSESSIVE-COMPULSIVE STATES

Full-blown cases of obsessive-compulsive states present a dynamic equilibrium in which obsessive preoccupation with ego-alien fantasies (incestuous, coprophilic, sadistic-homicidal ideas) are precariously balanced by rituals representing an exaggeration of social standards, such as cleanliness, punctuality, consideration for others. The obsessive ideas are mostly asocial in nature, whereas the compulsive rituals are caricatures of morality. The dynamic formula is similar to bookkeeping, in which on the one side of the ledger are the asocial tendencies which the patient tries to balance precisely on the other side with moralistic and social attitudes. The 50-50 ratio is characteristic of these patients and explains their central characteristic: doubt, indecision, and ambivalence. Every asocial move must be undone by an opposing one. Many of the complicated touching and washing rituals can be explained by this peculiar polarity in the emotional household. The endless hand-washing is a response to coprophilic tendencies. Touching is a symbolic substitute for hurting; the left hand must undo the sin committed by the right hand.

Psychodynamically, the compulsive-obsessional states differ from the hysterical conditions primarily in respect to the defense mechanisms. In the hysterias the principal defense is repression. In the compulsive-obsessive states the repression is not successful —the ego-alien ideas appear in consciousness sometimes without any distortion whatsoever. The defense consists in allaying anxiety and resolving the conflict by compensating measures (overly moralistic rituals), by which the asocial tendencies are undone, and by isolation of the ego-alien tendencies from the rest of the mental content. The objectionable ideas are de-emotionalized; they appear disconnected and almost as abstractions, like foreign bodies for which the patient does not feel responsible. Displacement, too, may play an important part in obsessive-compulsive symptomatology. This could be demonstrated in a 65-year-old patient who developed a mild, lifelong counting compulsion which suddenly became aggravated to an almost psychotic degree a week after his sixty-fifth birthday. Formerly a wealthy man, the patient was then forced to realize the precariousness of his financial situation. Instead of facing the hard financial facts and his future economic problems, which required some calculation, he began to count everything in his environment and was unable to free himself from this compulsion for even a few minutes during his waking hours. Meaningless counting of any countable objects substituted for his facing the highly disturbing numerical facts of his future economic existence. Counting objects is one of the most primitive forms of mastery—bringing some order into the chaotic world. A regression to this form of mastery when all other methods of controlling one's life-situation fail is a not uncommon form of neurotic evasion.

The preponderance of anal-sadistic impulses is well established in compulsive states. The defensive measures employed are particularly suited for dealing with the conflicts aroused by hostility.

The following is an illustrative case of obsessive-compulsive neurosis, showing the presence in consciousness of incestuous, coprophilic, and sadistic fantasies, as well as the ego's constant preoccupation with making restitution, isolating, or undoing the above-mentioned ego-alien impulses. This clinical example also demonstrates the psychodynamic difference in the defense mechanisms of the obsessive-compulsive state as contrasted with the hysterias.

A 31-year-old married white woman who had always been a compulsive and scrupulously clean housewife was forced by financial reverses to seek her father's help. He lived with two older sisters of the patient, one married and childless, the other single. The patient consciously resented the relationship of the father to the older sisters and frequently referred to them angrily as her father's "wives." Conscious hatred was felt for her father and the two sisters. The patient felt guilty about these hateful emotions but did not admit into consciousness any of her hostile death wishes. Instead, they appeared in consciousness in the form of acute anxiety or panic states whenever any disaster occurred. She was unable to read the newspaper headlines or listen to the radio for fear she would hear of some recent disaster. If this happened, she was then plagued with doubt that she had not performed her compulsive mental rituals correctly. If the disaster was a fire, then she wondered if she had not said "long life" the last time she saw the word "fire." If she had been talking to someone or looking at someone, she felt she must go over and over in her mind certain ritual phrases that were designed to deny the presence of any hostile wish that someone should drop dead, or burn to death, or come down with some dread and crippling disease. For example, she would repeat such phrases as "I mean she should not get sick" or "there should be no fire" or "I mean there should be no war." Frequently, doubt would arise in her mind as to whether she had got the phrase right, thus indicating quite clearly the breaking-through of the hostile wish.

Sometimes this tendency to undo or negate was directed against anal-sadistic impulses. For example, thinking about a man or being in his presence might force her to mumble to herself, "I don't mean kiss my behind." Further evidence of her anal-erotic fixation is indicated by her sexual responses to her husband's advances. She was unable to enjoy sexual activity with him unless she guiltily indulged in fantasies about spanking. In these, some other woman was always being spanked. It is interesting to note that the patient's father, a surgeon, was frequently plagued with a compulsive doubt regarding his preparation for the sterility of the surgical field, or he wondered if he had made all his sutures tight enough.

Being forced to return to her father's home for help threw the patient back into the unsolved oedipal conflict of her childhood. Her mother had died when she was six, and she and the two older sisters were reared by this father with the aid of housekeepers. At the time of the mother's death the child developed some kind of rectal trouble requiring frequent enemas. There was some regressive soiling at that time, with frequent punishment by her father.

It is not difficult to see that this patient resented her father's "wives" and wished them dead; but fear that her magical death wishes might cause their deaths, just like the real mother's, aroused intense anxiety and led to the displacement and spreading of the hostility to cosmic proportions. The compulsive cleanliness and anal-sadistic fantasies are obviously a regression to a previously overstimulated erotic zone that was accidentally fixated by the constant enemas and spankings.

DEPRESSIONS

In depressions, also, ego-alien impulses—in this case, hostile tendencies—can no longer be excluded from consciousness by repression, and the ego has to use other modes of defense against them. The principal method is to turn the hostile impulses originally directed against other persons against one's own self. The melancholic patient indulges in an orgy of self-accusation which substitutes for destructive wishes toward others. The original target of hostility is always an ambivalently loved and hated person. Because of the love component, the hostility cannot be vented freely and must be turned back against the hating person himself. This is a suitable defense, because to hate a person whom one also loves is the source of the most intense sense of guilt. Attacking one's self—a kind of self-punishment—not only drains off the aggressive impulse but also serves at the same time as an atonement for wanting to destroy the beloved person.

The picture is further complicated by another important dynamism, which is of specific significance in depressions—identification. The love relationships of the depressive are tenuous and easily regress under frustration to a precursor of mature object love, that is, to identification. The lost object is reconstituted within the ego by the process of identification. The ambivalent conflict originally entertained toward the object now continues intra-psychically toward the person introjected. The process of identification thus favors the retroflection of the hostile impulses toward the self.

The quality of the impulses which participate in this dynamism are primarily of oral-aggressive nature. The tendency to incorporate the object as a part of the ego corresponds to that early period of development in which the interpersonal relations are of oral-dependent and oral-aggressive nature. According to Freud (5) and Abraham (1), the depressive patient has a fixation to the early oral phase of development and regresses to it whenever his tenuous object relationships in later life are disturbed. The dynamics of the depressive reaction are identical with those of mourning. In a depression the ambivalent character of object relationships is more pronounced, and the whole process is more intensive and prolonged. Because there is ambivalence in every object relationship, mourning is a universal phenomenon.

The following is an illustrative case of depression:

A 26-year-old white man developed a severe depression following the death of his wife. His depression was typically accompanied by feelings of guilt and ideas of a self-accusatory nature. He hated himself for not being kinder and blamed himself for her death because she had died in childbirth. During his depression that lasted about nine months, he suffered from frequent bouts of nausea and was unable to eat anything but baby foods. Analysis revealed that their $3\frac{1}{2}$ years of married life had not been very congenial. His wife had wanted a baby soon after marriage, but he claimed it was not wise because of financial reasons. There were frequent quarrels between them because he did not care to go out with her socially except to visit his mother's home. He also fussed about his wife's failure to develop into as good a cook as his mother. When she finally did become pregnant, he was openly neglectful and frequently left her alone to visit his mother or to be with the "boys."

The oral fixation and the ambivalent attitude to the wife are obvious in this case. The depression lasting nine months and his nausea and vomiting are indicative of an oral incorporation of the dead pregnant wife. By this process of identification, the hostility that he felt for his wife was turned upon the introjected object. In this case it can be clearly seen how the principal defense of depression, namely, a turning of the hostile impulses originally directed against his wife against his own self, is made possible by the process of oral incorporation and identification. It is interesting to note that as a child he suffered from a severe eating problem and had to be placed in a boarding house for several months.

HYPOCHONDRIASIS

Only because it so frequently occupies the central place in different forms of neurotic conditions does this syndrome deserve discussion under a special heading.

Anxious preoccupation with one's own body and fearful expectation of a disease are always manifestations of a deep-seated need for suffering which derives from unconscious guilt feelings. A further important factor is that the preoccupation with a supposedly diseased part of the body can serve as a particularly suitable excuse for withdrawal of interest from the external world and for concentration of all love and attention to one's own self. The fact that this excuse consists in suffering allays guilt feelings, which a mature adult feels because of an excessive degree of self-concern.

A third factor is that the preoccupation with a concrete disease symptom allows the patient to displace a more intensive form of anxiety (such as castration fear or its feminine equivalent), as in the phobias, to one circumscribed area. The important role which narcissistic withdrawal and guilt play in these cases explains why the hypochondriasis syndrome is usually either the substitute for or a component of a depressive state.

BEHAVIOR DISTURBANCES

Behavior disturbances are "neurotic character," "fate-neurosis," "psychopathic personality," and "impulse-ridden character." The outstanding feature of these conditions is that ego-alien impulses find outlet in actual behavior rather than in neurotic symptoms. As we have shown, neurotic symptoms are symbolic substitutions in fantasy for co-ordinated activity. Neurotic characters, however, are not satisfied with such tenuous gratification; they "act out" these impulses. Their life, in contrast to the neurotic, who suffers from typical symptoms, is dramatic; it is not just a private affair of the patient, it involves the environment. Because the ego-alien impulses are often of an aggressively antisocial nature, these patients often get into conflict with the law and form the major portion of the delinquents. Other neurotic characters express their unconscious impulses in eccentric behavior. Many famous adventurers, collectors, mountain climbers, and daredevils belong to this category. Neurotic acting-out of an impulse is the equivalent of a neurotic symptom. The difference lies in its alloplasticity.[1]

1. Ferenczi differentiated between autoplastic and alloplastic adaptations at the disposal of the organism: (1) changes within the organism (for example, development of heavy fur in the Arctic regions); (2) changes in the environment (for example, building fire or homes as protection against cold). Neurotic symptoms exemplify the first category because subjective needs are satisfied merely by internal processes, such as fantasy. Neurotic characters, on the other hand, gratify their alien drives by full-fledged activity which directly influences the environment, such as delinquent or unconventional behavior.

However, like neurotic symptoms, such symptomatic behavior is still only a substitute for realistic gratification of the repressed tendency, which is only rarely acted out in unadulterated form by severely disturbed psychotics.

This group of behavior disorders has long baffled psychiatrists, and the diagnosis "psychopathic personality" has come to be considered a wastebasket diagnosis. From the psychodynamic point of view, however, this diagnosis is not more difficult to make than any other diagnosis of a neurosis. The differential criterion is "neurotic acting-out" versus neurotic symptoms. The presence of an unconscious neurotic conflict can easily be recognized. It manifests itself by the following phenomena:

a) Irrationality of behavior, which is ill-motivated so far as conscious awareness of motives is concerned.

b) Stereotyped repetitive acting-out of unconscious motive forces which are not accessible to the modifying influence of conscious inhibition. This explains why, for example, neurotic delinquents repeatedly decide to start a new life and end their irrational behavior, only to fail again and again in their determination to reform. The opinion of most people, including many psychiatrists, that this inconsistency is a deception leads to the faulty view that these patients lack a superego and are fundamentally—indeed, constitutionally—asocial. There is no evidence that constitution is of greater significance in these patients than in those suffering from any other form of neurosis.

c) Marked self-destructive tendencies which express the neurotic conflict. Neurotic delinquents always manage to be caught, as a result of a strong need for punishment, an outcome of guilt feelings, which themselves arise from the asocial impulses.

d) The actual neurotic behavior is a distorted substitute for unconscious fantasies. The actual crime, for example, is often a substitute for incestuous or patricidal impulses. The criminal who is acting from a guilty conscience, as described by Freud (7), attempts by a more or less trivial delinquency to express his crime, and in this way he appeases his unconscious guilt and makes a bargain. He suffers consciously for a smaller crime, while in his unconscious he secures substitutive outlet for his deeply repressed asocial tendencies, for which he would be punished much more severely. In fact, he exchanges the unconsciously dreaded castration as the expected punishment for his oedipal guilt with a more trivial form of suffering, such as imprisonment or, at most, hard labor.

The following case is illustrative of the acting-out neurotic character and demonstrates the features so typical of this condition, namely, the acting-out of ego-alien impulses, suffering being experienced by those in the environment because of the aggressive, antisocial nature of the impulses.

This is the case of a 27-year-old white male who is the youngest of three children. Both the older brother and sister are now hospitalized for schizophrenia in a state institution. His father, a very aggressive and successful business promoter, who was somewhat unscrupulous and inclined to alcoholism, died several years ago. The patient was attached to his mother, who was an indulgent and weak-willed woman who failed to exercise any discipline. The father was a bully, so that the patient was thrown between the spoiling of the mother and the bullying of the father. Although his intellectual capacity was adequate, he did poorly in school because of his truancy and defiance of male schoolteachers. He quit after two years of high school and then showed an even poorer work record. He was inclined to get into frequent quarrels with others and would then show traits that were imitative of his father. He would talk in a "big" and grandiose manner, scold, and act in a physically threatening manner. He most often associated with people of questionable character, because he felt ill at ease with those of his own set. He was easily affected by small amounts of alcohol and would evince the picture of pathological intoxication at times, approaching a confusional state. These periods lasted from only a few days to three weeks. Twice during such periods he became married to scheming women who had to be paid off and the marriage annulled. From one of these women he contracted syphilis.

This case reveals the unconscious competition and identification with the powerful and bullying father and the guilt about his incestuous attachment to his indulgent mother. But the neurotic conflict, instead of being discharged autoplastically, is drained off alloplastically in acting out the role of the superior and bully toward his inferiors and in choosing the indulgent prostitute as both a denial and a gratification of his incestuous attachment.

ALCOHOLISM AND DRUG ADDICTION

These conditions deserve special classification for practical reasons because of the combination of the physiological effect of the drug with an unconscious emotional need.

The essential factor is that, by means of their narcotic effect, both alcohol and the different forms of drugs favor the possibility of regressively escaping conflictful life-situations. Through the narcotic effect, alcohol and drugs give physiological support to the regressive tendency to re-establish the carefree, passive state of Nirvana, of early infancy, when the child's needs are satisfied at the mother's breast. On the other hand, the initial stimulating effect of the drugs, which sooner or later is followed by the sedative effect, permits the patient to overcome his psychological inhibitions. The latter factor is particularly important in alcoholism. Alcoholics are often recruited from neurotics who are particularly inhibited in their human relationships and suffer from intense feelings of insecurity. The physiological effect of alcohol allows these patients to express themselves more freely and to feel effective and superior.

In the second phase of the intoxication the effect of alcohol dulls the pains of self-depreciation and insecurity. In other words, narcotics are pain-killers not only in the physical but also in the psychological sense.

The fact that indulgence in alcohol is socially sanctioned and that it offers pleasant, although temporary, relief from emotional stress explains its widespread use and partially explains the difficulties of therapy. In fact, alcoholism—both in theory and in therapy—is one of the most puzzling problems of present-day psychiatry. The question is: What makes certain persons become victims of this drug, from which other people derive only temporary relaxation from the tribulations of everyday existence? Some hidden allergic sensitivity of the organism has often been postulated, but no objective findings have been presented for the support of this hypothesis. On the other hand, there is indication that a psychological susceptibility, a basic weakness of ego control, might be the crucial factor.

SEXUAL PERVERSIONS

One of Freud's early formulations was that a neurosis is the negative of a perversion (8). In other words, what a neurotic person represses and can gratify only symbolically by symptoms, the pervert expresses directly in his sexual behavior. Little can be added to this formulation, but the factors which are responsible for one person's developing a sexual perversion and another a psychoneurosis are still largely unknown.

In perversions either the quality of the sexual strivings or the object of the sexual striving is abnormal. In sadism, masochism, exhibitionism, voyeurism, and transvestitism the nature of the sexual striving is disturbed. In homosexuality, pedophilia, and zoöphilia the normal object is replaced by an unnatural one. In fetishism the object of the sexual striving as well as its quality is abnormal.

Etiologically, it is of primary significance that perversions show fixation to early pregenital forms of gratification. Regression to points of fixation is often manifest, but usually the perversion can be traced back as a continuous inclination of the patient from early childhood. There may be exacerbations and remissions, and occasionally there may be a long interval between fixating childhood experiences and the manifestation of the perversion in later adult life.

Because of the significance of the fixating childhood experiences, one should consider perversions as manifestations of an interrupted sexual development rather than as a disintegration of mature sexuality into its pregenital components. Although disintegration may play a certain role, in pronounced cases sexual maturity has never been firmly established. This fact might be responsible for the unusual difficulties which these patients offer to any form of treatment.

In sadism, inflicting of pain is the main content of the sexual urge. This aggressive impulse is completely dissociated from any utilitarian goal, such as the elimination of an enemy or an obstacle. Inflicting pain is an aim in itself and the source of sensual gratification. The same is true of masochism. Here the suffering of pain is the content of the sexual sensation. Voluntary endurance of pain is an important component of rational adaptive behavior. In order to achieve a cherished goal, a person may often willingly subject himself to all kinds of suffering. This, however, is not masochism. In masochism the endurance of pain is not subordinated to any goal but is a pleasurable aim in itself.

In exhibitionism, the showing-off becomes an isolated aim and the source of sensual gratification. Voyeurism can be described as the sexualized form of curiosity. Curiosity, too, is an integral component of purposeful behavior. When curiosity becomes a goal in itself, it assumes an erotic quality.

These forms of perversions, in which the quality of the instinctual strivings retain their pregenital form, substantiate the thesis that sexual gratification does not depend upon the quality of the instinctual urge but upon the mode of discharge. Every emotional tension, such as aggression and endurance of pain, curiosity, or vanity, can be expressed in sexual and nonsexual form. What is characteristic of the sexual expression is that here the emotional tendency is not subordinated to a self-preservative function but is an aim in itself. Object love also can be expressed in a nonsexual and in a sexual form, as is demonstrated by the double meaning of the word "love."

In the group of perversions in which only the object of the sexual tendency is disturbed—homosexuality, pedophilia, and zoöphilia—the sexual maturation is more advanced than in the group mentioned above. Here the influence of the oedipal conflict manifests itself in the replacement of an incestuous object by another one. Accordingly, homosexuality is often a defense against an intensive mother- or father-fixation. Another common mechanism in male homosexuality consists in identification with the original forbidden object of the sexual striving, for example, with the mother. At the same time, the person's own role is projected onto the homosexual partner. The sexual relationship re-establishes the mother-son relationship in which the patient plays the role of the mother and enjoys vicariously the pleasures of the partner who has the role of the son. The same mechanism is equally common in cases of female homosexuality.

In fetishism the main function of the perversion is to bind intensive castration fear. This is borne out by the fact that fetishism is restricted to the male sex. The fetish, usually a part of the female body or some article of female apparel (for example, shoes), represents the male genital, which the fetishist insists on attributing also to the female sex. By this he denies the existence of a castrated being (a body lacking a penis), which would arouse his own castration fear to an unbearable degree.

It is not intended to give illustrations and clinical examples of all the various perversions. However, the following case of homosexuality in a male is cited to illustrate some of the salient factors noted above. Analytic study of this case revealed that the perversion had been expressed by the patient from early childhood and at no time had been completely absent. This case also demonstrates the fact that perversions are a manifestation of partial interruption in the sexual development, partial because some degree of heterosexual development took place. This patient also shows that his homosexuality was not only a direct expression of libidinous striving of that nature but that this avenue of discharge was also used to drain off frustrated emotional striving arising from other sources.

This is the case of a 31-year-old married white male who came for treatment only after he had been picked up by a plain-clothes policeman for attempting a sexually perverse act. He is a well-built and handsome man but has a somewhat effeminate appearance. His mother is a very dominating and domineering woman, who came from a wealthy family. The patient's father, a soft-spoken, passive, timid creature, who was always browbeaten by his wife, worked in the father-in-law's business. A younger brother had to be hospitalized in a state institution for the feeble-minded.

This patient's homosexual experiences go back to the age of eight, when he seduced a colored man servant into fellatio and mutual masturbation. From then to his present age he has actively sought homosexual partners. He usually tries to find large muscular men, with whom he engages in mutual embracing or fellatio. When he was fifteen, his parents were quite conscious of his difficulty, sought help, and sent him to a military school. The behavior of the patient's mother in regard to sex was traumatic to him. The patient remembers awakening to find his mother examining and handling his genitals.

It is interesting to note that his libidinal organization influenced his vocational choice. He became interested in women's hairdressing and is now engaged in a thriving business. Although the idea of heterosexuality nauseated him, about two years ago he married a soft-spoken, mild sort of a woman, who can, however, be hard and firm upon occasion. This was shown by her ability to stand up to his dominating mother (her mother-in-law). The patient has always been contemptuous of his father but has been fearful of his mother.

When he came into therapy he revealed a boyish and infantile sort of orientation. He was still "mother's boy" and often spoke petulantly of his wife's ill-treatment of him. Sexual relations with her were only a matter of form. His desires often led him to such places as men's lavatories in hotels. This tendency on many occasions increased under any kind of stress. Quarrels with his wife, troubles in business, or difficulties with his mother often led to homosexual release. In his fantasies he often pictured himself being hugged and made love to. It was understandable that this man's trouble was greatly aggravated when his child was born and that he got into particular difficulty with the child's nurse.

This case of male homosexuality is illustrative of intense "mother-fixation," with the solution being a regression from the oedipal conflict because of fear of incest to a passive, oral position. Fear of the tyrannical mother made him turn to men for his passive oral gratification. He then sought for male lovers who would love him as he wanted and feared to be loved by his mother. Unconsciously, he established a love relationship with these men and played the role of the young child, giving the mother role to his male partners. A female creature was unthinkable because of his disgust and fear of the tyrannical mother. His feminine identification was further enhanced by his intense longing for the strong father whom he had never had in childhood.

BIBLIOGRAPHY

1. ABRAHAM, K. "Manic-depressive States and the Pre-genital Levels of the Libido," in *Selected Papers* (London: Hogarth Press, 1927).
2. DEUTSCH, H. *Psychoanalysis of the Neuroses* (London: Hogarth Press, 1932).
3. FREUD, A. *The Ego and the Mechanisms of Defence* (London: Hogarth Press, 1937).
4. FREUD, S. "Analysis of a Phobia in a Five-Year-Old Boy," in *Collected Papers*, Vol. 3 (London: Hogarth Press, 1924).
5. FREUD, S. "Mourning and Melancholia," in *Collected Papers*, Vol. 4 (London: Hogarth Press, 1924).
6. FREUD, S. "Notes upon a Case of Obsessional Neurosis," in *Collected Papers*, Vol. 3 (London: Hogarth Press, 1924).
7. FREUD, S. "Some Character Types Met with in Psychoanalytic Work," in *Collected Papers*, Vol. 4 (London: Hogarth Press, 1924).
8. FREUD, S. *Three Contributions to the Theory of Sex*, in *The Basic Writings of Sigmund Freud* (New York: Modern Library, 1938).

IV

ACUTE NEUROTIC REACTIONS

Leon J. Saul, M.D., and John W. Lyons, M.D.

UNUSUAL external stresses may elicit acute reactions. These stand in contrast with those chronic neuroses which are reactions to long-standing difficulties and are, by comparison, more independent of the external life-situation.

If a number of people are exposed to the same stress, only certain ones develop neurotic reactions. Earlier psychiatrists attributed this to constitutional weakness, while others stressed the reactivation of repressed infantile experiences by the trauma. More recent formulations (12, 28), born of the experience of World War II, utilize the concept of "specific emotional vulnerability" —how and when *any* individual will succumb depends, in the main, on the violence, duration, and nature of the stresses bearing on the specifically vulnerable parts of his personality. An individual's vulnerability is determined in part by constitutional factors, of which little is known, and in part by his emotional development, of which considerable is known.*

* These relations have been schematized in the following formula (28):

$$Vs \times Ss \propto \frac{Ad}{F} \times \frac{R}{P} \propto \frac{T}{E} \propto N,$$

where

Vs = Specific emotional vulnerability;
Ss = External stresses, especially in relation to specific emotional vulnerability;
Ad = Difficulty of adjustment, internal and external;
F = Flexibility, adaptability, including capacity for temporary and partial regression;
R = Regressive forces, including fixation (toward childish dependence or infantile attitudes or reactions);
P = Progressive forces (toward independence, responsibility, productivity, maturity);
T = Emotional tension;
E = Ego strength (especially control and integrative capacity);
N = Degree of neurosis.

Since war, with its unusual physical and emotional hardships, is probably the most fertile source of the acute reactive neuroses, most of the literature deals with reactions to the stresses of war, and this chapter is based chiefly on the study of war neuroses.

Freud considered the central feature of traumatic neurosis to be a psychic fixation to the moment of trauma (9). The neurosis then becomes a reproduction or a repetition of the situation, because the task of mastering and digesting it is still to be accomplished. Freud stated that constitution and infantile experiences are complementary and that minor traumata might reactivate infantile responses in a predisposed individual. This observation helps to explain the wide range of breaking points in various people to specific traumata.

In 1921 Freud (11) wrote that, if previous research had not substantiated the sexual theory in war neurosis, neither had anyone shown it to be incorrect. Freud, of course, used the term "sexual" in a broad way to mean (1) "sensual" and (2) "love" in its widest sense. The experience of World War II bore this out, in showing that prolonged frustration of emotional needs was a central factor in many cases of war neurosis.

Freud felt that the intra-psychic representative of reality may consist not only of genuine superego (that is, roughly, "conscience"—the internalization of parental ideals and standards) acquired in childhood but also of later and more superficial identifications with various other authorities. War, with its rigorous training and living conditions so dissimilar to peacetime, may create a "war superego" which permits the expression of forbidden impulses and tempts the ego with demands intolerable to the real superego. Freud felt that in many of the war neurotics a "peace ego" arises in defense against the "war superego." This view was confirmed by Abraham, Ferenczi, and Jones (11). Freud wrote (9) that the individual is impelled by a self-seeking, egoistic motive, and his quest for protection and self-interest maintains the conflict, once the symptoms occur. This aims at protecting the ego from a repetition of the trauma and persists until the danger is no longer present or until some compensation has been received.

Ferenczi (11) believed that not only love of others (mature love, "genital attitude," "object interest") but its precursor, love of self (narcissism), was affected by war. The symptoms of terror, depression, instability, etc., arose from increased ego sensitivity as a result of the withdrawal of libido from the object into the ego, in other words, from a retreat from the usual mature interests in others to preoccupation with one's self. This is the tendency under stress—to abandon other considerations and take care of one's self. Thus those predisposed by a high degree of self-centeredness (narcissism) will be susceptible to traumatic neuroses. Because of the universality of the narcissistic stage, no one is immune. Children only gradually outgrow their self-centeredness and become capable of adult parental responsibility and sacrifice.

Abraham (11) agreed that men who developed war neuroses were predisposed before the trauma. Since their previous adjustment was dependent on self-interest (narcissistic concessions), they were ill-prepared for the selfless sacrifices demanded by war.

Jones (18) wrote that the conflict was between fear and the adaptation to war. Conflicts over killing, dirt, and discipline, combined with fear of being maimed or killed, tend to overwhelm the ego.

In the traumatic neurosis the dream life continually goes back to the disaster situation, indicating a "fixation" to the trauma. Freud felt that, if the wish-fulfilment theory of dreams were to be maintained, then dreaming suffers a dislocation along with other functions and is sidetracked from its usual purpose. He postulated a "repetition compulsion" for powerful experience that goes beyond the "pleasure principle" (8). According to this hypothesis, the dreams represent a regression to a more primitive mode of mastery. Through repeated reliving of the trauma, control may be slowly regained by the gradual discharge of energy and relief of tension. Recent work (29), without contradicting this hypothesis, indicates that some, if not all, catastrophic nightmares of the traumatic neuroses fit perfectly into Freud's well-established theory of dreams.

Freud believed that the ego developed in part at least for the purpose of avoiding traumatic states by its ability to anticipate expected trauma and prepare the individual so that the effects are softened. Economically (quantitatively), such preparation consists in making ready amounts of "countercathexis" (countercharge of emotion) to bind the expected excitation. To be forewarned is to be forearmed. Unexpected traumata are experienced more forcefully. Pathological and archaic attempts at mastery may be utilized to stem the painful incoming stimuli. An incident may have a traumatic effect in direct relationship to its unexpectedness.

Simmel (32) stated that there were no appreciable differences between the neuroses of World War I and those of World War II. He felt that the dynamic conflict lies within the ego itself, in its attempt to mediate between instinctual demands and external reality. The ego in its struggle for survival is undermined by the prospect of annihilation from the external world. The symptomatology results from the ego's use of the mental mechanisms of defense in transforming real anxiety (fear of death) into neurotic anxiety.

A nation at war, as an external representative of the parents, permits a return of the repressed aggressive impulses and sanctions them if used against the enemy. However, if relations to the parents were bad, then there is a tendency to be hostile against all authority. Soldiers indoctrinated in a military unit are joined libidinally and are collectively identified with a leader, who becomes the externalized superego (10). Thus the soldier is in the old child-father relationship and feels secure and even immune to death as long as the relationship with the superior is good. However, discrimination, poor leadership, and disappointments tend to isolate the individual and render the authority unsuitable as an externalized superego. Since he feels released from the group, the man's original conscience and standards function again. The ability of the ego to withstand trauma now depends on the strength and normality of the soldier's peacetime superego.

War symbolizes the ambivalent conflict with the father in a specific manner. Where the self-esteem is hurt by authority, the authority becomes the hated father. The aggressive destructive tendencies previously aimed at the authorities are turned inward and tend to augment the strictness of the inner superego. This guilt may then paralyze the personality by phobic reactions and may cause overt aggression or pathological heroism. In other words, repressed hostility to superiors can reach such intensity and cause such guilt as to generate neurotic symptoms. To the predisposed, war can also represent the original oedipal situation in the form of the enemy symbolizing the father and the home country the mother.

As Simmel saw it, the symptoms of war neurosis are mechanisms of escape from an unbearable situation, as in psychosis. These mechanisms turn into neurotic symptoms through the interference of the superego, which is able to turn the external danger into an internal, instinctive danger. Thus the symptoms are not converted erotic longings but destructive impulses. That is, they are powered not by sensual feelings but by anger, hate, and hostility. By forming symptoms, the ego avoids a complete psychotic break with reality and brings about a release of the tensions toward the superego. By protecting himself against the danger of his own hostile aggressiveness, the person maintains his stability.

In treatment Simmel stated that, if the war neurotic can turn anxiety into rage and aggressive action, the ego will find its way back to reality. Consequently, he introduced and encouraged the venting of rage on dummies and recommended the assumption of a benevolent superego (kindly, tolerant, permissive) attitude on the part of the therapist.

Kardiner (19) finds that there is no specific neurosis created exclusively by war conditions but that war offers an opportunity for the development of neuroses in greater concentration and frequency. He discusses inhibition as the major force, operating broadly and disordering the various mechanisms of adaptation. The neurosis becomes the organism's attempt to adapt itself under the circumstances of vastly reduced resources. The continuous conflict necessitates constant control and inhibition. This tends to change the individual's conception of himself and the outer world. It produces a feeling of helplessness and a tendency to give up and to be parasitic (regression). His altered conception of the outer world as a threatening place inhibits vital psychological functions, in part as a defense against further traumata. His regression to infantile helplessness in the face of the threatening world engenders further fear and hostility. Catastrophic dreams then occur because of the feared retaliation for his own hostility. Though his regression may give him some inner security, it may also tend to perpetuate the neurosis.

A sudden loss of control over the situation causes lasting damage to the adaptive capacity. Rado (24) postulates an emergency control mechanism which tends to remove the individual from dangerous situations. The basic pattern is described as being a conflict between military duty and self-preservation, with an ensuing flight into illness, fixation on the trauma, and a secondary gain from the illness. The emergency control mechanism, spurring toward flight or blind attack, is in conflict with the sense of duty, which requires calmness and rational thinking. The traumatic period becomes the last straw, and the man finds relief from tension in a flight into illness, especially if it can last for the duration of the war.

In the post-traumatic period the anxiety perpetuates itself by creating the illusion that he is still in battle. There are sporadic resurgences of rage and anxiety as the personality relaxes its subjugation to the emergency control mechanism. As time goes on, the process gradually subsides. If, however, the traumatic phobic factor is too strong, the fear of recurrence becomes dominant, and the patient regresses to dependency and unconscious appeals for support. The sexual function is vulnerable because of its susceptibility to anxiety since childhood (castration fears).

Grinker and Spiegel (12, 13) find the nuclear problem of war-induced neuroses to be anxiety, much of which results from the stresses of war bearing upon the integrative functions of the ego. War, equated with potential injury or death, stimulates every emergency biological mechanism for flight. The conflict between the desire for flight and the fear of punishment from officers floods the ego with emotion. Further sources of anxiety are the individual's feeling of helplessness and the unusual situation of actually having approval for hostile and destructive behavior. Anxiety springs also from the liberation of primitive reflexes and its associated energy, such as the noise, sight, and smell of battle. Thus the ego is flooded with anxieties from external reality, from the man's own instinctual drives, and from the reactions of the superego. On the other hand, the ego is protected from anxiety by a number of factors: the individual's ability to identify with a group, approval of war aims, sense of invulnerability, and ability to express hostility outwardly.

Ego-exhausting factors, such as fatigue, hunger, pain, sensory overstimulation, traumatic identification, guilt, and expected injury and death, tend to undermine the ego from without. At the same time, previous neurotic trends and traumata bore from within. As the pressure on the ego continues, its inhibitory and intellectual functions weaken. Signs of free-floating anxiety, confusion, and poor concentration result. The process may go on to complete disintegration, as in fugues, stupors, or schizoid dissociated states. This loss of ego function appears to be a biological regression to more primitive levels of adaptation. Anxiety may subside also by being bound to conversion symptoms, leaving the rest of the ego to function normally.

In a later publication (2) Grinker states that "in the interval before returning to the U.S. war neurosis seems to undergo a change of pattern; the newer reactions are engulfed by old patterns and the total picture stands out sharply, showing the reactions to war to be a repetition of old reactions to previous conflicts."

Saul (28) proposed a theory of acute neurotic reactions to cover the highly individual factors as well as the general causes. He combined the concept of "specific emotional vulnerability" with the concept of emergency physiologic mobilization for fight or flight. The specific vulnerabilities, in addition to the various general factors discussed above, such as superego conflicts and ego depletion, account for the individual variations in symptomatology; the psychophysiologic "fight-flight" reaction accounts for the similarity of the syndromes.

INCIDENCE

Acute neurotic reactions are seen also in civilian life following catastrophes, such as automobile and train wrecks, mine cave-ins, and other accidents. Emotional shocks can produce similar effects. As an example Adler (1) has reported a study of survivors of the Coconut Grove holocaust in Boston. Here the suddenness of the calamity, along with the panic and the fact that large numbers were trapped in the blazing café, served to place many in sudden danger of death. Many of those who became so disturbed emotionally as to develop neurotic symptoms had escaped unscathed physically. The symptoms of most of the survivors subsided in a relatively short time, but many were left with residual neuroses. The most common memories of the group studied were fear of imminent death and of being choked and trampled.

It is in wartime that the acute neurotic reactions of various kinds and degree are seen most profusely, not only at the front, but in rear areas and in civilian life. The transformation of the individual from his peacetime life into one of war, with all its dangers, hardship, and stresses, tends to make unusual demands on the ego.

During the last war (according to statistics compiled by W. C. Menninger) (21) 382,000, or 34 per cent, of all the medical disability cases were neuropsychiatric. These occurred in a well-screened group. Obvious neurotics and misfits had been rejected. Of the 15,000,000 men examined, 1,846,000, or 12 per cent, were rejected for neuropsychiatric disorders. These were 38 per cent of the total number rejected for all causes. Of the remainder, 250,000 were later discharged administratively. Furthermore, 3–7 per cent of all trainees consulted the mental hygiene clinics; of this number, only 7 per cent had to be hospitalized. Unknown but large numbers consulted division psychiatrists and flight surgeons. These needed no further care or hospitalization.

ETIOLOGY

It cannot be too strongly emphasized that the etiology of acute reactive conditions is not a matter of the individual's neurosis, latent or otherwise, but of his "fit" (Alexander) or adaptation to the particular environment. Every "normal" has vulnerabilities and may break under stress upon his specifically vulnerable spot. Conversely, a severe "neurotic" may adjust very well if his neurosis happens to fit the particular stressful situation. Thus individuals with frank chronic neuroses, such as compulsives, mild paranoids, schizoid personalities, neurotic characters, can and did adjust to combat and other situations where the external stress did not excite their specific vulnerability. Indeed, certain situations were such that a person with a certain kind of neurosis could adjust much better than a normal mature individual. For example (28):

Two professional men came into the service together. The one held to very high standards and was very adult in all his relationships. He was warmly interested in people, very much in love with his wife and children and devoted to his work. When obstacles arose to the accomplishment of what he deemed right, he invariably sought to overcome them. He was a strong, loyal man of high type and unusually mature.

The other man, although able, was of much easier virtue. Also a family man, his eye nevertheless sometimes roved. His interest in his work was noticeably overbalanced by his enjoyment of relaxation, and he never fought through obstacles or for the maintenance of standards if he could possibly avoid the trouble. In the service, as things turned out, both men went overseas and were subjected to considerable stress. The former persisted in his faithfulness to his family, strove to do the job with the utmost effectiveness and consideration and refused to compromise on his standards. As a result, he missed his family painfully but could not forget them with other women, and he had many battles to fight on his job. At the end of a year, although he maintained full control and performed efficiently, the underlying tension had so mounted that he developed disturbances of both heart and stomach and had to be evacuated.

The second man, however, took the easier way. He freely sought refuge from the frustrations of his job and personal life in wine, women and song—in his duty did no more than was expected of him, while after hours he totally forgot his troubles in the pursuit of whatever pleasures were available wherever he happened to be. A relatively lazy, irresponsible child as compared with the former upstanding, responsible, productive, independent man, he nevertheless, through his ability to escape into play, avoided enough frustration and gained enough pleasure and surcease to continue to function on this level. His ability to regress protected him, while the former man, maintaining his high level and unable to regress, broke down.

As indicated by J. Appel (3), it is probably true that every individual, if subjected to enough stress, will break down. Also many men will endure successive combat campaigns and then break down for other reasons. If the stress is sufficiently intense and prolonged, even the strongest will succumb. Some break sooner than others. Although there are basic similarities in what men feel and can stand, there are individual differences in kind and in degree of sensitivity. Everyone has vulnerabilities and breaking points.

It must be remembered that a man who breaks under a specific stress would not always do so, had he not been sensitized and his controls weakened by other experiences. This point may be clarified by the following examples (28):

A young officer complained of anxiety, irritability, and insomnia after 3½ years of extensive combat duty aboard ship. His symptoms had developed suddenly at the termination of his leave as he was preparing to return to his ship.

Actually combat did not unduly upset him. In a way it held the same thrill as hunting. True, his emotional tension mounted continually aboard ship but not because of fear. Further exploration revealed that one of the sources of his increasing stress was being told how and when to get his hair cut. This was significant of all the restrictions aboard ship which he found eventually to be unbearable—changing his clothes for meals, standing inspection in whites after a night of enemy action, and similar infringements of his personal liberty.

He could discuss his combat experiences freely and with little discomfort, but even the memory of these minor impairments of his freedom enraged him. His resentment increased until, just before returning to his ship, he literally trembled with rage. He did not understand this and did not realize the intensity of his feelings. He was terrified only by these mysterious symptoms.

To understand this man we must go into his personal history. He was raised in the Canadian Rockies, where he enjoyed freedom beyond the realm of that known in urban or even most rural areas. At 13 his parents died and he went to live with a rigid restricting aunt, where he found conditions intolerable. Instead of giving in to her restrictions, he went off to live in a small town where he was well acquainted. He set himself up in a small cabin, worked in his spare time and went through high school. Self-reliant, and loving the freedom of the mountains, his was the personality of the independent frontiersman. It became clear why he could face danger and violence coolly but could not stand four years of supervised hair cuts. His sensitivity was restriction. He would not have broken under fear alone. In civil life he had similar but milder symptoms. Generally good natured, he had a violent temper when his freedom was impaired. Like typical combat fatigue, he suffered with insomnia and nightmares, but his dreams were not of battle. Instead, they were repeatedly of being "held down" or "fenced in."

Another man had his symptoms precipitated when his ship hit a mine. Half the crew was killed, and he was hurled 30 feet through the air. His anxiety persisted for three months, along with stomach distress and repeated nightmares, in which the scene was almost exactly the same, but the screaming of wounded shipmates noticeably worse.

He came from a poor financial background in which the necessary frugal living was a source of distress to him. In high school he was able to earn enough to have the things he wanted. He felt more comfortable and secure and resigned himself to hard work in order to get what he wanted. He thought his father could have been a better provider.

As the patient talked, it was evident that strong hostile feelings toward his father and brother were checked and controlled by a very loving and gentle attitude. This latter came from identification with his mother, who was a kindly and religious woman. He never had a fist fight, nor was he cruel to animals. He could not stand violence or bloodshed of any kind.

Here we see a young man with considerable repressed hostility which had long been inhibited because of love of his parents and careful upbringing. He could not indulge it even in reading or fantasy. In his own mind hostility could not be acted out externally but only turned against himself. Aroused by combat he could not become aggressive. His violently aroused emotion went not into hostility for others but into fear for himself.

In spite of the many complications and variations, the etiology of the acute reaction seems to boil down to a variety of internal and external factors, both physical and psychological (danger, exposure, disease, separation, anxiety, morale, etc.), which exert stresses on the individual and cause (1) general weakening and sensitization, (2) reactions resulting from specific emotional vulnerabilities, and (3) weakening and impairment of the powers of control over the symptoms.

Once a person is threatened by increasing pain, frustration,

anxiety, and weakening forces of control, he reacts by physiologic and psychologic mobilization for fight or flight. This
manifests itself in the various symptoms and behavior patterns
common to war neuroses.

TYPES OF STRESS AND REACTION

World War II afforded psychiatry an excellent opportunity
to study the effects of stress and strain on the average person.
Screened individuals from all walks of life were thrown into the
common experience of military life and combat. The individual
reaction to this experience depended, in a large part, upon the
person's makeup and the particular kind of stresses to which he
was subjected.

Combat was found to be only one of the stresses common in
breakdowns. It can be a completely dissimilar experience under
different conditions. A man who has been on a ship doing routine
patrol, out many months without touching port, may find occasional action to be a relief from tension and boredom. On the
other hand, combat can also loom horribly, and in time everyone,
no matter how strong, will crack.

War affects men differently. It stirs up repressed tendencies
which previously exerted some influence on a man's emotional
life but by no means necessarily caused neurotic reactions. These
tendencies become intensified by the stresses of war, and adequate control is lost or weakened. Irritability becomes belligerency; mild anxiety dreams become nightmares; accustomed tension becomes unbearable anxiety with startle reaction; the latent
predisposition or vulnerability becomes a full-blown neurosis.

It is a matter, as we have said, of adaptation. Many very neurotic persons adjusted themselves adequately to the stress of war
because their neuroses fitted the situation. A relatively normal
person may succumb to neurotic illness if he finds himself unable
to adapt to a particular situation. Instances of men performing
heroically under tolerant officers and later breaking down under
rigid discipline in the rear area are numerous.

Stresses other than those resulting from (1) combat can be
roughly grouped as those arising from (2) the service itself, such
as discipline, isolation, inferior assignments, and lack of recognition; (3) relations to family, such as worries about finances,

marital faithfulness, illness, etc.; and (4) other relationships as to career, friends, etc.

In general, men whose emotional problems arise from aggression, guilt, and anxiety are more susceptible to breakdowns precipitated by combat or other forms of violence. One who severely inhibits his hostility is likely to have more fear and anxiety than those who accept freer expression of hostility. On the other hand, some individuals with too free hostility became murderously hostile and developed acute anxiety when their forces of control weakened.

The Achilles' heel of guilt was often seen by military psychiatrists, and frequently it was noted that the amount of guilt feelings was all out of proportion to the reality involved. Closer study often revealed that this self-blame (manifested by guilt) was because of wishes rather than deeds. For example, the death of a buddy in combat sometimes was followed by more than the usual amount of depression. The feeling tone often became one of extreme guilt, self-condemnation, and blame. Investigation frequently revealed that the accidental death of the buddy had gratified unconscious death wishes toward him.

Thus external stress acting upon the internal makeup and current emotional state of the individual can precipitate a neurotic reaction. The final appearance of the symptoms is further dependent upon the man's forces of control and his ability to cope with the reaction.

This can be summarized in the following outline which is by no means complete:

I. The intensity of the reaction is determined by:
   A. External factors
      1. Various stresses and combinations of stresses, such as loss of a buddy, decimation of a unit, severe damage to a ship
      2. The suddenness, violence, and duration of the situation
      3. Inability to express excitement by activity
   B. Internal factors (including current emotional state)
      1. Primitive instinctual impulses, such as excessive dependence or hostility
      2. Rigid superego, causing excessive guilt and fear of hostility

3. Weakness of the ego, with consequent lack of independence, self-reliance, and self-confidence

II. The strength of the forces of control and the individual's ability to cope with the reactions are determined by:

A. His internal makeup, such as his adaptability, strength of ego, and tolerance for anxiety and hostility

B. External factors, such as physical hardship, boredom, training, and indefiniteness; personal factors, such as understanding the reason for fighting, quality of leadership, relations with his outfit

III. Secondary reactions

Once symptoms begin to develop, the individual reactions are diverse—from minimizing the situation and hiding to complete surrender and even exaggeration

SYMPTOMS

As with other disease processes, there may be an incubation period for emotional disorders. But, unlike certain of the acute infections, there is no specific time interval between exposure to stress and the development of symptoms. It depends upon the person's makeup and current physical and emotional state, upon the kind, amount, and duration of the stresses, and upon the outlook for the future.

The symptoms of the acute neurotic reactions are of two kinds. There are those which seem to be basic to the condition and which occur in combination in practically every case. In addition, any individual may have any other symptoms known to psychiatry. Most writers (6, 17, 22, 25) agree that the basic constellation of symptoms is as follows: (1) anxiety, (2) irritability and belligerency, (3) easy fatigability, (4) startle reaction, (5) insomnia and repetitive nightmares, and (6) difficulty in concentrating. In addition to this constellation, any individual is likely to show vegetative disturbances, depression, paranoid trends, compulsiveness, schizoid reactions, and any other symptoms which he is accustomed to developing under stress of any sort.

The typical picture seen in the last war is a fighting man recently returned from combat or the front areas. His features are distorted with fear and wan with fatigue. His normal co-ordination is troubled with gross tremors, and excessive perspiration dampens his body. Even in the quiet of the rear area, his biologic mobilization for fight or flight remains. He overreacts to ordinary noises; a low-flying commercial plane sends him into a frenzied dive for shelter. The sudden ringing of a telephone may send him leaping out of his seat, followed by hysterical crying and extreme rage at himself for such an emotional display. He is alternately passive and clinging and equally aggressive and combative on slight irritation. War movies and usual civilian noises send him into a panic, so that he becomes seclusive and prefers to remain in the ward rather than take part in the rehabilitation program. Night becomes a time of terror, when every shadow threatens danger. Even the escape into sleep is hampered by insomnia, or, when sleep does come, it ends with nightmares of his horrible experiences. His waking hours are further plagued by tension, indecision, difficulty in concentrating, headaches, gastrointestinal disturbances, dizzy spells, and other psychosomatic disturbances.

DYNAMICS OF SYMPTOM FORMATION

Under stress every person reacts, as does every animal organism, with physiologic and psychologic mobilization for fight or flight. This may be felt subjectively as anger and/or fear. The fight impulses are manifested outwardly by irritability and belligerency. When they are repressed, they probably always generate anxiety and flight reactions, with all kinds of subsequent psychologic and somatic symptoms. These may include anxiety, paranoid trends, nightmares, cardiac palpitation, gastrointestinal disturbances, and numerous other physiologic disorders. When the flight impulses are expressed outwardly, they may become manifest in actual blind fleeing from the trauma or more unconscious and face-saving flight, such as malingering. When repressed, they may motivate misbehavior, produce physiologic symptoms designed for escape, or they may find expression in physiologic and psychologic regression to childish and infantile reactions. This may be expressed in eating disorders, enuresis, speech disturbances, motor inco-ordination, evasion of responsibility, and increase in passive-dependent-receptive demands.

Thus drives to fight and to flight, aggressive and regressive, may combine to produce any variety of impulses and tensions to reactivate childhood patterns and cause neurotic symptoms. Every neurosis, and possibly every neurotic symptom, is motivated in part by a combination of fight and flight impulses in various proportions. Long ago Freud stated that some day our psychologic understanding would rest on a physiologic basis. The understanding of hostile aggression and regression and their interplay is aided by the recognition of the physiology and biology of the fight-flight reaction (5, 31).

The basic constellation of symptoms appears to be a manifestation of the biologic fight-flight reaction, which is a mechanism common to all people and seen in one form or another throughout the animal kingdom (27). The differences are explained by the various individual ways of handling these reactions. These ways are the result of each individual's particular, highly personal endowment, training, and experience.

The study of war neuroses has contributed to a clearer understanding of the acute neurotic reactions and of the nature of neurosis in general. From it we can conclude that, if the emotional development of the individual is relatively complete, then his adaptability is high, his regressive tendencies are low, and his vulnerability is minimal. Susceptibility to neurosis thus appears to be a disturbance in the emotional development which causes specific vulnerabilities to stress and impairment of adaptability.

For a dynamic interpretation of his symptoms and as a basis for successful treatment, it is necesary to have an understanding of the man's personality and his emotional vulnerabilities, combined with the form and degree of regression, along with his characteristic methods of defense.

GENERAL FORMULATION

An individual's adjustment is the result of his personality makeup interacting with his environment.

1. His makeup depends upon his heredity and congenital endowment interacting with the training, experience, and emotional influences to which he is subjected, particularly during the earliest years of childhood.

2. Every individual has certain special strengths and weaknesses in his emotional makeup.

3. These depend in large part upon how fully he matures emotionally.

4. His adjustment in any given situation depends upon how well his particular makeup fits the particular situation. If the situation fits, then an infantile or neurotic personality may adjust to it better than a mature one.

5. Breakdown can be caused by internal stresses (conflicts) or

by external ones. This chapter is concerned only with the latter, that is, the acute *reactive* neuroses.

6. When the person's makeup does not fit a given situation, the stresses of the environment generate tensions. The stresses may be general, such as overexertion and consequent fatigue; but in most cases breakdown can be understood only in terms of specific stresses acting in certain ways upon the personality makeup. Every individual has specific emotional vulnerabilities, and in most cases symptoms develop when particular stresses bear upon these.

7. Under this pressure the organism reacts to the threat with the basic biologic emergency mobilization for fight or flight. Usually, neither direct fight nor flight is possible, nor is either one a solution of the intolerable situation. Tendencies to fight and to flee must then be repressed, and they then interact to cause symptoms. The tendency to fight generally brings about powerful conscience reactions, with guilt and anxiety.

8. Psychologic regression is one form of flight. The combination of repressed impulses to fight and to flee, along with the conscience reaction and regression, give the typical picture of combat or operational fatigue—anxiety, irritability, startle reaction, catastrophic nightmares, fatigability, and a variety of other psychologic and somatic symptoms.

9. The individual struggles consciously to control his reaction (ego control).

10. The strength of the control depends upon various general factors, such as fatigue, and upon various specific factors, both internal and external.

11. As the force of the reaction exceeds the ego's capacities for control, anxiety mounts, and the symptoms are intensified.

12. Whatever the original stresses and causes of the symptoms, once they are developed, the individual can react to them in different ways. He can continue to fight against them, or he can try to exploit them for certain purposes, such as sympathy, escape, or compensation. This is called "secondary gain."

SEQUELAE

Probably the most important complication of the acute neurotic reaction is "secondary gain": a fancied or real reward for perpetuating the illness. Theoretically, one would expect a group of symptoms precipitated by a specific stress to subside, once the stress had ceased to exist. But in every illness there is a tendency to exploit it for ulterior purposes to justify dependence on others, tyrannizing over them, and so on. Commonly this is to secure compensation. This wish is not usually a primary cause of the illness but a secondary utilization of it. It can be a very powerful motivation, however, and a long-lasting one, as is only too well known to the Veterans Administration and insurance companies, as well as to others. The secondary gain can prolong a psychologic regression from which the individual may never recover. This must be sharply distinguished from neurotic symptoms which persist for the primary reason that a man's balance of emotional forces has been upset and equilibrium never regained—for example, where so much hostility or guilt has been aroused that they are not again adequately repressed.

DIAGNOSIS

Usually there is no difficulty in the diagnosis of the acute neurotic reaction. One can see the stress and the individual's reaction to it. Sometimes, however, it may not be simply an acute reaction but a reactivation of a latent psychosis brought on by the stress. Usually, careful observation and the working-out of the major dynamics will reveal the true condition.

It is necessary to work out, so far as possible, the full dynamics—the patient's personality structure and major psychodynamics as they were prior to the stress and the effects of the stress upon these. It is then often found that the obvious and apparent stress was by no means the one that caused the break, but rather something quite unexpected. For example, classical war neuroses were sometimes precipitated in returning combat veterans without previous symptomatology, when they discovered evidence of infidelity, heard of the wife's pregnancy, family and financial difficulties, death of a relative or friend, and other disturbing situations.

It is well to watch for a concurrence of organic disease and psychological difficulties. Frequently, a wound was accepted with equanimity because it served as an escape from the immediate stress of combat. Soldiers were known to hope and pray secretly for a wound which would serve to initiate evacuation without loss of face. Malaria and other diseases also acted similarly and no doubt helped materially to decrease the number of psychiatric casualties by giving a rest from stress before the controls of the individual were weakened.

The syndrome "blast concussion" (20) underwent a period of popularity in the Pacific, like "shell shock" in World War I, before it was recognized to be largely psychogenic in origin. Fighting men, subjected to a near-by blast, suffered a short period of unconsciousness and, upon reviving, found their controls to be almost completely lost. The symptoms varied from regression to infantile helplessness (flight) to maniacal outbursts of completely undirected rage (fight). After a few days the patient would suddenly "awake" with a complete amnesia for all his dissociated behavior. Investigation with sodium amytal or hypnosis usually revealed the amnesia to be psychogenic and the process an acute neurotic reaction (traumatic neurosis) having the same dynamics as discussed above.

An invaluable instrument for diagnosis is dream interpretation. The dream is "the royal road to the unconscious" (9) and usually leads directly to the central theme of the acute neurotic reaction. Accurate dream interpretation, however, requires a knowledge of dynamics and special training.

DREAMS

In acute neurotic reactions the dreams are typically repetitive catastrophic nightmares, which represent the traumatic scene. In war, with so many traumatic experiences, the repetitive scene is usually the one that precipitated the breakdown. The nightmares show the fixation to the trauma and the individual's attempt to digest it. *These dreams, which may persist indefinitely are analyzable in exactly the same fashion as any other dreams*

A common feature is violence usually directed against the individual but also very often or regularly against others. This violence, upon analysis, is always found to spring from the man himself. It is usually the expression in his dreams of his attempted defense by fight or flight. Often it represents mobilized hostility It usually shows a conscience reaction aroused by the trauma For example, a 21-month-old child was painfully injured on the leg by a falling object. That night he apparently had nightmares whenever he fell asleep. His serene features would become distorted with fear, and his arms and legs would flex. Wakened by the pain from the movement of the injured limb, he would immediately slap his father, who was trying to comfort him. One could suspect that the child was reliving the trauma repetitively in an attempt to digest it. However, his aggressive behavior o awakening is suggestive of a mobilized fight reaction as a consequence of the trauma.

Persistence of traumatic neuroses and of the nightmares signifies a failure of psychological digestion—a failure of adaptation. The reason for this failure to overcome trauma can usually be found from the dream itself in the following way: Although the nightmare typically represents the traumatic scene with great accuracy, yet some detail is usually altered. Why the individual alters this detail nearly always gives the clue to his emotional vulnerabilities and to what keeps the neurotic reaction going.

For example (28), an anxious Marine, exhausted, underweight, and jaundiced by many attacks of malaria, had become too tense to carry on. He had extensive combat service and gave a good account of himself in hand-to-hand fighting. In telling his life-story he revealed nothing which cast much light on the severity of his condition. He had a repetitive nightmare. He was in a fox-hole, and the enemy were coming at him. He reached for his rifle, but it was gone. He reached for his revolver; it was gone. He reached for his knife, but it, too, was missing. He was in a panic because he had nothing to fight with.

The dream repeated a battle scene exactly, except for the detail that the patient in reality never was caught without a weapon. The central theme of the dream is being attacked and not having weapons with which to fight. When asked to talk about this detail which differed from the reality, he revealed further facts about himself. In school he was a fine athlete. He had an athletic scholarship to a large university and an offer from a big-league baseball club. His heart was set on an athletic career, and now all his hopes were dashed by malaria. Twenty-five pounds underweight, periodically racked by chills and fever, he saw his career shattered. Without his athletic prowess he felt defenseless, and now he was reminded of the dream. He started with sudden emotion. With a burst of insight, he saw that in the dream, while asleep and off-guard, he had repeated the anxiety which tormented him *now*. As he slept and felt anxiety, rather than facing its true source, in his shattered health, career, and security, he attached it to past danger, which was no longer real.

Another Marine (28) with typical combat fatigue symptoms dreamed repeatedly of making a landing where a large number of his companions were killed, including two buddies. The dream ended with the patient himself being caught in machine-gun fire. Except for this ending, the dream repeated in minute detail the invasion scene, which, in reality, left the patient unscathed. By dreaming of being caught in machine-gun fire, this man made the scene even more terrible than the reality. A dream of killing and being killed is certainly likely to represent hostile feelings toward those who are killed, and guilt can be so great that one feels that he deserves to be killed in turn. The patient admitted that, in reality, he did wish to be killed himself, and the reason for this was that he felt so terrible about his dead buddies.

Further investigation revealed that the patient had never been at ease in his relations with people as a result of early maternal overprotection and impaired masculine freedom and security. Because of feelings of insecurity about his background, he felt uneasy and not accepted by the above-average people with whom he desired to associate. The same pattern carried over into military service, where he did not achieve the promotions he desired. He felt inferior to his buddies. This heightened his resentment, and he developed an intense underlying hostility toward his friends which he kept concealed even from himself because of his need for recognition by them. When the buddies were killed, this satisfied his unconscious hostility toward them. However, the unconscious guilt over this was overwhelming and precipitated his breakdown.

The endings of dreams are of special importance. The dream is an expression of the dreamer's feelings. Because the feelings are conflictful, the scenes are usually distorted. The ending of the dream tells something of the outcome of the patient's conflicting feelings and the kind of solution he seeks for his emotional problems.

PROGNOSIS

The prognosis in the acute reactive neuroses is dependent on the following factors: (1) the previous emotional makeup, (2) degree of disruption of the balance of emotional forces, (3) extent of the regression, (4) promptness and adequacy of treatment, (5) secondary gain, and (6) present life-situation and future prospects.

The personality structure of the individual, with his aggressions, guilt, dependency, narcissistic needs, and other instinctual demands, and *how he handles them* in relating to reality contain the essence of the neurotic predisposition. The closer the individual was to emotional maturity prior to his illness, the better is his prognosis with rapid and accurate treatment. Individuals with low adaptability, marked regressive tendencies, and many vulnerabilities have, on the other hand, a relatively poor prognosis. The man with marked passive-dependent needs who finds gratification in his illness has little stimulus to get well. Even he often gets a therapeutic push from the hurt masculine pride which rebels at the dependency.

Frequently, people who have been able to emancipate themselves from dependency on the parents and to establish a mature independent existence will regress to childhood dependence under stress. The extent of this regression is prognostically important. It depends on the force of the trauma, the stability of his maturity, and, again, the gratification found in the regression. Long years of childhood leave a taste for carefree dependence in all of us. If a person, new to the pleasures of independence, is traumatically forced into a regression, he may never again find the confidence to leave the security of his reawakened childhood patterns.

The rapidity with which accurate treatment is instituted is also important prognostically. Men often failed to seek help because of the hurt pride involved in having a psychiatric disability and carried on in spite of severe subjective suffering. Finally, as the process progressed and they became less and less effective, they were turned in by their superiors. Many of these were found to be quite refractory to any psychotherapy. Also, the slowness of evacuation or the large number of casualties because of military exigencies often allowed weeks to go by before skilled psychiatric help was available. By that time the complications of secondary gain had set in, and this handicapped any short-term therapy. The shortage of skilled psychiatrists in the last war was another major factor in preventing rapid, accurate treatment of the acute neurotic reactions. These factors, plus many others, served to allow and to encourage regressions in these reactions. The delay in treatment allowed both conscious and unconscious recognition of the secondary gain involved and precluded any real desire on the part of the man to get well, lest he be returned to the precipitating trauma.

PROPHYLAXIS

An excellent study by Appel and Beebe (3) involving an epidemiologic approach to prevention of the acute neurotic reactions was incorporated into the Army procedure prior to termination of the war in Europe. The senior author made a first-hand study of psychiatric casualties in Europe and concluded that practically all men in rifle battalions who are not otherwise disabled ultimately become psychiatric casualties. The average point at which the break came was from 200 to 240 aggregate combat days. The study indicated that a man reached his effective peak in 90 days and suffered a gradual fall of efficiency from then on.

It was believed that proper incentive was an important prophylactic measure, and specific measures were recommended to encourage proper motivation. It was suggested that a specific limit be set to the number of combat days, that more appropriate awards for achievement be given, that the method of evacuation screening be improved so that men still able to perform in combat would not be lost through evacuation and that the replacement system be improved so that only men trained for combat be sent in as replacements. Further suggestions included morale and emotional training, with added emphasis on independent thinking under combat situations. The importance of adequate leadership was also emphasized, especially along lines of proper maturity and attitudes, of the leaders.

The authors state that psychiatric casualties represented the result of particularly heavy enemy opposition, incompetent unit commanders, deficiencies in supply, improper training, and untoward morale influences. Similar conclusions were reached by other psychiatrists who were concerned with these problems (14). Long-range prophylaxis can aim to develop a nation of individuals with high adaptability, low regressive tendencies, and a minimum of emotional vulnerabilities. This can be achieved through the proper rearing of children emotionally so that they reach full emotional maturity.

TREATMENT

The basis of treatment of these conditions is the same as for any neurotic condition. This can be expressed in three words—

understand the person. This means that one must understand the patient's emotional makeup, the stresses acting upon it, and his reactions to these stresses. With these understood, a therapeutic plan can be outlined.

The treatment of the acute neurotic reaction depends on the stage in which it is first observed and the nature and intensity of the reaction. The procedure of Grinker and Spiegel (13) was first to remove the patient from the immediate battle area. Then sodium amytal was administered, under which the patient relived with intense emotion the traumatic events. This time, however, it was only in fantasy, as he was actually in a safe place and, most important of all, he had the support and understanding of the physician. Interpretation was used where it was indicated. These authors used narcosynthesis as an adjunct, their treatment being based on psychodynamic understanding.

In the subacute stage, treatment depends chiefly upon judicious insight therapy. Interpretation, however, must be accurate. This means understanding, so far as possible, the patient's emotional makeup, his vulnerable points, and the effects of trauma on these. *The core of the emotional dynamics must be hit, since the main therapeutic objective is to help the man to understand his problem and to help himself.*

Dramatic effects can often be achieved in one to three interviews. The insight gained continues to operate for many months to come. A man's progress may even continue beyond his pre-illness adjustment. If the central theme is clearly delineated, then this insight may be enough to start him on his way out.

The therapeutic effect is largely due to the fact that a mysterious affliction is suddenly turned into an understandable problem. The terror of an unknown illness with the stigma "mental," "NP," or "psycho" turns into an understandable emotional problem that can be dealt with. The patient sees a solution if he will shift his emotional attitudes. He uses this insight for weeks and months thereafter. This can be supported by infrequent short interviews in the ensuing months. This "working-through" period is important. The insight gained must be worked over, in order to be consolidated, to insure the gains in the shift toward maturity in attitudes and satisfactory adjustment to life.

It would seem that the longer the neurotic reaction persists, the closer it comes to expressing current typical neurotic problems. The treatment then approximates the usual psychotherapeutic handling.

A great variety of accessory methods of treatment has been tried. Reference has been made to the use of dummies for the abreaction of rage (17). Prolonged sleep, electric shock, group psychotherapy, repeated sodium amytal interviews, insulin subshock, supportive therapy with rest, quiet, and diversion have all been used (for detailed discussion see Grinker and Spiegel, 10). Many of these are of great help in individual cases. Fundamentally, however, it is a neurotic reaction which is being treated, and the same basic type of accurate understanding and psychological treatment is required as for any other neurotic condition.

BIBLIOGRAPHY

1. ADLER, ALEXANDRA. "Neuropsychiatric Complications in Victims of Boston's Coconut Grove Disaster," *J.A.M.A.*, 123:1098, 1943.
2. ALEXANDER, F.; FRENCH, T. M.; *et al. Psychoanalytic Therapy* (New York: Ronald Press Co., 1946).
3. APPEL, JOHN, and BEEBE, G. W. "Preventive Psychiatry: An Epidemiologic Approach," *J.A.M.A.*, 131:1469, 1946.
4. APPEL, K., and STRECKER, E. *Psychiatry in Modern Warfare* (New York: Macmillan Co., 1945).
5. CANNON, W. B. *Bodily Changes in Pain, Hunger, Fear, and Rage* (New York: Appleton-Century, 1929).
6. DUNN, W. H. "War Neuroses," *Psychol. Bull.*, 38:497, 1941.
7. FRENCH, T. M. "Insight and Distortion in Dreams," *Internat. J. Psycho-Analysis*, 20:287, 1939.
8. FREUD, S. *Beyond the Pleasure Principle* (London: Hogarth Press, 1922).
9. FREUD, S. *A General Introduction to Psychoanalysis* (Garden City, N.Y.: Garden City Publishing Co., 1943).
10. FREUD, S. *Group Psychology and Analysis of the Ego* (London: Hogarth Press, 1922).
11. FREUD, S.; FERENCZI, S.; ABRAHAM, K.; and JONES, E. *Psychoanalysis and the War Neuroses* (Vienna: Vienna International Psychoanalytic Press, 1921).
12. GRINKER, R. R., and SPIEGEL, J. P. *Men under Stress* (Philadelphia: Blakiston Co., 1945).
13. GRINKER, R. R., and SPIEGEL, J. P. *War Neuroses in North Africa* (New York: Josiah Macy, Jr., Foundation, 1943).
14. HANSON, F. R. (ed.). *Combat Psychiatry* (Bulletin of the U.S. Army Medical Department, November, 1949).
15. HASTINGS, D. W.; WRIGHT, D. G.; and GLUECK, B. C. *Psychiatric Experiences of the Eighth Air Force* (New York: Josiah Macy, Jr., Foundation, 1944).

16. HEATH, R. G., and POWDERMAKER, F. "The Use of Ergotamine Tartrate as a Remedy for 'Battle Reaction,'" *J.A.M.A.*, 125:111, 1944.

17. JASKIN, M. "Psychodynamic Aspects of the War Neuroses," *Psychiatry*, 4:97, 1941.

18. JONES, E. "War Shock and Freud's Theory of the Neurosis," *Proc. Roy. Soc. Med.*, 1918.

19. KARDINER, A. "The Neuroses of War," *War Medicine*, Vol. 1 (March, 1941).

20. LYONS, J. W. "The Blast Concussion Syndrome," *Pacific Fleet M. News*, December, 1944.

21. MENNINGER, W. C. "Facts and Statistics of Significance for Psychiatry," *Bull Menninger Clin.*, 12:1, 1948.

22. MILLER, E., et al. *The Neuroses in War* (London and New York: Macmillan Co., 1940).

23. MURRAY, J. M. "Psychiatric Aspects of Aviation Medicine," *Psychiatry*, 7:1, 1944.

24. RADO, S. "Pathodynamics and Treatment of Traumatic War Neuroses," *Psychosom. Med.*, 4:362, 1942.

25. RAINES, G. N., and KOLB, L. C. "Combat Fatigue and War Neurosis," *U.S. Nav. M. Bull.*, 41:923 and 1299, 1943.

26. SARGENT, W., and SLATER, E. "Acute War Neuroses," *Lancet*, 2:1, 1940.

27. SAUL, L. J. *Bases of Human Behavior* (Philadelphia: J. B. Lippincott Co., 1951).

28. SAUL, L. J. *Emotional Maturity* (Philadelphia: J. B. Lippincott Co., 1947).

29. SAUL, L. J. "Psychological Factors in Combat Fatigue, with Special Reference to Hostility and the Nightmares," *Psychosom. Med.*, 7:257, 1945.

30. SCHWARTZ, L. A. "Group Psychotherapy in the War Neuroses," *Am. J. Psychiat.*, 101:498, 1945.

31. SELYE, H. "The General Adaptation Syndrome," in *Textbook of Endocrinology* (Montreal, Canada: Acta Endocrinologica, Inc., 1949).

32. SIMMEL, E. "War Neuroses," *Calcutta M.J.*, 43:269, 1946.

V

EMOTIONAL DISORDERS OF CHILDHOOD

Margaret W. Gerard, Ph.D., M.D.

A N ADEQUATE description and analysis of childhood problems and their treatment would require at least a volume. In this chapter an attempt will be made only to point out the more important general principles in respect to the kind, the cause, and the treatment of childhood problems. It is hoped that the information presented here will be sufficient to stimulate readers to follow through the sources of our knowledge of emotional disorders of children in the literature now available on this subject (see references at the end of the chapter).

Historical Notes

Just as psychoanalysis developed a dynamic approach to the study of psychic disorders in adults, so it stimulated a similar change in the study of disorders in children. Previously, childhood problems were thought to be caused by constitutional deviations, about which little more than diagnosis could be accomplished. The discovery of Breuer and Freud (21) that, in the adult hysterical neurosis, the symptoms stemmed from reactions to previous experiences stimulated a re-evaluation of the causes of childhood neuroses and behavior disorders, since they, too, are related to environment and experiences.

In the same way, Freud's recognition that the adult personality represented a stage in a developmental continuum inevitably focused the attention of investigators upon the various stages of childhood in the search for the anlage of personality characteristics or difficulties. As Freud had related adult problems to various sexual experiences in childhood, the early psychoanalysts of children tended to interpret child problems only in terms of the sexual causes found in allied adult neurosis. Much valuable information concerning childhood sexuality was thus unearthed, which gave evidence that children did pass through various stages in which pleasurable experience had erotic elements and was focused in oral, anal, and genital areas. The importance of the genital problems of the oedipal period was emphasized in the investigation of childhood neuroses (59), just as Freud's early investigations of adult neuroses were focused on the causative role of sexual difficulties of the oedipal period.

Anna Freud offered the stimulus to investigators in Vienna to analyze the symptoms of children by means of a modified technique, which she used and taught (37). Concomitantly, Melanie Klein (67) in Berlin developed a method for the treatment of childhood disorders based upon analytic theory but quite different from that of Anna Freud. Klein's method involved hypothetical interpretation of the child's play activity as symbolic expression of inner conflicts, whereas A. Freud's method approximated more closely the more empirical method of adult analysis, in which one interpreted the meaning of an act or a fantasy only after it had been made clear through further information. This information, gained in adult analysis through "free association," was collected in child analysis through play, conversation, fantasy, etc., since the child cannot and will not associate freely in the same way as an adult. Because of the difference in the two methods, the Vienna school has produced more information concerning psychic development, which one can check in observing children and from which one can understand the causes of symptoms and of deviate activities of children of various ages.[1]

From the stimulus of the work of both schools, the child-guidance movement in this country flourished and has adapted the methods of investigation and treatment to the clinic setting. The child-guidance clinics, in turn, helped to influence education, pediatrics, and parental upbringing of children, so that, although child psychoanalysis was initiated in Europe, American child psychiatry and child care are at the present time thoroughly infiltrated with psychoanalytic knowledge.

Although most of our knowledge has been gleaned from the study in a treatment situation of children of various ages and

[1]. Melanie Klein has produced theories of development which deviate markedly in major points from those which are generally accepted and which are based upon collected evidence (56). Klein's theories hypothecate the occurrence of certain psychic phenomena in the early months of a child's life. There are no methods as yet to confirm or disprove these hypotheses, but one may hope the future will bring forth evidence to determine whether or not they are valid. In the meantime, the present chapter will omit discussion of her theories and thus avoid confusion.

with various problems by psychoanalytically trained therapists, in recent years various studies involving observation of infants and older children in their everyday activities have added much information to previous knowledge and have modified concepts which had been formulated by the recapitulation from memories of the early years of older children and of adults (3, 38, 39, 47, 61, 84, 89). These studies have been particularly valuable in elaborating our accurate knowledge of the environmental and constitutional influences which are responsible for the child's choice of methods of adjustment (ego mechanisms) to the variety of life-problems which he must solve at various stages in his development. The kind and quality of these early problems and the early methods of their solution form the groundwork for the beginning of childhood psychic difficulties and determine in part the constellation of adult character and its aberrations. In other words, studies of the child have aided in explaining the child and also in explaining the adult: the reverse of the original situation in which the child was described and explained by information gained through the childhood traces found in the adult. Both methods have yielded valuable results and check each other for accuracy in timing developmental events and in evaluating the importance in character formation of the quality and quantity of any one experience or of any one constitutional factor.

ETIOLOGY

When we speak of psychic disorders in childhood, be they classified as behavior problems, neuroses, or autonomic symptoms, we are concerned in general with the disorders in adaptation to the environment in which the child finds himself. For this reason, some behavior may be considered abnormal in one environment and not in another. Anthropological studies have exposed these differences as they occur from one culture to another. Similar differences occur within a culture from one social group to another and are superficially evident in differences in manners, sexual behavior, and so forth. In even greater degree, differences occur from one age to another. What may be a serious symptom in an adult may represent normal behavior for a two-year-old and only questionable behavior for a five-year-old, as, for example, nocturnal bed wetting, temper outbursts when thwarted, fantastic lying, genital exposure. It is obvious that consideration of a disorder must always be undertaken in view of the expected or "normal" behavior of a child at the age of occurrence and with recognition that environmental demands and expectation change with the age of any child. The environment to which the child must conform not only varies from child to child but from age to age.

In chapter iv there is a discussion of the role played in personality development by the conflict between instinctual drives and environmental demands, between instinctual drives and superego standards, and between opposing instincts. When methods of solving conflicts are reached which satisfy instinctual needs, environmental expectations, and superego demands, successful and healthy adjustment follows. Symptoms, on the contrary, represent methods of solving conflicts which are unsatisfactory, because the methods do not sufficiently satisfy either the instinctual needs or the rules of social behavior or both. Any disorder, then, may be considered as evidence that the process of "structuralization" of the personality has deviated from the "norm" or from the expectancy for the particular age, to such an extent that the purpose of adaptation is only partially realized, and thus the functioning of the individual is handicapped.

These deviations are due to a variety of causes, which may operate at any or all stages of development. In chapter iv, it is pointed out that development occurs as "the interaction between the maturational processes and environmental influences." In the discussion of the development and treatment of any abnormal condition, one must consider the role which each element plays in its creation. Both the conditions of maturation and the environmental situations are changing from time to time. Yet there are certain relative constants which form the framework around which these changes occur.

One of these constants is the constitutional inheritance of the child. In 1932, Freud (42, p. 296) stated: ". . . we are not as yet able to distinguish between what is rigidly fixed by biological laws and what is subject to change or shifting under the influence of accidental experience." And our methods of measurement are still not sufficiently refined to differentiate accurately between a constitutional element in the production of a symptom and the modification of an inherited factor by environmental influences. However, certain basic capacities and defects are generally believed to be inherent in the individual's endowment and to influence the direction of development. Intellectual capacity—at least taken in extremes of superiority and defect—body-build, and talents of special artistic or creative superiority are generally accepted as inherited and determined by genetic patterns.

Probably there is also a constitutional variation in an individual's capacity for ego development. The development of a "strong" or well-functioning ego and superego may be partly inherent in an innate capacity. In the same way, variations in the strength of instinctual drives between one person and another may possibly be due to constitutional differences. The strength of sexual strivings as well as of aggressive tendencies, then, will play an important role in the way in which an individual can or chooses to adjust the expression of these drives to the pressure of social demands.

On the other hand, since so many other factors enter into these formulations and since it is impossible to evaluate the constitutional elements involved, practical analysis of symptom formation in this chapter will assume that variations in innate ego capacity and strength of instinct may be possible, if not probable, but are too problematic to discuss dynamically.

Of less constancy than the constitution of an individual are the personalities of the child's mother, father, and other people in his environment. Since the mother is usually the most constant individual in the child's life, particularly during the most formative years, her personality, her behavior, and her attitudes toward the child and in his presence are usually the important influences in the infant's choice of modes of impulse (instinct) satisfaction. In the absence of the mother, the person (or persons) who "mothers" or cares for the child's needs takes over this role. Other members of the family or home group come second in their influence upon his development. Thus, the family plays the role of interpreting to the developing child the rules which society expects him to obey, and teaches him the ways in which he can direct his energy to conform and still gain satisfaction for his needs. As each mother's personality is different from others', as each family's standards and habits are different, so does each child experience social pressure in different ways.

Besides the constitutional and family environmental factors which represent continuing influences on personality development, other accidental and less predictable influences also play important roles. Traumatic experiences, considered at first by

Breuer and Freud as the essential causes of the neuroses, no longer hold such prime position in the theories of causation, though they are still recognized as significant influences in the development and fixation of the pattern for certain neurotic constellations. Dynamically, an event becomes traumatic to the child when the ego is incapable of mastering the suffering and anxiety which the experience produces or of resolving the emotional conflicts created by it. This situation occurs either if the ego is weak and the event overpowering or if there is not sufficient help from parental persons in resolving the conflict. Therefore, the younger the child and the weaker his capacity for mastery, the more possible it will be to traumatize him and the more protection he needs to support his inadequacy.

Another factor which may determine the injury to the personality which a traumatic event may cause is the capacity of the event to revive a conflict which was inadequately solved at an earlier age. Hartmann (61, p. 15) has stated that the intensity of the castration fear in the oedipal phase is in direct proportion to the intensity of the oral deprivation felt at weaning.

As the child becomes older, the ego develops more adequate methods of mastering the anxiety produced by conflicts and of overcoming suffering. Hence events which could have been destructive to him when younger are no longer disturbing and may even aid in the production of adaptive techniques rather than symptoms. For example, separation of several days from a loved mother will usually cause anxiety and regressive symptoms in a one- or two-year-old child but will offer to a child of six or older an opportunity to discover that he can master many situations from habits which had previously seemed to depend upon the mother's presence. Instead of fear and regression, he gains the courage to experiment with new and even better techniques.

These more or less accidental experiences which may operate as traumas to personality development are manifold. They may occur as the result of physical illness or bodily injury; of parental losses by death or separation; of sibling births or deaths; of economic deprivation; of sexual experiences; of strong instinct temptations before the child has developed the strength to master them; of school misplacement or rejection; and so on. The way in which a child reacts to any trauma is determined by the total constellation of constitutional trend, his status of physical maturation, his integrative capacity, his previous experiences, and the type of trauma.

A final factor in the development of any symptom which must not be ignored is the influence of other symptoms and their causes which have occurred in earlier stages of development and remain as facets of the personality constellation. New symptom habits which form to meet new problems are superimposed upon old habits, the pattern of which remains interwoven with the new. Thus new symptoms partake of old symptoms, just as new skills are aided or handicapped by old skills or ineptitudes.

In childhood disorders, as in those of adults, in no instance will one cause be found for one neurotic symptom; but acting together in the production of neurotic illness are constitutional and environmental factors, degree of maturation, and previous symptoms and traumata.

Problems of the "Oral" Period (Early Infancy)

As was discussed in chapter iv, in each phase of development the individual must solve conflicts specific for that phase, such as weaning and temporary separation from the mother in the oral phase; excretory and motor control in the anal phase; rivalry and genital fears in the oedipal phase; and so on. Only when the solutions are not adequate for self-expression and not satisfactory to meet the environmental demands do problems develop which cause the internal stress of neuroses or the external conflict of behavior difficulties. Emotional difficulties, therefore, may be differentiated according to age, as more or less inherent in the problem solving of each of the ages.

Investigations in recent years have enriched our knowledge of the importance of the early months of life in normal and abnormal personality development. Studies in the direct observation of babies under various conditions have accumulated data correlating the reaction of the infant to the type of care, or lack of it, he receives. Theoretical conclusions from the findings have added greatly to our previous understanding which had been gleaned from recapitulation in the psychoanalysis of adults.

O. Rank (82) emphasized the influence of the traumatic experience of birth upon the developing infant. Recently, speculations concerning the effect of prenatal experiences upon the postnatal personality carry the concept of environmental influence even further back and offer interesting modifications to our theories (57). Some confirmation that prenatal effects may occur was offered in a study by Sontag (85), in which correlations were found between excessive hyperactivity of the newborn (crying, sleeplessness, regurgitation, etc.) and maternal emotional stress during pregnancy, as well as between infant serenity and a normal contented pregnancy. Since it has been shown that reactions at each age are dependent in part upon the status of personality development which has grown out of reactions to previous experiences, these studies suggest that the infant probably enters the world with constitutional trends already modified by the impingement of the environment upon him while he was still in utero. In any case, there is much evidence that occurrences in the early postnatal months are very important in forming the basic patterns of reaction within which all later changes take form. It is within the security of the mother-child "symbiosis" (11) that the child's primary narcissism flourishes. Later differentiation of the concept of self from that of the mother and her breast separates love for the mother and breast from love of the self, and object love is initiated. When this "symbiotic" security is lacking, various pathological conditions develop.

Spitz (86) has shown that infants deprived of mothering in the early months of life develop a type of behavior which he calls "anaclitic depression." The child is irritable to stimuli of all kinds and develops no appropriate responses to different stimuli, becomes emaciated and marasmic. If the condition is not changed within the months of the oral phase, Spitz believes the condition is irreversible and treatment impossible. Such conclusions need to be tested by further studies directed toward adequate therapy of the child who has been so deprived, which consists of educative and ego-building techniques within the framework of affectionate personal relationship, as described by B. Rank with very disturbed children (79). However, Spitz's observations (87, 88) have clearly shown how necessary is the relationship to a mother-person for the early development of the ego. It is clear that the motherless infant, he reports, lacks any signs of adaptive mechanisms and seems to have lost even the capacity for certain reflex adaptation, such as sucking, grabbing, and pushing away.

Severe disorders in later years have been traced back, in several studies, to a pathological condition of these early months. Levy (73) and Bender (9) and more recently Bowlby (20) have described children in the latency age and in adolescence with various conduct disorders in which symptoms of extreme narcissism with affective "emptiness," defects in standards, and ego inadequacy were prominent. These children were reared in institutions with only routine care and were completely deprived of mothering.

B. Rank (80) adds a similar cause for disorganized behavior in younger children who, because of severe emotional deprivation, show indications of arrest in development such that diffuse excitability follows any sensory stimulus. For these children, object relationship is primitive and associated with the production of body sensation, as skin rubbing, rocking, sucking, etc. She has been able to relieve these conditions by a therapeutic program in which the child is given a relationship to the therapist similar to that in very early development and then led forward through the various stages as they should normally have been traveled.

Besides these severe character disorders resulting from maternal deprivation, recent researches indicate that other severe disorders—psychoses and schizophrenias in particular—and many vegetative disorders (5) can usually be traced back to markedly pathological parental attitudes, exhibited in excessive neglect, cruelty, and gross inconsistency. However, perhaps in lesser degree, the farther back our information is carried in the study of the neuroses and the behavior problems, the more we find that both psychopathological conditions and adequate personality characteristics have their roots in the experiences of the first year of life and are closely related to the types of maternal behavior to which the child is exposed or to the lack, in varying degrees, of any mothering.

This is quite understandable when we consider the factors involved in ego and superego development taken in conjunction with the fact of the organism's tendency toward repetition, which is described as the "repetition compulsion," "inertia principle," or "habit formation." If the infant in the early months has no consistent pleasant stimulus from a mother who is tender and caressing and if he is not protected adequately by her from the pain of hunger, cold, skin irritations, etc., one can easily relate to the deprivation the development of symptoms of narcissistic withdrawal, poor interpersonal relationship, and inadequate social adaptive habits described by Spitz and Bender. In the absence of a mother, the child must master his feelings of discomfort alone and satisfy his needs through autistic rather than objective activity. Once initiated, these methods become fixed through repetition into habits and ego trends, so that each new difficulty is met by turning back to one's self and thus avoiding at each step the learning of new methods of adjustment through the help of a trusted person.

A cruel and inconsistent mother offers a kind of necessity for self-sufficiency in an infant. To overcome the pain and anxiety resulting from these experiences at the mother's hand, it is possible that the child must avoid the discomfort by denying reality and avoiding object contact, at the same time creating in fantasy a world closer to "his heart's content," which forms the fabric out of which schizophrenic delusions may later be formed. Or he may localize suffering in a part of his body, the organ cathexis in psychosomatic disorders; or he may ward off awareness of pain by gross defensive motor activity, as in various hostile aggressive behavior disorders. The baby is too helpless yet to develop, on his own, adequate social habits of countering cruelty or of caring for himself independently.

In recognition of the importance of a secure, reliable, and pleasant mother-child relationship for the development of a healthy personality, concepts of child rearing have veered from the spartan ritualistic routines of the early twentieth century to immediate indulgence of the child's longing for food, for holding, for rocking, for sleeping, etc. (3, 84, 91). The term "demand feeding" is an expression of this trend. If the mother is "motherly," showing tenderness and loving gentleness, such attempts to save suffering and to foster dependence in the early months of life have proved successful for the development of emotionally secure and outgoing babies, most of whom settle soon into self-imposed routines of feeding and sleeping. If demands are then made upon them slowly to postpone bodily pleasure and gradually to modify behavior according to social needs, a continuous healthy development ensues. Difficulties occur if the demand indulgence continues too long and adaptive habits are not encouraged. Enjoyment of physical pleasure then becomes the most important goal for the child, the relationship to the mother the means toward that goal; and the pleasure of object love for the mother and from her does not grow stronger. It is pleasure from such love for the mother rather than simple sensory pleasure which encourages him to postpone physical pleasure or give it up and to master his antisocial impulses, thus avoiding the mother's displeasure and increasing her affectionate behavior. Only within this framework of love, as she differentiates for him unacceptable and acceptable behavior, does he have a guide and the incentive for ego and superego development.

Unchallenged instinct gratification continuing into and beyond the training or "anal" period deprives the child of incentives for the formation of standards (superego) and of methods for behaving according to those standards (ego). It is an important cause for later symptoms in impulsive children whose lack of ego defense mechanisms exposes them to constant anxiety produced by environmental conflicts as well as by inner instinctual conflicts which they have not the skills to resolve. The condition is similar to that of a younger child to whom a too difficult task is given; the infant is unable to meet the task because of physical immaturity; the older impulsive child cannot meet the task fitted for his chronological years because of emotional immaturity.

Another discrepancy growing out of the tendency to rely upon indulging the infant as a prevention of later difficulties lies in the role played by the mother's actual love or hostility toward her child. If she loves him, her handling is likely to be tender, painless, and unfrightening; if she rejects him or is neurotically anxious about him, no amount of indulgence can prevent the handling of her child from being painful and threatening. She hurts him or frightens him by unconscious mishandling, due to various actions—the tightness of her muscles, the awkwardness of her movements, the querulousness of her voice. To aid mothers to a better relationship to their newborn infants, closer early contact with them is encouraged more and more in obstetrical hospitals, by the "rooming-in" projects, in which prenatal and postnatal education in baby care is offered (63). Such projects help in avoiding mishandling because of maternal anxieties due to strangeness or lack of knowledge and in nourishing biological maternal love in these mothers who do not have neurotic difficulties which produce defective "motherliness." Neurotic mothers, however, who reject their children either consciously or unconsciously cannot learn adequate techniques of loving care and may even reject their children more intensely if they are expected to care for the baby during the hospital period, when they long for relief from responsibility. For the babies of such mothers, neither "rooming in" nor "self-regulating feeding" will make infancy serene; only therapy for the mother to overcome her rejecting feelings for her child will answer his needs.

Since so many emotional difficulties have their beginning in disorders of the first months of life, it is important to recognize initial symptoms, that one may know when to undertake corrective measures early before the symptoms become too fixed, and also to recognize and to understand early causative factors in later disorders, even though, at first, they may seem quite unrelated. It is important also to be able to differentiate between behavior which is normal for the maturational level and that which warns of dysfunction.

Crying in the infant is the biological response to discomfort, the purpose of which is undoubtedly to cause changes which will relieve the discomfort. It presupposes a mother-child symbiosis such that she may respond to the cry. Crying is an early action in nonspecific relationship to secure someone in the environment to relieve the suffering and satisfy the infant, and only later is it directed toward a specific person, the mother. Crying, thus, is quite normal when it is a warning and stops when appropriate relief is offered, such as feeding, warmth, or other bodily need. It is also normal, and to be expected later, when the child not only cries to gain relief of discomfort but to indicate his longing for the repetition of pleasure. This occurs often when the child has enjoyed the warmth of being held, the pleasure of caressing and rocking, both for skin and muscle sensation, and later after specific object relationship to the mother has developed. The fear of loss of pleasure and comfort then develops in separation periods, and the baby cries to bring back the loved person.

It is only when crying occurs in the absence of discomfort or in the presence of the mother or when it is excessive that one may consider the crying as a problem which has symptomatic meaning. Soon after birth, it may be indicative of trauma, both psychic and physical, resulting from difficulties during birth or possibly during the intra-uterine period, leading to what one might term "anxious expectation." In most instances, with adequate care for the infant's bodily needs, this postpartum instability passes within the first or second week. When excessive crying continues, it indicates difficulties which should not be ignored. If physical pathology is ruled out, the "emotional climate" of the mother's attitude and behavior is usually found to be at fault and may result from a variety of neurotic attitudes: frank rejection of the child with roughness in handling; impatience and forced feeding; ignoring and neglecting its needs; excessive adherence to, or marked neglect of, routine. It is common knowledge that a very young infant may cry and appear irritable and uncomfortable in its mother's arms or in her presence but will quiet down almost immediately when picked up, caressed, and spoken to gently by an experienced motherly woman, even though she be strange. This is an indication that the mother's handling is causing discomfort to the child, that the cry is in response to this discomfort, and that the infant is striving for relief from the suffering rather than for the comfort of the mother's presence which occurs later. Kris (68, p. 33) names this early relationship "anaclitic" in differentiation from true "object" relationship, which develops slowly during the first months of life.

This early period is that of "primary narcissism," in which the world seems to be accepted by the child as an extended part of himself. It is understandable, then, that discomfort and pain, if not relieved, may produce intolerable anxiety, since he has not yet learned that he alone is not responsible for his safety and that pain may be relieved by another person. Unrelieved discomfort then may start a habit of expectant anxiety, in the presence of pain or suffering of any kind. Symptoms which develop to allay this anxiety are varied. Excessive crying has been mentioned. Autistic pleasures, such as thumbsucking, head rolling, rocking, rubbing, and so forth, are very common, as if the child tries to distract attention from pain by an excess of pleasure. The danger to normal development when excessive indulgence in autistic pleasure occurs is found in the realm of object relationship and of social adaptation. Such infants grow into children and adults who turn back to themselves at the slightest frustration and difficulty; burden themselves with the task of handling life's problems alone; distrust others; are constantly anxious, with many symptoms and with restricted pleasures and restricted realms of activities.

To prevent the development of such a state, one can recognize the value of the excessive indulgence of the young infant, mentioned above, which has been in vogue for the last few years, coining the term "demand" schedule or "self-regulating" schedule to mean feeding, sleeping, caressing at the first sign of wish from the infant. A cry, then, is an "alert" to the mother to busy herself in satisfying her baby's wishes or needs. This present-day change in infant care is in direct contrast to the previous rigid schedules of almost ritualistic routine, in which the child was expected to "cry it out" and continue to fight off his discomforts until the moment arrived for his feeding or play period or other pleasure.

This change in procedure is sound certainly for the first three or four months of life. Like so many partial truths, however, it has become accepted by many physicians and parents as an essential preventive measure for later ills. To relieve early anxiety and thus to prevent severe trauma to a sensitive organism, avoidance of discomfort is essential, and the serene and healthy development of most "demand" babies substantiates the value of it. On the other hand, it is certainly not a "prevent-all," as one can recognize by the fifth or sixth or later month when the baby, now differentiating itself from his mother, is influenced by many subtle situations in this relationship. The "climate" or atmosphere produced by the mother's attitudes, in her affection, her rejection, her anxieties, her distractibilities, or even her absences becomes as essential in producing or relieving anxiety as body discomfort or its relief had been previously.

Since eating is one of the essential activities in infancy, there is need for warning that discomfort in this sphere is the most common cause of crying. However, other symptoms of feeding difficulties begin to arise early and are forewarnings of more difficult problems to come if relief is not forthcoming. The most common early symptoms are food refusal and vomiting. In both instances, if the child is physically well, the symptoms represent defense mechanisms against feeding discomfort (36). Such avoidance of an instinctual pleasure surely indicates suffering of intensity. Roughness of a mother, forced feeding beyond satiety, or too fast feeding may cause conflict between the wish for pleasure in eating and the wish to avoid suffering, in which the latter often wins out. Only by alleviating the environmental cause of the conflict—the mishandling of the child—can the symptom be resolved.

If the symptom has become fixed through automatic repetition and the mishandling occurs at the hand of the mother who cares for the child, the dawning object relationship to her becomes associated with the symptom. In such cases the first object love is ambivalent. The negative side shows up in hostility provoked by discomfort at feeding and by the consequent narcissistic suffering involved in self-denial of the satisfaction of eating. The reactive and defensive nature of this hostility becomes evident when one observes and treats such an infant. If treated in the first few months of life by substituting for the mother (or nurse) at feeding times a nursing person who is relaxed and gentle, sensitive to the baby's indications of sufficiency, one who holds him caressingly and speaks or sings gently, the symptom seems to disappear like melting ice.

As an example, a baby boy of six months entered the children's ward of a hospital with the tentative diagnosis of pylorospasm for the consideration of surgery. Since the diagnosis could not be confirmed with x-rays, the pediatrician suggested further observation on the ward in a warm emotional climate. The baby did not vomit after admission, ate and slept well, and gained weight until normal for age. He has continued well since return home under the mother's care, who, during the child's hospitalization, was given some psychotherapeutic insight into the child's conflicts and into her own attitudes and behavior which produced them and has received continued supportive and advisory aid from a social worker. The symptoms in this case were arrested during their developmental stage before fixation into a habitual defense occurred and before true object love or hostility toward the mother was well established and before the anxious attitude toward the mother who forced the food was generalized into an anxious attitude toward all people. One may hope that the early correction of this pathology may prevent further feeding difficulties.

In some instances, vomiting may occur initially as a physiological reaction to a disturbed organic condition, such as pyloric stenosis or other obstructive conditions, allergic sensitiveness to certain foods, and the like. If the organic condition is allowed to continue for months, so that vomiting is the usual sequence to food intake, an infant protects himself from the experienced discomfort by refusal to eat at all or to eat more than a minimal amount. Even if the organic condition is relieved later, an anxious expectation may be maintained and feeding continue to be invested with anxiety. This pattern of reaction to feeding and its associated experiences as to a danger is similar to the pattern produced by the rejecting mother already described. In both instances, if the baby is still within the first year of age, prevention of later neurosis with food symptoms or various symptoms derived from the "intaking" process is possible. In the one instance, correction of the organic condition must be accompanied by sensitive care in feeding, such that the child is allowed to eat at his own speed, with his own measure of quantity, and with accompanying pleasurable experience, such as tender words and caresses. In the second, similar feeding care by a motherly person may relax the baby sufficiently that the neurotic pattern is given up in favor of acceptance of food, a pattern more fitting to the "corrected" experience. Rarely does this approach fail in the early months. However, if symptoms persist in spite of physical therapy and convincingly adequate environmental change, the neurosis probably has already become integrated into the developing personality. In this case continued alertness must be used to avoid further trauma and to maintain pleasant feeding conditions. Psychotherapy may later be necessary to resolve the conflicts producing the neurotic attitude.

Thumbsucking, previously so offensive to many mothers, has become respectable in recent years. Levy's (70, 71) study of the relation between thumbsucking in infants and the length of the interval between feedings led him to conclude that sucking in itself represented a pleasure entity for which the infant strove. If insufficient satisfaction was obtained in the feeding periods, the child sucked at other times, fingers, lips, tongue, etc. The fact that babies on four-hour schedules sucked their thumbs or fingers almost universally and that those fed more frequently or whenever restless did not seek accessory sucking, he explained as due to a sucking need. This confirms Freud's description of the mouth as an erotic zone.

One does not question that stimulation of the lip and mouth mucous membrane is associated with pleasure. For the infant, it is undoubtedly the area where most pleasure is obtained, although recent studies indicate the importance of skin, muscle, and joint sensations as essential in the production of satiety reactions of the infant. Certainly, the infant may suck his thumb if he experiences insufficient pleasure in sucking at feeding. However, he sucks his thumb also for substitute pleasure when other pleasures are lacking or for solace when anxious if alone and separated from a loved person, or when actually in pain. The author has seen an eight-month-old infant, previously not a thumbsucker, suck his thumb so violently that it was cut by his teeth when he was suffering intense pain from an acute appendicitis. Following the operation, he returned to his nonthumbsucking status and did not resume the habit. Extra-feeding sucking, thus, may not always be a benign autoerotic indulgence but may be a warning that all is not well and that the child is attempting to allay the distress of undesirable experiences. The admonition so common nowadays, to let the child suck his thumb as much as he seems to wish, is certainly wise in helping a mother to overcome her own fears that sucking is evil, but if the baby is no longer a small infant and still using thumbsucking as the only pleasure in waking life, one would be as remiss to omit searching for dissatisfactions in his life which encourage the habit as to ignore vomiting or other obvious symptoms. The solution is not to let the habit continue late into latency any more than to prevent it forcefully, but to correct the cause.

Sleep disturbance often observed in early infancy is rarely or perhaps never an isolated symptom. As in later years and in adulthood, it is an indication of anxiety. The anxiousness may be from physical pain, and then sleeplessness is usually accompanied by crying; or the child may be sleepless or an excessively light sleeper because he is on his guard against an environment which has been made frightening by a neglectful, cruel, or rejecting parent. Later, sleep disturbances may be more severe or be accompanied with terrifying dreams because the dangers have been internalized. But, in general, they have their beginnings in anxious insecurity of these early months. Hence it is important to attempt to unearth the causes for the restlessness early and to relieve them before the symptom becomes habitual in order that internalization of the danger may be prevented.

PROBLEMS OF THE "ANAL" OR TRAINING PERIOD
(LATE INFANCY)

The influence of experiences in infancy upon the development of the "normal" personality and upon the kind and character of later disorders has been discussed. The child's reaction to bowel training will in part depend upon his reactions to people, especially the mother or nurse, which have become habitual in infancy. Symptoms developing in the anal period will partake of elements of symptoms which developed out of oral problems.

As the months bring maturation of the neuromuscular system, such that the anal and urethral sphincters can be voluntarily controlled, the anal phase is ushered in. At the same time, purposive activity of the skeletal muscles becomes gradually more co-ordinated into grasping, pushing, crawling, and walking. Therefore, not only is the child asked to control his excretory activities at the mother's behest, but self-expression in all aggressive[2] activity is encouraged or prohibited, as the child is taught

2. "Aggressive" is used here to mean "physically active" rather than hostile destructive aggression as is the frequent connotation in psychoanalytic literature in which aggression is used as a direct translation from the German (62).

not to touch dangerous objects or to break precious ones and to walk and crawl in circumscribed areas for his own protection.

The emotional conflicts which develop in the anal period are inherent in the prohibition and direction of the child's excretory and muscular activity which the parent as the surrogate of society imposes.

If the object relation to the mother is a pleasurable loving one, the child easily solves the conflict between his instinctual wish for free self-expression and his dependent wish for his mother's love, by modifying his activity according to the mother's demand. He defecates on the toilet and, later, urinates there instead of on the spot where the urge arises. Also, gradually he controls his grasping, walking, and other actions to accord with the permission of the mother. This is the first sign of ego development, and it represents a part of the ego described by Hartmann as "nonconflictual" (60). It is concerned with the development of adaptive skills rather than with defense against instinctual drives. The heightened pleasure which the child feels in response to his loved mother's approval of his action makes the choice of substitute outlets fairly easy. His wish to avoid her disapproval intensifies the wish to conform.

However, if the relationship to the mother has not been satisfactory either because of neglect, which intensified the need for narcissistic autistic pleasures, or because of suffering at the mother's hand, which transformed normal self-preservative aggressiveness into hostile destructive aggression toward the mother, added problems may begin to show in this training period. Negativism and stubbornness against suggestion and direction are common. The so-called "temper tantrum" becomes a reaction at each point of minor or major frustration, and the need to maintain one's will seems to be the child's concept of maintaining his integrity. He may remain incontinent and stubbornly refuse to be trained. This incontinence may be preceded by constipation, by which the child refuses to part with the product of his body until forced by physiologic bowel reflex. Playing with the stool and smearing is a common sequela in these children, who not only express hostility and rage against the unloving or severe parent by refusal to conform but actually attack with the "dirty" feces. The excreta thus become invested with value as a personal creation which affords power to ward off danger and also become an instrument of attack against the love object who has become ambivalently hated.

Less common, but sometimes beginning in this early training period, is the attempt at solution of the feared dangers by an excessive conforming obedience, in contradistinction to the aggressive temper and stubbornness. This occurs usually when the positive arm of the ambivalence toward the parent outweighs the negative hostility. The wish to maintain the love fosters conformity, but, to overcome the ever resurging hostile element of the ambivalence, the nascent ego strengthens the process of conformity so that the child may ritualize toilet activities, aggressive play, dressing, and all the other routines of life. Then, like a full-blown adult compulsion neurotic, he becomes anxious and upset if the ritual is disturbed.

In this training period one observes a dawning conscience or superego. The child with a loving dependent relation to his mother begins to differentiate "right" and "wrong" according to the mother's designation of acceptance or disapproval of his behavior. He usually can conform in the parents' presence and occasionally when alone. It has been suggested that the parent and his standards have not been truly integrated into the child's personality at this tender age, but ease of hallucinatory experiences due to his lack, as yet, of adequately differentiating reality from fantasy, brings the mother's image to him to aid in controlling his action. In those children showing exaggerated compulsive conformity, the superego seems to have a true, if precocious, existence, and in many instances the child behaves as if these standards of behavior were a separate part of himself, the parent introjected but not yet integrated. A fairly typical example of this condition was exhibited by John, a boy of twenty-six months about whom the author was consulted. He was an only child of successful parents, both of whom were perfectionistic, fairly rigid, serious persons, who believed that, with consistent discipline, one could train a child early and well. In general, John was a very obedient, friendly, serious, and undernourished child, who had been somewhat of a feeding problem from the time of the introduction of semisolid food, when he began to be fussy about the new foods and spit them out when they were forced into his mouth. He was trained for bowel control by seven months and for day wetting by ten months; he was overly clean, insisting upon hand washing with even small amounts of soiling, and had begun to be anxious at bedtime if his toys were not in a particular arrangement which he had contrived. I visited him in his own home, and, at first, he did not know anyone was there when from the hall I observed him in the family living-room where small breakable objects were placed on a low coffee table. He started to reach with his right hand for a glass dish—drew back, reached again—drew back, reached again several times until, finally, with a quick grab he picked up the dish and crashed it to the floor. He looked startled, began to cry, then with his left hand he slapped his right hand very hard, saying "Bad Johnny! Bad Johnny!"

This self-punishment indicated a precocious conscience which denied misbehavior, but a weak ego which could not control impulsive behavior. The solution then was a compromise which demanded punishment for the unacceptable act. Most children in these years can avoid disobedience when in the presence of the disciplinarian but show no sign of compunction when alone. It is as if the presence of the loved, training adult acted as both the ego and the superego. This indicates that the child as yet had not accepted as his own the standards and behavior demanded by the parents; or, in psychodynamic terms, there was a minimal internalization of the parental commands to form the superego or conscience. When the training has been too severe and too rigid for the child's maturational level, as occurred in Johnny's case, the fear of punishment and of loss of love produces control of impulsive behavior by inhibiting and punishing it before skills can be developed to express the wishes in substitute or sublimated activities. Punitive control at this stage initiates ritualistic regulation of sufficient strength for nascent compulsive symptoms, such as excessive cleanliness, orderliness, and routinization of play and toy arrangements. If the routinization is disturbed, anxiety symptoms—crying, muscle tenseness, and other symptoms—appear and indicate the fearful need for self-control which the parent has created in the infant.

Sleeping difficulties (18, 31) are not very common at this age, but they appear quite frequently in markedly conforming children. These children exhibit fear of going to bed and of being left alone and frequent wakeful crying during the night. Sometimes true night terrors occur, with dreams of injury, particularly from animals—bears and lions or tigers which eat or squeeze them. In sleep, the child is away from the protection of parental admonition, and impulses are uncontrolled by reality reminders. The superego, even though precocious, is too weak to function entirely alone, and fear that misbehavior can break through in sleep creates wakefulness or clinging to the parents in order to guard against sleep temptations. Punishment dangers then appear in the hallucinatory dream creation when sleep is yielded to.

The integration of symptoms carried over from maladjustment in the oral-dependent phase into training-period symptoms may determine the method of the resistance against training or the form of expression of hostility against the parent, or even the direction of rituals that the precocious superego takes for controlling impulses. The mouth and eating then become the areas of hostility, with malicious biting of the mother or substitute figures and objects, even biting, chewing, and swallowing toys, blankets, clothes, and all manner of objects. Feces may be eaten at this time, an indication that the continued and exaggerated investment in oral pleasure has become fused with the narcissistic meaning of the feces, the child's first "creative" production. In eating his stool, the child integrates several pleasures: eating, defying the mother whose disgust he stubbornly resists, keeping by ingestion his creative product for himself, avoiding the sense of loss which all children feel at first in the training period when they must comply with bowel control, but which deprived and severely controlled children feel severely.

A symptom one sees occasionally is interesting because it integrates eating, associated nursing movements, destructiveness, and self-punishment, that is, the twisting of hair clumps (associated with nursing), pulling the hair out (destructive and painful), chewing and swallowing it (eating). If this symptom becomes habitual, it continues into latency and may be the most noticeable symptom of a severe autistic compulsive neurosis.

PROBLEMS OF THE "OEDIPAL" OR SEXUAL PERIOD

The oedipal period (beginning around three and lasting roughly until six years of age) is characterized by a turning of the developing sexual impulses toward the parent of the opposite sex and by an increase in sexual curiosity. Behavior difficulties which begin at this time grow out of the child's incapacity to deal with the conflicts, both environmental and instinctual, which are created by the increase in sexual impulses. The capacity to develop acceptable methods for handling the conflicts of this period is directly related to the emotional security with which the child enters this stage. If the experiences of the dependent (oral) and training (anal) periods have been wholesome and healthy and a minimum of symptoms has developed, the child meets the new conflicts with ease and with adaptive reactions. If he has been deprived, rejected, neglected, rigidly trained, or the like, his insecurity increases the problems of adaptation. Feelings of castration fear, penis envy, inferiority, and rivalry are complicated by exaggerated rage, stubbornness, dependent longing, and greed (4, 61).

Disturbing environmental experiences occurring at this time may further complicate adequate solution of oedipal conflicts, and thus aid the causation of symptoms. The birth of a sibling which may produce dependent rivalry for the mother adds to the total rivalrous feelings created by the triangular oedipal jealousy (see chap. iv) and intensifies rivalry to neurotic proportions. If the father is unusually punitive, cruel, or, in reverse, seductive toward the child, fears and exaggerated sex feelings are intensified and problems to solve are increased. Inconsistency in training and too rigid training cause trouble for the child also, for he needs help from the parent in restricting direct expression of his instincts and in guiding their expression into acceptable methods of action. That is, he needs his parents to offer superego standards and ego training. Many other experiences, familial or extra-familial, to which the child may be exposed can add to the production of neurotic symptoms. Among those most commonly found are seductive experiences, such as introduction to fellatio or sodomy; adult genital exposures; genital tampering; primal scene exposure; cruelty from other children or adults; exposure to accidents and death; and the loss by death or long absence of a loved one, such as mother, father, sibling, nurse.

The genital sensations turn the child's interest toward the pleasure he experiences in this area. Masturbation begins often as a result of exploration and may then be repeated, from time to time, by any normal child for the autistic pleasure itself, or as a momentary solace, when lonesome, bored, or in pain. Masturbation may become excessive and take on all the characteristics of a compulsive neurotic habit. In this case, it serves the purpose of allaying anxiety which may stem from a variety of causes. Frequently the rejected or neglected child who has solved his fear of insecurity and discomfort by various infantile autistic pleasures, such as thumbsucking and fecal smearing, will turn to masturbation as a more satisfactory solace. The average mother finds it often more difficult to sanction masturbation than other autistic indulgences, but the rejecting mother is likely to be extremely incensed with the child for the act. This increased rejection intensifies his need for masturbation to relieve his fear, and as a result he stubbornly continues to indulge himself.

In other instances, compulsive masturbation may result from a fear of injury; persistent handling of the genitals is a reassurance of their intactness. This fear may result from threats of injury, which parents and nurses so frequently offer if the child is seen to handle himself, or from some traumatic experiences, such as fellatio or rough play with the child's genitals by another child or adult; or from the poor reasoning of a little boy who first sees a girl and thinks her injured; or from an expectation of retaliation from the father whom he wishes to displace in his mother's exclusive love.

A little girl also may masturbate compulsively for reassurance, but with less evidence to comfort her. She, too, becomes more interested in her genitals with increasing hormonal production. Exploration of the area discloses that she has less than her brother or little boy playmate. Repetitious compulsive handling of her genitals seeks for the missing penis. Since it is never found, excessive masturbation may continue because the pleasure offers some relief from the anxiety which arises from the feelings of inferiority and envy. As has been described previously, under healthy conditions for normal feminine development, these feelings are fleeting and are resolved in the little girl by an identification with her mother, who accepts the advantages of feminine love and maternity. Penis envy and inferiority feelings, however, may become intense and obvious symptoms in the little girl who is already disturbed in her relationship to her mother (4, 61). Insecurity which was initiated in the oral-dependent phase and continued into the training period expresses itself in the oedipal stage through an added despair of personal inadequacy. Oral envy or deprivation thus reinforces penis envy or feeling of genital incompleteness. The person she has turned to for love, that is, herself, when she was unloved or rejected by her mother, thus is believed to be an injured or imperfect person, unworthy of love. Despair develops again when her dawning sexual feelings long for love from her father. She who was unloved by her mother now finds herself unlovable, and in her childish reasoning must be completely incapable of competing for her father's love.

These feelings of unworthiness and these fears of injury may get out of bounds and lead to the exaggeration of other activities, normal for the age in mild form but presenting disturbing symptoms when intensified, as "peeping," exhibiting of genitals, "tomboy" behavior of girls, or "sissy" behavior of boys, and excessive rivalry and jealousy. These symptoms are usually part of an attempt to deny the knowledge of genital anatomy and to get reassurance that all is not as inadequate or as dangerous as experience has seemed to indicate. The peeper keeps looking and looking compulsively, after he has seen enough to know the facts, because of the persistent wish to find evidence to assure him that he is not injured or inferior. Similarly the child persistently exposes his genitals as if to say, "See, I am all right, adequate, and uninjured." But his belief to the contrary discredits reassurance, so that the act is continued again and again.

Denial of genital facts is carried even further in fantasy when the little girl insists that she has a penis, acts like a "tomboy," and refuses to accept her feminine status. The roots of later serious masculine identification are seen in her excessive aggressiveness, her competitive hostility toward boys, and even in attempts to urinate like a boy. As one little four-year-old girl confided to her therapist, "I am sure I have a 'peenie,' for I can make my 'wee wee' go straight into the toilet like Johnny does—if I stand close and pull my skin tight in front." The little boy denies his feelings of inadequacy by fantasying himself with enormous genitals to match his father's, bragging of strength and bigness, and, like the girl, expressing his fantasied exaggerated masculinity in excessive aggressiveness and competitive hostility, a forewarning of aggressive, destructive behavior problems in years to come. His denial, when fear of injury is excessive, may take the opposite form, and he fantasies himself a girl with no penis to be injured. Concomitantly, he gives up masculine aggressiveness; becomes passive, shy, and feminine, a "sissy" who is afraid of all boyish activities and prefers a feminine role. As a boy of five and one-half shyly said to his mother, as he tucked his penis between his legs, "See, mom, I look just like Mary!" When questioned further he answered, "I do it when I am afraid at night, or when Dad scolds me, or any old time."

Anxiety symptoms may begin to be excessive at this period, with repetitious nightmares and fear of the dark, of new situations, and of strange persons. Phobias with special objects to fear may arise to displace the more generalized anxiety. Anxiety is always in evidence when conflicts are not yet solved. It is, therefore, present always in one form or another during childhood, a period of continuous need for new solutions of new problems. Anxiety may become excessive in the oedipal period when circumstances historical and present make an acceptable solution impossible. The anxiety produces protection against danger of injury or punishment by creating a wariness which aids in the avoidance of dangers. This wariness may be so intense that the child becomes more and more withdrawn and autistic, with regression to thumbsucking, fecal play, and such. More common, however, is the allaying of free-floating fearfulness by the production of symptoms, which, if they offer some comfort by partial solution of the conflict or conflicts, become habitual. In latency one finds these symptoms organized and integrated into the personality as habits of living, so that the conflicts are allayed in part by repression and in part by other defense mechanisms involved in the symptom formation. Further healthy development, however, is handicapped by the fact that much energy must be expended in maintaining the symptom, energy which should be available for the development of adaptive skills, and by the fact that the symptom itself interferes with normal behavior.

These neurotic symptoms which begin to show embryonic organization in the oedipal period become obvious handicaps in the latency period. Phobias and compulsive rituals are early symptoms. Pathological motor activities, such as stammering and tics, may begin. Some autonomic symptoms commonly arise early, such as asthma, enuresis, constipation, colitis, and a variety of feeding difficulties, such as food sensitivity and aversion, neurotic vomiting, and anorexia, as well as bulimia with obesity. Indications of some unacceptable behavior symptoms are often found at this time, such as sadistic cruelty and masochistic submission, uncontrollable stealing and lying, insatiable demanding with concomitant selfishness.

Problems of the "Latency" Period

The term "latency," originally used to delineate those years between the sexual period of the oedipal phase and the sexual maturation of adolescence, assumed that sex impulses remained latent during this time. Freud (44) described the period as one in which the recession of instinctual drives is accompanied by the consolidation of the superego; and Anna Freud (33, 35) elaborated this description by emphasizing the role of ego development in which the ego gradually assumes superiority, directing the behavior of the child according to the exigencies of reality, while the sex drives remain latent. The study of neurotic manifestations in these years, between about six and twelve, indicates that there is not truly a recession of sex impulses at this time (23), but an increasing tendency toward their repression, with renunciation of erotic activity. This change results from the gradual strengthening of the ego, which directs sexual energy into substitute and sublimated channels according to the behest of the superego, which becomes increasingly organized, and of the environment, which makes increasing demands for conformity to social rules.

Latency, then, may be considered for practical purposes as that period in which the child develops standards of behavior, which he accepts as his own (superego) and in which he gradually develops skills, mental and physical, to serve the purpose of adaptation (ego). This process passes through various experimental attempts, so that symptoms may occur transiently and then give place to more adequate behavior. Only when a symptom remains fixed in spite of its adaptive inadequacy do we consider the condition pathological in childhood. It is an indication that the ego can find no solution more satisfactory and that the repetition compulsion has crystallized the symptom into a habitual reactive pattern, more or less permanent.

Just as neuroses in adults have their origin in unsolved—or one might say "mis-solved"—conflicts in childhood, so do the neurotic and behavior problems of latency stem from prelatency conflicts. One will find the same neurotic constellations in childhood as in adulthood. Analyzing the dynamic structure of the childhood conditions, one finds the same causative conflicts, the same defense mechanisms involved, the same standards enforced as are known to occur in comparable adult neuroses. Various differences, however, are disclosed when one compares, in detail, similar neuroses of different age periods. These differences are directly related to the stage of maturation of the individual, which, grossly, is related to his chronological age. Hence, in the adult, the neurosis is much more firmly integrated into the character of the patient; and the younger the child, the less fixed has it become as a mode of reaction. In the young child both ego and superego are still influenced by the behavior of the parents and others in the environment, so that a change of environment may modify the strength or kind of superego-ego actions. The older the child, the firmer is the character pattern, the less influence has the environment in changing it, and the closer is the total neurotic constellation to that of the adult. This variation is significant both in the prognosis and the responsiveness to therapy and in the modification of treatment techniques to fit the needs of the particular age, as well as the needs of the particular neurosis.

Just as the neurosis is less fixed in childhood, its dynamic pattern is less complicated by secondary defense mechanisms which may have developed to resolve secondary problems created by the neurosis itself. For that reason, the analysis of childhood symptoms can offer clarification as well as confirmation of the dynamic mechanisms involved in the production of the similar adult neuroses.

In childhood one finds in one form or another, or at one time or another, all the adaptive and defense mechanisms which are revealed in adults. These appear weaker and more vulnerable, however, in the nascent forms of childhood, and, as the neurosis progresses, one or another mechanism may be displaced or complicated by more efficient mechanisms, or at least more adequate to the solution of the problems. This change occurs as needs vary according to problem changes during maturation and as the integrative capacity of the ego is strengthened through education as well as through growing ability to adapt both mentally and physically. Symptoms may therefore be transient or may be replaced or enhanced by other symptoms; mechanisms may change; and superego standards vary so that latency displays a slow kaleidoscopic change, but always with inherent trends traceable to early infancy which form the framework within which the variations are built.

The earliest mechanisms observed are denial and inhibition, which show in the prelatency period in lying and in control of impulsive activity, particularly in the presence of adults. A small child may raid a prohibited candy box when no one is around but never touch it during a parent's presence, or innocently insist he had not touched it later when evidence of a candy-smeared mouth reveals the act.

Repression which progresses from denial and inhibition may

be observed first in the oedipal period, as destructive impulses and sexual impulses are found to be unacceptable to the child, since they are incompatible with each other and are unacceptable to those whose love he wishes to maintain. In latency, repression becomes increasingly firm and forms the basis from which other mechanisms form and then produce neurotic solutions of the repressed instincts, feelings, and superego standards.

Projection also begins early, at first as conscious lying, i.e., "Johnny broke the chair, not I," and later as true projection seen so commonly in latency, when the child, already guilty from the pressure of his standards of behavior, never lets himself feel responsible for fights, sex play, or other misbehavior and really believes "Johnny started it!" or "Johnny made me do it!" Re-action formation—a frequent defense against hostility and un-requited love—is typical of the late oedipal and early latency periods, either as a normal phase of development or in exagger-ation as a symptom. The child then "adores" the rival siblings or "hates" the parents of the opposite sex. Substitution of activity or of objects occurs early at the behest of others, but only well into latency does it become a technique integrated into the personality and voluntarily accepted. It represents the effect of a fairly consistent and firm superego and an ego strong enough to enforce renunciation of intense wishes.

Sublimation occurs as an even later refinement of substitution and may indicate sturdy adjustment or a too restricted adaptation with many concomitant symptoms. Displacement, also, arises in the oedipal period, and at first it is seen in simple form, as when the little boy becomes fearful of losing a leg or a finger instead of a penis or indulges in nose boring instead of anal or genital play. One child of four, a nose-borer whenever he was anxious, said once, when fantasying smearing feces all over the world, "I have no bowel hole, none at all; I don't make 'B.M.' at all; if I had a hole, I'd push it back up." In latency, displacement becomes in-creasingly an important method of solving conflicts growing out of unacceptable body wishes, and forms an important part of all the autonomic symptoms of this period as well as of adulthood.

The use of a part for the whole, as seen in fetishism, is quite common in childhood both as a phase in normal development and also in problems of compulsive rituals. A little girl of seven, to ward off dangers of "murdering burglars" at night, took to bed with her a pine-needle pillow of her mother's; she said, "the small and firm feel of it makes me feel safe and cozy." Introjection—perhaps one of the earliest methods of solving the discomfort arising out of separation from the mother—becomes an important way in latency of solving and accepting the demands of the parents. It is responsible also for depressions seen frequently in late latency or preadolescence.

Causative factors in the emotional problems of latency are multiple. The same attitudes of parents which produced problems in infancy, if unchanged, continue to interfere with normal or adequate development: lack of love, neglect, rejection, cruelty, perfectionistic demand for good behavior, inconsistency, and the like. Added problems grow out of personal inadequacies of physical and mental ability, traumatic experiences, and, particularly important in latency, differences in moral and behavior demands between those of the parents and those of the larger environment into which the child enters at five or six. Finally, one should emphasize again the handicaps of earlier neurotic difficulties with which the child enters latency and which form the foundation on which he builds new habits to meet new experiences.

In this short chapter, it would be impossible to describe and discuss in detail all the problems and their kaleidoscopic configurations which occur in latency. An attempt will be made only to designate the more common difficulties, their general causes, and the more important dynamic factors involved in their organizations. As is well known, disorders do not occur in isolation, nor do they result from one cause. Any one child may present a variety of problems, any one of which may seem in the ascendancy at one time, another at another time, but all of which are interrelated and interdependent. For practical purposes, the psychic disturbances of childhood are classified here according to the realms of interference rather than according to classical symptom categories or even dynamic constellations. Groupings chosen are (1) infantile phenomena or marked developmental immaturity, (2) motor disorders, (3) conduct problems, (4) common neuroses, (5) vegetative disorders, and (6) psychoses.

Infantile phenomena include various mouth activities of thumb or finger or object sucking or biting, anal or urine incontinence, and excessive masturbation. Causes of these activities have been discussed earlier. If they continue into latency when the attitude of persons, such as parents, teachers, and friends, in the child's environment tends to disapprove and criticize, it usually indicates a marked insecurity in respect to love and protective needs and to self-esteem. He clings to old autistic pleasures for solace and stubbornly refuses to give them up for more mature satisfactions because he is afraid of loss or suffering. Sometimes incontinence continues not only from unwillingness to give up the pleasure of excretion at his own will but because there has not been sufficient incentive to control himself. Mothers who allow "self-regulation" of the excretions as they wisely allowed self-regulation of feeding earlier and offer no special approval as incentive for cleanliness may be responsible for prolonged incontinence, which, in turn, fixes pleasure-seeking at the anus and urethra. Such fixation then causes withholding of interest in the pleasure of substitute activities acceptable in latency, as play, learning, exploring. In reverse, incontinence may result from negativism, a defense against pressure from a too rigid, too demanding parent, in an attempt at survival and for self-esteem or narcissistic wishes. The conflict is simple instinct versus environment, with instinct conquering when environment offers no comparable gratification or when other gratifications are too dangerous because they are punished. Nocturnal enuresis, however, if not simple incontinence and not accompanied by diurnal wetting, is a conversion symptom and represents a substitute for masturbation. It may occur as a regressive phenomenon after training for cleanliness has been accomplished (7, 52, 53, 66).

Various infantile activities, such as thumbsucking, incontinence, or excessive masturbation, occur as regression phenomena in a child who may have achieved development up to his age expectation of five, six, seven, or older, when traumatic experiences are severe enough to break down his feeling of personal adequacy or his expectation of parental love and protection. Such trauma may be sudden loss of a loved parent through death or disaster, the birth of a sibling who monopolizes the mother's care and love, serious physical illness or operation, with separation from a mother by hospitalization. These regressions often cause sufficient disintegration of the still weak and insecure ego to retard development and to give access only to neurotic solutions, which build cramping symptoms rather than healthy adaptive techniques.

Motor disorders may occur as generalized: excessive purposeless activity, inhibition of movements, awkwardness, and repetitive organized, purposeless movements like rhythmic movements, tics, and stammering.

Hyperactivity often occurs as one phase of other serious difficulties in conduct or in neurosis. It is usually accompanied by lack of concentrated thought and always indicates an anxiety state in which the underlying fear is near the surface and is not resolved by organized symptom formation or goal-directed activity. One common cause of this excessive motion is inconsistency in training accompanied by cruelty and often neglect. The child is constantly afraid of his own instincts, the expression of which may bring punishment. He is afraid of suffering from deprivation or just from irrational, unexplained rage in a parent. He can learn no defense against this suffering either from precept or from experience, and he moves constantly, as if to move is to get away from suffering, partly to drain off unacceptable instinctual energy, and partly to avoid pain. Neurotic hyperactivity must be differentiated from that found in organic disorders, in which other signs of organic involvement will be found (10), and also from the hyperactivity often seen in epileptics (55), in which both the convulsive occurrences and electroencephalogram tracings will aid in the differential diagnosis.

Inhibitions of movements and awkwardness often result from fear of various instinct expressions in which the parental restrictions are consistent and firm, and inactivity is rewarded by various signs of acceptance. Such inhibitions may cause slowness in walking, in the use of hands in skills, and is usually accompanied by psychic withdrawal into fantasy when impulses may be surreptitiously indulged in autoerotic satisfactions. In extreme cases, such inhibitions may interfere seriously with social adjustment and reality adaptation.

Rhythmic movements of various kinds may result from movement restrictions in infancy (74). Such restriction interferes with more versatile movement and directs motor impulses into the one or more possible movements, such as rocking and head rolling. In latency the child may continue the habit for solace or to express, through displacement, new but unacceptable wishes like masturbation, so that erotic satisfactions become so combined with infantile muscle pleasures that the one movement expresses through condensation two primitive needs. Many so-called "bad habits" fall into this category, such as nail biting, ear pulling, hair twisting, nose boring, teeth grinding.

Tics are inappropriate movements similar to the rhythms mentioned above but are different, in that they are usually defined as fleeting spasms of small muscles representing a physiological unit movement, such as eye blinking, grimacing, tongue clicking, head jerking. Since psychotic mannerisms are often confused with tics, various dynamic explanations have been suggested (30, pp. 161–65). Those cases carefully analyzed in which the precipitating experience was known disclosed the tic as a part of an inhibited grosser defensive movement which occurs at a point of excessive trauma in children with fairly severe superegos, who are inhibited in large-muscle activity by restrictive but warm parents. The partial movement, then, later takes over the meaning of a defense in other anxious situations to which it is not appropriate (54). An example is that of the little boy with eye blinking initiated as a defense against seeing, first, an uncle with an empty eye socket and, second, a little girl's genitals with a slit instead of a penis. The blinking at first represented an attempt at denial of the unacceptable fearful knowledge, and later occurred whenever he was frightened. Stammering is probably a form of tic. It has been variously described as a displaced anal constipation (25, 26, 29), a partial inhibited obscenity of verbal hostile aggression. But, whatever the conflict may be against which stammering defends, the form of partial spasmic motion is ticlike.

Conduct problems cover a variety of difficulties which interfere with the child's social living both at home and in the larger world of school and neighborhood. Withdrawn behavior, in which the child avoids as much as possible relationship with persons, both adults and children, and acts more or less as an automaton, is a problem which one sees occasionally. When severe, it may be the precursor of a psychotic state, or, when only an occasional occurrence, it may indicate a tendency toward a fantasy solution of problems when a reality solution is too difficult. It has its roots in the autistic pleasures of infancy, intensified by deprivation of pleasure in the relationship to the mother. When analyzed, such children show a strong narcissistic tendency, with poor affective relation to others. They conform outwardly to demands made upon them but live in a rich fantasy life involved with both destructive activity and pleasurable indulgence. Such children are often described in such terms as "I can't seem to get close to him" or "nothing I do or say seems to affect him, but he's a good enough child." The superego in such children seems to be only a reflection of those in his environment at the time. His standards for reality behavior change from good, to bad, to indifferent as a chameleon changes his color. He is imitative but not creative except in his fantasies. Because so much energy is absorbed in autistic fantasies, skills develop slowly, and school achievement is far below ability. As causative, neglect is found to be the most pertinent factor. Levy called it "affect hunger" (73); Rabinovitch (78) described such cases as resulting from maternal deprivation; and one can believe that many of the deprived children described by B. Rank as "atypical" (79) continue to develop the autistic inaccessibility of these withdrawn children. In some cases, if the child is not allowed to withdraw into fantasy but some strong stimulus from the outside forces him to respond for protection, explosive destructiveness or sexual indulgence may break into action with all the energy previously used in fantasy creation. Such a child then changes from passivity to a severe impulsive behavior problem. When the defense is broken, the capacity for mastery is impaired. It is probable that some of the adult criminals described by Alexander belong to this category (6). When this occurs, anxiety reasserts itself, and the child becomes fearful of the consequences of his untamed impulses.

A withdrawn boy of ten, when attacked by a gang of boys who teased him by whipping him with ropes, calling him "sissy," "goody, goody," suddenly became violently aggressive, kicking, punching, and screaming. At home, later, and until taken into a protective institution for treatment after several months, he hit at everyone who came near him, had screaming nightmares, and evidenced excessive sweating and palpitation at sounds or movements. Previously fairly moderate in eating, he began to eat excessively and wolfishly, and soiled and wet himself occasionally. This extreme regression occurred in a child when his only defense was broken, because he could depend in no way for help and comfort upon parents who had always neglected him and given only necessary routine care, without love.

Aggressive conduct disorders range from those mild ones of disobedience and stubbornness to more serious delinquencies. The dynamic factors in the milder disorders are similar to those in the delinquencies, with similar, if more exaggerated, symptoms. It is pertinent, therefore, to outline some of the more common delinquent symptoms, with the psychodynamics involved, and say only for the less extreme symptoms that they may occur as reactions to a provocative environment; but if they remain untreated or if conditions continue to provoke the child, these milder symptoms may be only the precursors to the development of delinquent character and delinquent behavior.

Delinquencies may occur as a result of the pleasure-seeking of children incapable of controlling a wish to steal, to burn, to destroy, and in some instances to kill. The impairment of ego control may or may not be accompanied by a rigid or corruptible superego. In the case of the rigid superego, the delinquency is likely to be followed by self-punishment, either in depressive phenomena or in self-destructive activities, such as observed in the child who always stumbled, hit his head, or was otherwise hurt when he beat his little sister. More often, however, the child's standards are corruptible, and consequent behavior is likely to be directed toward avoidance of punishment and continued delinquency. Lack of superego patterns altogether is most unusual.

Delinquencies from neurotic reasons are fairly frequent (6, 46, 64). Stealing may be compulsive, a defense against the feeling of deep oral deprivation, when the object stolen is only a symbol for the love wished from the mother. It may occur also as an attempt to obtain objects to substitute in a symbol for the longed-for penis in the case of the little girl, or the more potent father's penis in the case of the little boy. One boy who stole fountain pens for this purpose had accumulated 113 before he was apprehended. The delinquent act had become the means of allaying temporarily the anxiety created by the oedipal conflict.

Destructive cruelty, such as beating a playmate or a dog, may similarly express destructive wishes toward a sibling, a father, or a mother. The satisfaction of the act then fuses the cruelty with love wishes which may also be directed toward the same pattern, and a sadist is born.

Sexual delinquency is rarely serious in the latency period, except as it may indicate a method of solving conflicts and allaying anxiety which, if maintained, may cause serious consequences in adolescence or adulthood. Peeping may be the normal result of unanswered questions, or it may be a compulsive and repetitive method of attempting to overcome a castration fear. The same may be true for exhibitionism and other perverted activity. The dynamics are similar to those of the adult perverts' exhibitionism and peeping, sodomy, and fellatio. In the child, however, the erotic drive is less intense, and, through wholesome education or through adequate treatment, the symptoms are less malignant than of those of the adult in whom the perversions have become a fixed pattern.

Under common neuroses are included the various neurotic constellations which are described under adult neuroses: phobias, compulsions, hysterical phenomena, learning inhibitions, etc. The description of symptoms and dynamic analysis need not be repeated in this chapter. It should be mentioned, however, that in the latency period symptoms may occur transiently as temporary methods of problem solving, but may be discarded in favor of more adequate methods when and if they become available. An example of a transient neurotic symptom is the compulsive avoidance of cracks in a sidewalk entered into by many children at a time when conflicts involving hostility versus tender feelings for a mother are being solved. This crack-jumping is accompanied by a revealing poem, "If you step on a crack, you will break your mother's back." Such experimental solutions, however, may remain permanent and a childhood compulsion neurosis develop, quite similar to that in the adult.

Disturbances of the vegetative functions (5) are also found in childhood. Allergic disorders occur and exhibit various manifestations at different times, disclosing the same mechanisms of causation as have been found in adults. Change in symptoms with change in maturation levels is particularly interesting and probably due to changes in the problems the child must solve. The change from eczema to asthma is an example. Although the majority of the vegetative symptoms investigated have been found to have their onset most commonly at adolescence or later, still instances are unearthed quite frequently in any large pediatric practice or clinic. One sees ulcerative colitis, diabetes, asthma, skin disorders, alopecia areata, rheumatoid arthritis, hyperthyroidism, and duodenal ulcer.

The psychoses, like the organic disorders with emotional etiology, are less common in childhood than among adolescents and adults. However, cases with classical symptoms disclosing severe pathological ego defects, disorientation to reality and delusional life have been described and analyzed. They show mechanisms similar to those of adults (8, 28, 50, 51), and have been described as occurring in children with basically disturbed relationship to the mother (76). Whether or not these conditions represent lack of development beyond primary narcissism or regressive phenomena is not yet clear. However, accuracy in diagnosis and analysis of the total development of the child may aid in better understanding of the conditions described by various authors and lead to a more accurate differential diagnosis between psychoses and organic brain symptoms, a subject still confused in the literature.

TREATMENT

Psychoanalytic treatment of children, like that of adults, is based on the uncovering of the unconscious psychic conflicts which, in the ego's attempt at solution, are responsible for the development of the symptoms. The more mature ego is capable of finding more adequate methods of adaptation. Anxiety initiated in infancy is easily resolved after it is disclosed and recognized as inherent in the infant's incapability of avoiding suffering but as no longer appropriate to the abilities and facilities for adaptation accessible to the mature human being. The child's ego is still in the making, and the younger the child, the less fixed the patterns and the less secure the standards to guide him. It is this difference in ego capacity which is responsible for an important difference between the technique of child analysis and that for adults. The analyst must not only aid the patient in resolving the unconscious conflicts which cause difficulty, but he must educate the child in methods of adaptation for use of the free energy in skills and social life. The child's superego, unlike that of the adult's, has not arrived at true independence and still relies upon adult guidance and precept. He cannot find more acceptable standards of behavior methods of adaptation without help. The analyst may be called upon to set standards and goals.

Anna Freud (37) discusses the importance of the analyst in education of the child's ego during the analytic process and describes various educational aids. By her honesty, her consistency, her understanding of the child's wishes, and by offering him acceptable ways of satisfaction she temporarily functions as a parent, a wise parent in lieu of the unwise real ones. Therefore, as the pathological patterns are broken down and the impulses freed from repression, re-education into healthy expressions and standards takes place. The educational process is improved by manipulation of school, home, and recreational facilities, to create new impressions and new outlets for the child and to revise the demands made upon him by the outside world. Often the parents are encouraged to seek treatment for themselves, so that they no longer have the original neurotic attitudes toward the child and may create more easily a new home environment. At times, "collaborative therapy" of two analysts, one for parent, one for child, is recommended (65, 95).

Another significant difference between the child and the adult which influences the technique of treatment is the difference in mode and capacity of communication. Free association in the sense of adult analysis is impossible to the child except in late latency, when verbal facility is advanced. When the child recognizes suffering as coming from internal rather than external circumstances, his therapeutic wish may be sufficiently great to aid him in co-operation with the analyst. Most children and particularly those with emotional problems distrust adults as a result of past experience and therefore refuse the confidences inherent in verbally free associative activity. Not only the fear of adults but also the child's fear of his own impulses which have been "tamed" so recently and with such difficulty offer another resistance to free speaking which might easily uncover those wishes he fears. For most children, however, the analyst unravels the elements of the neurotic constellation as they are revealed in the child's play or verbal and pictorial fantasies, in his attitudes toward the analyst, the parents, other adults, children, animals, and the like.

Different also is the role of the analyst in the psychoanalytic process. Although Melanie Klein (67) contends that the relationship to the child analyst is that of a transference neurosis similar to the transference of the adult, the experience of most analysts has shown that it is only in part a transference neurosis and is also in part a new realistic relationship, as described by Anna Freud (37). This difference is due to the fact that, in general, children in treatment are still living with and reacting to their own parents and have not yet such fixed patterns of reaction that they transfer them to each new person. The younger the child, the less fixed the pattern and therefore the weaker the transference neurosis.

It has been shown that this new relationship must be one in which the analyst is found to be sympathetic, friendly, and useful, different from the destructive characteristics of the parents.

To be confidential, the child must have a minimum of hostile feelings toward the analyst. A positive, dependent relationship is the most auspicious for cure (37). To create this positive feeling in the child, it is not only essential that the analyst behave differently from the parents, but he must also like the child, since the child is dependent upon the feelings of adults in his environment for security and comfort and he is more sensitive than most adults to the actual feelings of other people. He senses intuitively and quickly ambivalence, rigidity, rejection on the part of the analyst. An introductory period for the development of this positive relationship is usually necessary in each child analysis. Anna Freud suggests that this period vary from one to several months, depending on the specific child's fear of persons. In this period the analyst makes himself as useful and necessary to the child as possible, as a good companion in play, as an aid in making equipment, models, dolls' clothes, or the like, and as a teacher of skills when the child so wishes. Once liking and confidence have been achieved, the little patient can confide more easily his fears and his attitudes and so work through feelings and conflicts which have developed through his relationship to his parents under whose influence he is still suffering. In the framework of this good relationship he avoids a major part of the transference neurosis and acts out his feelings toward the original objects upon whom he is still dependent.

Sickness insight on the part of the child, if it may be obtained, is an advantage in the progress of treatment. A very young child is incapable of such insight, for his intellectual capacity is not yet developed sufficiently to differentiate adequate and inadequate social techniques, or relative suffering. The older the child, however, the greater capacity he has to understand that his suffering stems from within and from unsuccessful behavior habits. His insight then creates a longing for change and a willingness to suffer the discomfort of further communication for the purpose of future happiness. To help the child to this sickness insight, a good relationship to the analyst is essential; for, before he is willing to face his weakness, he must know that, unlike the parents, the therapist will sympathize with rather than criticize his difficulties.

Sickness insight aids the child in understanding the relationship of the symptom to the conflict at its root, and in facing the original anxiety which grew out of it. As with the adult, to understand is the first step in the resolution of an infantile conflict and is the basis for viewing it as no longer pertinent to the present stage of development. Thus before the child's energy can be freed for use in adequate adaptation, interpretation is as essential as for freeing the adult. Direct interpretation may be possible in some instances if the evidence is clear, when, either because of his age or previous analytic aid, the child's ego has become sturdy enough to face the anxiety which he could not face at the time of the onset of the symptoms, and when his wish to get well is great enough to give him courage to view previously unacceptable facts abou himself. This situation rarely occurs, and, until nearly the end of treatment, most children shy away from a direct interpretation until it has become palatable by indirect methods. The indirect methods used are many and varied and depend to some extent upon the skill and bent of the analyst, partly upon the interest of the patient. Sometimes a story may be used in which the situation of the patient is portrayed in the characters of the tale. In other instances a correlation is made between the child's fantasies and his own life, and yet again a comparison between others' experiences and those of the patient, or a generalization that all children "feel that way sometimes" may introduce an interpretation. But, eventually, as in adult analyses, the interpretations will include explanation of origins and causes leading the child back to the forgotten traumas of earlier years and to the recognition of the present unreality of the anxiety.

The frequency of treatment periods and the duration of treatment tend to vary much more in recent years than when child analysis was first developed. The five periods a week has been modified, depending on the optimum frequency and also on the actual difficulties of time taken in transportation, taken out of school or out of other healthy activities. To maintain an optimum condition for a good relationship and analytic progress, the child must not give up so much that he feels deeply deprived. He must not sacrifice too much of companionship or suffer too much of ennui and discomfort, to make him dislike going to the treatment. Therefore, the optimum frequency is sometimes sacrificed for optimum co-operation. If not too infrequent, however, thorough analysis may be entered into even if the child is not seen daily. The author has found that at least twice a week is the minimum for progress. In general, one finds that the young child progresses better, the greater the frequency. The frequency necessary for the older child varies according to the kind of difficulty and to the capacity of the child to maintain a continuous analytic relationship during intervals.

The details of analytic techniques will vary from age to age, as has been indicated. The younger the child, the more play will be used for communication and the less complicated will be the interpretations; the older the child, the more likely that the analysis will be conducted verbally in conversation, fantasies, dream retailing, and the like, even though play or constructive activity may occur concomitantly, and the more direct and inclusive the interpretations. Other modifications also are necessary in the treatment of the child and will depend upon the variations in the constellation of the character. Only a few may be mentioned here. Aichhorn (2) has described in detail the modification he developed for the treatment of delinquents who possessed corrupt superegos and weak or criminal egos. He found the creation of a loving, dependent, needful relationship even more necessary in these cases, and thus made himself not only a desirable person but an absolutely necessary person to such a child. For other forms of defective ego problems, as with many acting-out impulsive children, modifications also are used, in which the analyst, for a long time, acts in place of the ego for the child, protects him by kindly restriction and direction from acting out directly either destructive or erotic impulses. Also in the treatment of psychotic children the analyst may play a very active role, attempting to make reality sufficiently interesting to lure the child from his narcissistic and unrealistic autism.

DIAGNOSIS

Although, for practical purposes, classification of the child's problems is made according to the area of disturbance, such symptom diagnosis is not all that is necessary for the planning of treatment. Of even greater importance is an evaluation of the dynamic causes of the symptoms, including the basic conflicts involved; the ego mechanisms used in attempted solution; the historical experiences which produced the conflicts; the development of the symptoms and concomitant personality characteristics; and, finally, the effectiveness of the ego and superego functions relative to the normal expectation for the age of the child.

From these data one can evaluate the capacity of the child to relate himself to the therapist, his capacity for insight, the severity of the illness, and the strength of resistance to treatment he may offer.

For such a dynamic diagnosis, a careful developmental history from the parents is valuable. Many projective tests, based on psychoanalytic principles, such as the Rorschach, Szondi, and Thematic Apperception tests, may be useful, for they give detailed information concerning kinds of fears, conflicts, and automatic solutions. Finally, and probably of greatest value, is the preliminary period with the child, when the analyst may explore the child's social attitudes, his fears, and his methods of self-protection as they occur in the new situation.

PREVENTION

A word on prevention should not be omitted. The more we know of the emotional experiences during development which initiate psychic disorders and of those which maintain the pathology, once it is started, the wiser we can be in promoting healthy development and avoiding personality distortion. Obviously, healthy, loving parents are essential in our society, in which the child is reared in the family unit. Therefore, anything which promotes adult mental health is a cornerstone in the building of child mental health, be it adult education, adequate facilities for work and play, economic security, or psychotherapy.

Equally important is knowledge of the child's needs, which the loving parent, the teacher, and the physician can use to avoid the traumata of sudden pleasure deprivation, painful separation, demand of performance beyond his capacity, physical pain without protective sympathy, and the like. The more wisely the child is fed, is trained, is guided and taught, the greater his facilities for learning social skills to expend his energy; the fewer catastrophic experiences he is exposed to; and the more likely he is to grow into a sturdy, happy, creative person. It is obvious, however, that one cannot offer any child ideal conditions, and, in spite of good preventive measures, problems may develop. If they do, prevention then of future difficulties is possible if early diagnosis is made and treatment is provided, before the patterns are so fixed that the crippling is only partially reversible.

1. ABRAHAM, K. "Contributions to the Theory of the Anal Character," in *Selected Papers* (London: Hogarth Press, 1927), chap. xxiii.
2. AICHHORN, A. *Wayward Youth* (New York: Viking Press, 1945).
3. ALDRICH, C. A., and ALDRICH, M. *Babies Are Human Beings* (New York: Macmillan Co., 1939).
4. ALEXANDER, F. "Concerning the Genesis of the Castration Complex," *Psychoanalyt. Rev.*, 22:49, 1935.
5. ALEXANDER, F. *Psychosomatic Medicine* (New York: W. W. Norton & Co., Inc., 1950).
6. ALEXANDER, F., and HEALY, W. *Roots of Crime* (New York: Alfred A. Knopf, 1935).
7. ANGEL, A. "From the Analysis of a Bed Wetter," *Psychoanalyt. Quart.*, 4:120, 1935.
8. BENDER, L. "Childhood Schizophrenia: A Clinical Study of One Hundred Schizophrenic Children," *Am. J. Orthopsychiat.*, 17:40, 1947.
9. BENDER, L. "Infants Reared in Institutions; Permanently Handicapped," *Bull. Child Welfare League of America*, Vol. 24, No. 7 (September, 1945).
10. BENDER, L. "Organic Brain Conditions Producing Behavior Disturbances: A Clinical Survey of Encephalitis, Burn Encephalopathy, and the Traumatic States," in *Modern Trends in Child Psychiatry* (New York: International Universities Press, 1945).
11. BENEDEK, THERESE. "The Psychosomatic Implications of the Primary Unit: Mother-Child," *Am. J. Orthopsychiat.*, 19:642, 1949.
12. BERES, D., and OBERS, S. "The Effects of Extreme Deprivation in Infancy on Psychic Structure in Adolescence: A Study in Ego Development," in *The Psychoanalytic Study of the Child*, 5 (New York: International Universities Press, 1950), 212-35.
13. BERGMAN, P., and ESCALONA, S. "Unusual Sensitivities in Very Young Children," in *The Psychoanalytic Study of the Child*, 3/4 (New York: International Universities Press, 1949), 333-52.
14. BERNFELD, S. "Psychoanalytic Psychology of the Young Child," *Psychoanalyt. Quart.*, 4:3, 1935.
15. BLANCHARD, P. "Psychoanalytic Contributions to the Problems of Reading Disabilities," in *The Psychoanalytic Study of the Child*, 2 (1946) (New York: International Universities Press, 1947), 163-87.
16. BORNSTEIN, B. "The Analysis of a Phobic Child; Some Problems of Theory and Technique in Child Analysis," in *The Psychoanalytic Study of the Child*, 3/4 (New York: International Universities Press, 1949), 181-226.
17. BORNSTEIN, B. "Clinical Notes on Child Analysis," in *The Psychoanalytic Study of the Child*, 1 (New York: International Universities Press, 1945), 151-66.
18. BORNSTEIN, B. "Phobia in a Two-and-a-half Year Old Child," *Psychoanalyt. Quart.*, 4:93, 1935.
19. BORNSTEIN, S. "A Child Analysis," *Psychoanalyt. Quart.*, 4:190, 1935.
20. BOWLBY, J. *Maternal Care and Mental Health: A Report Prepared*

on Behalf of the World Health Organization as a Contribution to the United Nations Programme for the Welfare of Homeless Children (Geneva: World Health Organization, 1951).

21. BREUER, J., and FREUD, S. *Studies in Hysteria* (New York: Nervous and Mental Disease Publishing Co., 1936).

22. BURLINGHAM, D. "Child Analysis and the Mother," *Psychoanalyt. Quart.*, 4:69, 1935.

23. BUXBAUM, E. "A Contribution to the Psychoanalytic Knowledge of the Latency Period," *Am. J. Orthopsychiat.*, 21:182, 1951.

24. BUXBAUM, E. "Exhibitionistic Onanism in a Ten-Year-Old Boy," *Psychoanalyt. Quart.*, 4:161, 1935.

25. CORIAT, I. H. *Stammering: A Psychoanalytic Interpretation* (New York: Nervous and Mental Disease Publishing Co., 1928).

26. CORIAT, I. H. "A Type of Anal-erotic Resistance," *Internat. J. Psycho-Analysis*, 7:392, 1926.

27. DESPERT, J. L. "Play Analysis in Research and Therapy," in *Modern Trends in Child Psychiatry* (New York: International Universities Press, 1945), pp. 219–55.

28. DESPERT, J. L. "Psychotherapy in Child Schizophrenia," *Am. J. Psychiat.*, 104:36, 1947.

29. FENICHEL, O. *Outline of Clinical Psychoanalysis* (New York: Psychonalytic Quarterly Press and W. W. Norton & Co., 1934).

30. FERENCZI, S. *Further Contributions to the Theory and Technique of Psycho-analysis* (New York: Boni & Liveright, 1927).

31. FRAIBERG, S. "On the Sleep Disturbances of Early Childhood," in *The Psychoanalytic Study of the Child*, 5 (New York: International Universities Press, 1950), 285–309.

32. FREUD, A. "Aggression in Relation to Emotional Development; Normal and Pathological," in *The Psychoanalytic Study of the Child*, 3/4 (New York: International Universities Press, 1949), 37–42.

33. FREUD, A. *The Ego and the Mechanisms of Defence* (London: Hogarth Press, 1948).

34. FREUD, A. "Indications for Child Analysis," in *The Psychoanalytic Study of the Child*, 1 (New York: International Universities Press, 1945), 127–49.

35. FREUD, A. "The Latency Period," in *Introduction to Psychoanalysis for Teachers* (London: George Allen & Unwin, Ltd., 1931).

36. FREUD, A. "The Psychoanalytic Study of Infantile Feeding Disturbances," in *The Psychoanalytic Study of the Child*, 2 (1946) (New York: International Universities Press, 1947), 119–32.

37. FREUD, A. *The Psycho-analytical Treatment of Children: Technical Lectures and Essays* (London: Imago Publishing Co., 1946).

38. FREUD, A., and BURLINGHAM, D. *Infants without Families: The Case for and against Residential Nurseries* (New York: International Universities Press, 1944).

39. FREUD, A., and BURLINGHAM, D. *War and Children* (New York: Medical War Books, 1943).

40. FREUD, S. "Analysis of a Phobia in a Five-Year-Old Boy," in *Collected Papers*, Vol. 3 (London: Hogarth Press, 1946).

41. FREUD, S. *Beyond the Pleasure Principle* (London: Hogarth Press, 1948).

42. FREUD, S. "Female Sexuality," *Internat. J. Psycho-Analysis*, 13:281, 1932.

43. FREUD, S. "On Narcissism: An Introduction," in *Collected Papers*, Vol. 4 (London: Hogarth Press, 1949).

44. FREUD, S. "The Passing of the Oedipus-Complex," in *Collected Papers*, Vol. 2 (London: Hogarth Press, 1924).

45. FREUD, S. *Three Contributions to the Theory of Sex* (4th ed., New York: Nervous and Mental Disease Publishing Co., 1930).

46. FRIEDLANDER, K. *The Psycho-analytical Approach to Juvenile Delinquency: Theory, Case-Studies, Treatment* (New York: International Universities Press, 1947).

47. FRIES, M. "Interrelationship of Physical, Mental, and Emotional Life of a Child from Birth to Four Years of Age," *Am. J. Dis. Child.*, 49:1546, 1935.

48. FRIES, M. "Play Technique in the Analysis of Young Children, *Psychoanalyt. Rev.*, 24:233, 1937.

49. FRIES, M. "Psychosomatic Relationships between Mother and Infant," *Psychosom. Med.*, 6:159, 1944.

50. GELEERD, E. "A Contribution to the Problem of Psychoses in Childhood," in *The Psychoanalytic Study of the Child*, 2 (1946) (New York: International Universities Press, 1947), 271–91.

51. GELEERD, E. "The Psychoanalysis of a Psychotic Child," in *The Psychoanalytic Study of the Child*, 3/4 (New York: International Universities Press, 1949), 311–32.

52. GERARD, M. W. "Child Analysis as a Technique in the Investigation of Mental Mechanisms," *Am. J. Psychiat.*, 94:653, 1937.

53. GERARD, M. W. "Enuresis: A Study in Etiology," *Am. J. Orthopsychiat.*, 9:48, 1939.

54. GERARD, M. W. "The Psychogenic Tic in Ego Development," in *The Psychoanalytic Study of the Child*, 2 (1946) (New York: International Universities Press, 1947), 133–62.

55. GIBBS, E. L.; GIBBS, F. A.; and FUSTER, B. "Psychomotor Epilepsy," *Arch. Neurol. & Psychiat.*, 60:331, 1948.

56. GLOVER, E. "Examination of the Klein System of Child Psychology," in *The Psychoanalytic Study of the Child*, Vol. 1 (New York: International Universities Press, 1945).

57. GREENACRE, P. "The Biologic Economy of Birth," in *The Psychoanalytic Study of the Child*, 1 (New York: International Universities Press, 1945), 31–51.

58. GREENACRE, P. "The Predisposition to Anxiety," *Psychoanalyt. Quart.*, 10:66, 610, 1941.

59. HALL, J. W. "The Analysis of a Case of Night Terror," in *The Psychoanalytic Study of the Child*, 2 (1946) (New York: International Universities Press, 1947), 189–227.

60. HARTMANN, H. "Ich-Psychologie und Anpassungsproblem," *Internat. Ztschr. f. Psychoanal. u. Imago*, 24:62, 1939.

61. HARTMANN, H. "Psychoanalysis and Developmental Psychology," in *The Psychoanalytic Study of the Child*, 5 (New York: International Universities Press, 1950), 7-17.

62. HARTMANN, H.; KRIS, E.; and LOEWENSTEIN, R. M. "Notes on the Theory of Aggression," in *The Psychoanalytic Study of the Child*, 3/4 (New York: International Universities Press, 1949), 9-36.

63. JACKSON, E. B. "Pediatric and Psychiatric Aspects of the Yale Rooming-in Project," *Connecticut M. J.*, 14:616, 1950.

64. JOHNSON, A. "Sanctions for Superego Lacunae of Adolescents," in *Searchlights on Delinquency* (New York: International Universities Press, 1949), pp. 225-45.

65. JOHNSON, A. M., and FISHBACK, D. "Analysis of a Disturbed Adolescent Girl and Collaborative Treatment of the Mother," *Am. J. Orthopsychiat.*, 14:195, 1944.

66. KATAN, A. "Experiences with Enuretics," in *The Psychoanalytic Study of the Child*, 2 (1946) (New York: International Universities Press, 1947), 241-55.

67. KLEIN, M. *The Psycho-analysis of Children* (London: Hogarth Press, 1932).

68. KRIS, E. "Notes on the Development and on Some Current Problems of Psychoanalytic Child Psychology," in *The Psychoanalytic Study of the Child*, 5 (New York: International Universities Press, 1950), 24-46.

69. LEITCH, M., and ESCALONA, S. "The Reaction of Infants to Stress: A Report of Clinical Observations," in *The Psychoanalytic Study of the Child*, 3/4 (New York: International Universities Press, 1949), 121-40.

70. LEVY, D. M. "Experiments on the Sucking Reflex and Social Behavior of Dogs," *Am. J. Orthopsychiat.*, 4:203, 1934.

71. LEVY, D. M. "Fingersucking and Accessory Movements in Early Infancy," *Am. J. Psychiat.*, 7:881, 1928.

72. LEVY, D. M. "Maternal Overprotection," in *Modern Trends in Child Psychiatry* (New York: International Universities Press, 1945), pp. 27-34.

73. LEVY, D. M. "Primary Affect Hunger," *Am. J. Psychiat.*, 94:643, 1937.

74. LEVY, D. M. "On the Problem of Movement Restraint: Tics, Stereotyped Movements, Hyperactivity," *Am. J. Orthopsychiat.*, 45:644, 1944.

75. MENNINGER, W. "Characterologic and Symptomatic Expressions Related to the Anal Phase of Psychosexual Development," *Psychoanalyt. Quart.*, 12:161, 1943.

76. PIOUS, W. L. "The Pathogenic Process in Schizophrenia," *Bull. Menninger Clin.*, 13:152, 1949.

77. PÖRTL, A. "Profound Disturbances in the Nutritional and Excretory Habits of a Four and One Half Year Old Boy: Their Analytic Treatment in a School Setting," *Psychoanalyt. Quart.*, 4:25, 1935.

78. RABINOVITCH, R. D. "Round Table: The Psychopathic Delinquent Child," *Am. J. Orthopsychiat.*, 20:232, 1950.

79. RANK, B. "Adaptation of the Psychoanalytic Technique for the Treat-

ment of Young Children with Atypical Development," *Am. J. Ortho-psychiat.*, 19:130, 1949.

80. RANK, B. "Aggression," in *The Psychoanalytic Study of the Child*, 3/4 (New York: International Universities Press, 1949), 43-48.

81. RANK, B., and MacNAUGHTON, D. "A Clinical Contribution to Early Ego Development," in *The Psychoanalytic Study of the Child*, 5 (New York: International Universities Press, 1950), 53-65.

82. RANK, O. *The Trauma of Birth* (New York: Harcourt, Brace & Co., 1929).

83. RIBBLE, M. "Anxiety in Infants and Its Disorganizing Effects," *Modern Trends in Child Psychiatry* (New York: International Universities Press, 1945), pp. 11-25.

84. RIBBLE, M. *The Rights of Infants* (New York: Columbia University Press, 1943).

85. SONTAG, L. "Differences in Modifiability of Fetal Behavior and Physiology," *Psychosom. Med.*, 6:151, 1944.

86. SPITZ, R. "Anaclitic Depression: An Inquiry into the Genesis of Psychiatric Conditions in Early Childhood. II," in *The Psychoanalytic Study of the Child*, 2 (1946) (New York: International Universities Press, 1947), 313-42.

87. SPITZ, R. "Hospitalism: A Follow-Up Report on Investigation Described in Vol. I, 1945," in *The Psychoanalytic Study of the Child*, 2 (1946) (New York: International Universities Press, 1947), 113-17.

88. SPITZ, R. "Hospitalism: An Inquiry into the Genesis of Psychiatric Conditions in Early Childhood," in *The Psychoanalytic Study of the Child*, 1 (New York: International Universities Press, 1945), 53-74.

89. SPITZ, R. "Relevancy of Direct Infant Observation," in *The Psychoanalytic Study of the Child*, 5 (New York: International Universities Press, 1950), 66-73.

90. SPITZ, R., and WOLF, M. "Autoerotism: Some Empirical Findings and Hypotheses on Three of Its Manifestations in the First Year of Life," in *The Psychoanalytic Study of the Child*, 3/4 (New York: International Universities Press, 1949), 85-120.

91. SPOCK, B. *The Common Sense Book of Baby and Child Care* (New York: Duell, Sloan & Pearce, 1946).

92. STERBA, E. "Analysis of Psychogenic Constipation in a Two-Year-Old Child," in *The Psychoanalytic Study of the Child*, 3/4 (New York: International Universities Press, 1949), 227-52.

93. STERBA, E. "Excerpt from the Analysis of a Dog Phobia," *Psychoanalyt. Quart.*, 4:135, 1935.

94. SYLVESTER, E. "Analysis of Psychogenic Anorexia and Vomiting in a Four-Year-Old Child," in *The Psychoanalytic Study of the Child*, 1 (New York: International Universities Press, 1945), 167-87.

95. SZUREK, S.; JOHNSON, A. M.; and FALSTEIN, E. "Collaborative Psychiatric Therapy of Parent-Child Problems," *Am. J. Orthopsychiat.*, 12:511, 1942.

VI

CONTRIBUTIONS OF PSYCHOANALYSIS TO THE STUDY OF THE PSYCHOSES

HENRY W. BROSIN, M.D.

THERE is considerable psychoanalytic literature concerning the major psychoses, even though this has not been the primary working area for most psychoanalysts. With the wider dissemination of psychoanalytic training, especially in closed mental hospitals, we may hope for a much more intensive research-therapeutic program which will justify current assumptions that a large causative component of the psychotic process is psychological. It is notable that some of the leading analysts—Freud, Abraham, Schilder, Sullivan, and Alexander—do not subscribe to a total psychogenic etiology as an adequate explanation for ego weakness (11, 37, 62, 79, 95, 96). This was the situation in 1902–14 when Freudian concepts were first given a home in a closed hospital at Burghölzli in Zurich, Switzerland, by Bleuler, Jung, Ricklin, and Abraham, at a time when both neurosis and psychosis were generally regarded as without psychological meaning, since they were thought to be due to organic conditions such as anemias, infections, or irritations. The story of these early days when the psychodynamics of psychoses were eagerly studied has been told in part by Jung (70) and Brill (20). The productivity of this period is evident in the writings of this group in the *Jahrbuch für Psychoanalyse*, Vols. 1–6 (1909–14), which includes important essays by Bleuler, Bjerre, Grebelskaja, and Maeder. Unfortunately, this interest was not sustained. Sporadic essays and histories of cases continued to appear, however, with the result that most contemporary psychiatrists assume that the psychotic process is intelligible, even though they are uncertain about the etiology.

With the appearance of Freud's *Three Contributions to the Theory of Sex* (1905) (52) to reinforce the earlier writings, especially *Studies in Hysteria* (1895) (19), "Further Remarks on the Defence Neuro-psychoses" (1896) (45), and *The Interpre-*

tation of Dreams (1900) (46), students had enough evidence to permit them to grasp some of the psychotic mechanisms, especially in the spheres of reality testing, hallucinations, delusions, and illusions. The evidence for the existence of an active "unconscious," the logic of the emotions, the nature of repression and substitutive mechanisms, the purposefulness of psychotic behavior, and the direct relation of current symptom pictures to the genetic-dynamic development of the patient in the family setting became living concepts which stimulated workers to new efforts. This attitude was revolutionary, for, even though few patients showed marked improvement and an understanding of the etiology of psychosis remained incomplete, there was new hope that this psychological method would lead to better understanding and consequently to more effective therapy of the psychologic conflicts in the patient. Psychoanalysis furnished an instrument for the study of the underlying dynamics in the family organization in hospital policies and practices, and in the psychological meaning of physical and chemical therapies. The unfolding of these possibilities has been slow, but their potentiality remains large. Freud's papers on the Schreber case (1911) (51), "On Narcissism" (1914) (49), "A Case of Paranoia Running Counter to the Psychoanalytical Theory of the Disease" (1915) (44), "Mourning and Melancholia" (1917) (48), "Neurosis and Psychosis" (1924) (50), and "The Loss of Reality in Neurosis and Psychosis" (1924) (47) are perhaps his most important essays on the psychoses; but many of his other writings reinforce the general concepts which are useful in interpretation of psychotic behavior.

Though few in number, the contributions of Karl Abraham to this subject deserve special attention. Beginning in 1907–8 at Burghölzli with "The Psycho-sexual Differences between Hysteria and Dementia Praecox" (1908) (3), he continued with "Notes on the Psychoanalytical Investigation and Treatment of Manic-depressive Insanity and Allied Conditions" (1911) (2), establishing beyond doubt that some cyclic mood disorders could be favorably influenced by psychoanalytic therapy and could be understood in terms of the Freudian models for the neuroses. His major contribution, "A Short Study of the Development of the Libido, Viewed in the Light of Mental Disorders" (1924) (5), presents one of the few important psychoanalytic concepts not originating with Freud.

While still an enthusiastic Freudian, Jung wrote about twenty-five papers between 1902 and 1910, the most important of which deal with his association experiments and schizophrenia (1907) (70). He gives a 51-page report of a partial analysis of a paranoid woman which illustrates the Freudian approach. This account is more impressive than his efforts in the first half of the monograph to distinguish between hysteria and dementia praecox.

One of the most brilliant case histories in the literature on this subject is Victor Tausk's "On the Origin of the 'Influencing Machine' in Schizophrenia" (1919) (130). Here we find a step-by-step reconstruction of the probable phases of the development of a delusion from its primitive beginnings in childlike psychotic thinking to an organized pattern. It is assumed that these patterns enable a patient to maintain a precarious emotional balance with his distorted interpersonal relations and help him defend himself against a more regressive state. As in the lively descriptions of the horse phobia in "Little Hans" (43) and the delusions of multiple deities in Schreber (51), we are privileged in Tausk's presentation to see the origin, growth, and readaptation of these defensive idea-systems unfold as in a moving picture.

Storch (128), Ferenczi (38, 39), and Groddeck (59) are among those who opened up further potentialities for the comprehension of psychotic mechanisms during the second period of psychoanalytic development (1914–24), as described by Rickman (95). The observations that every man during some period of his early development has the potentialities for behaving, thinking, and acting in patterns much like those utilized by a schizophrenic, manic, obsessive, or phobic patient alter considerably the attitude of the investigator toward the phenomena of bizarre behavior.

HALLUCINATIONS

Gradually, by means of repeated observations, it was demonstrated that hallucinatory behavior, which seems so foreign to the well-integrated man, was not uncommon in various psychogenic, as well as in toxic or organic, deliria. A simple example is that of the desert prospector who, thoroughly dehydrated, hallucinates drinking water when he has only sand. Less severe is the projection of wishes into a mirage, so that the traveler thinks he sees an oasis but is only translating the heat waves into a desired picture. This illusion has the same goal as a hallucination, although less reality distortion is involved. Delusions and illusions are means of protecting the ego from dealing with painful perceptions. That the hallucinations could be fitted into a meaningful mosaic if one studied the current and past setting was another step forward in the understanding of psychosis. This was buttressed by Storch's and Freud's conclusions (and later from child psychiatry) that, in the early days of ego formation before the boundaries of the "me" and the "not-me" are firmly established, the infant is capable of gratifying his wishes by means of hallucinatory activity (128). As the ability of the ego to distinguish sharply between external and internal realities is weakened by toxic or emotional factors, there follows increased distortion of the external realities because of the intense personal needs. External realities which are unacceptable are falsified into something less threatening to the individual. Bleuler (14, 15), following Freud, was among the first to see that this propensity was present in the dreams of normal adults as well as in schizophrenics. Child psychiatrists furnish many examples of the similarities between infantile thinking and adult dreaming. In fact, hallucinatory wish-fulfilment may be thought of as an early crude form of abstract thinking which is later progressively modulated into daydreaming, imaginative construction of future events, and, at best, scientific thinking, utilizing abstract symbols (92). Fatigue, fear, or toxicity may cause regression in normal persons from the level of abstract thinking to that of the prelogical emotional thinking which employs concrete pictures as its vehicle rather than abstract symbols or words.

One aspect of this hallucinatory wish-fulfilment is the ability to deny unpleasant realities such as have been described in cases of general paresis, aphasia, severe tuberculosis, and lobotomy. Anna Freud has called this type of denial a "pre-stage of defense" (42). S. Freud believed that, when ego integrity is well developed through long practice in reality testing, regression to such complete falsification is not possible, but it is obvious from the examples given that the potentiality remains. In this connection there should be mentioned the selective hysterical hallucinations explained by Freud as "perceptions at the time of the repression" and differentiated from psychotic hallucinations (46, 50). Psychotic hallucinations are a category of primitive defense mechanisms which occur under many circumstances in different patients. One cannot make dogmatic assertions about their origin and purposefulness because of the multiplicity of determinants, although it is simple to define them as "substitutes for perceptions after the loss or damage of objective reality testing" (46, 47, 50) or "outward projection of inner feelings" (20). The experimental psychologists and physiologists must help determine the essential conditions which call for the Freudian mechanisms. Furthermore, the complexity of the content which is often anxious, self-accusatory, or guilty, but seldom concomitant with pleasure, needs much more careful study.

Herman Rorschach (99) attempts a description of the relation of the sense organ involved with the character structure and the age of the patient. He found in his series that only patients with a high capacity for "introversiveness" had somatic hallucinations and that these hallucinations decreased with age. Patients with visual hallucinations had an intermediate capacity for "introversiveness," and these diminished with time, to be replaced by auditory hallucinations, which also deteriorated with time. That the latter were by far the most common fits in with the fact that most persons have a relatively limited "introversiveness." Persons with a relatively empty "type of experience," that is, having neither strong introversive or extratensive qualities, had little or no capacity for hallucination. Rorschach further remarks that this is of interest in connection with the fact that some poets have marked color and sense-organ preference at various stages of their life. In examining an extensive analysis of the imagery of Goethe and Schiller, he finds that they follow the general pattern outlined above (99).

Hallucinations, like dreams, are intricate mental defense patterns occurring when the perceptive functions of the individual, owing to internal or external pressures, are under severe or disruptive stress. While some hallucinations are relatively simple attempts at creating acceptable substitute realities, many of them are representations of the repudiated forces of the id and the superego and are the projected expression of failure in repression of ego-alien material.

DELUSIONS, PROJECTIONS, AND PARANOIA

Delusions are based on ideas, not on sense-perceptions; these may contain elements of wish-fulfilment, anger, pain, fear, guilt, or reproach, just as in dreams. Reality is distorted in condensed symbolic fashion in order to satisfy the strong inner need to project painful inner ego-alien forces having their origin in both the id and the superego. They may be simple or extremely complex and are sometimes highly integrated into a tight, orderly system. They, too, have many component ideas which vary in their organization, as illustrated in Freud's Schreber case and in Tausk's "Influencing Machine." Delusions such as Schreber's were conceived by Freud as having a twofold purpose: (1) to serve as a defense against unacceptable homosexuality and (2) to provide a restitution (71, 72). Their fluid dynamic character can be seen in shifts from a phobic defense to a more primitive delusion, as in patients who alter their fear of contamination by dirt or bacteria to the fixed idea that they have been infected or poisoned. A dirt phobia may become obsessive when increasing pressure compels acting out avoidance patterns in a rigid way, but these remain on the "as if" basis, e.g., "I am compelled to act as if this were the case." When the patient actually believes that the sugar bowl or saltcellar contains poison, then the defense is delusional. Hypochondriacal delusions in psychoses are said to occur when the special investment of energy is attached to organ representations in the regressive process. These defenses along with others, such as literal cannibalistic fantasies, the belief in utter unworthiness and of being hated by everyone, commonly found in severe depressions, are transitional stages on the road to full-blown persecutory delusions.

Persecutory delusions may be seen in all stages of development from nondelusional delicate suspiciousness, with a tendency to interpret most events egocentrically, to the most bizarre constellations of deities. All these have the common property of projection of the conflictful elements from within upon the environment. "Not I, but *you*, are responsible" is a common formula. An overly severe conscience often makes the patient blame some significant person for his unconscious hostility or homosexuality. Often the hypersensitive person is keenly alert in his unconscious to the minute quantities of ambivalent or hostile feelings in others and blames them for his own reaction. Sachs's excellent metaphor, which is quoted by Freud at the end of *The Interpretation of Dreams*, is of special pertinence here: "What a dream has told us of our relations to the present (reality) we will then seek also in our consciousness, and we must not be surprised if we discover that the monster we saw under the magnifying glass of the analysis is a tiny little infusorian" (46). The paranoid magnifies his awareness of his own and other persons' drives out of context in an exaggerated fashion. Characteristics of one's own attitudes, usually from a punishing conscience, may be blamed upon the persecutor. Organs which are sources of conflict may be externalized as inventions. Freud was the first, in the Schreber case, to describe the development of a delusional system through the phases of denial, distortion, and projection from its roots, as in Schreber's ambivalent relation to his father and father-surrogates (doctor, God), and his castration fears. The progressive system of delusions was Schreber's attempt to deny his passive homosexuality, which stands developmentally between infantile self-love and genital love. He used the now familiar formulae:

1. I do not love him, I hate him   (denial).
2. He hates me   (projection).
3. I hate him because he persecutes me   (rationalization).

In the family of projections there are also ideas of reference and ideas of being influenced, usually in a severe, hypercritical manner, just as if the patient were being scolded by his conscience. It is probable that the patient's feeling that people are looking at him is a part of his wish to have relationships with them. Other types of projection are illustrated by the litiginous paranoid, who fights against a hated father; the person with delusions of jealousy, who used denial and displacement in the Freudian formula of "I do not love him, for she loves him" (when there is no justification in reality but because the patient is really interested in the third person).

Erotomania can be caused, according to Freud, by the logic of "I do not love him—I love her." Since there is the same need for projection, there is another step added to support the first thesis, namely, "I notice that she loves me," which enables the completion of the final proposition "I do not love him—I love her, because she loves me" (51, p. 449).

SCHIZOPHRENIC MECHANISMS

So far we have discussed mechanisms which might be described as attempts of an ineffective or damaged ego to defend itself against its own turbulent drives or against a harsh conscience. These are the commonly seen efforts at healing or restitution. There are schizophrenic phenomena which have been called "direct expressions" of this degradation of the damaged ego, now weakened through the loss of object relationships. It is a matter of interpretation which processes should be included in the category of direct expressions of the damaged ego, but fantasies of world destruction, somatic sensations, depersonalization, and confusion probably belong here. Archaic language, bizarre motility, delusions of grandeur, probably more complex, are better understood in the light of the ego, which under stress permits regression to the archaic processes of the first and second years of life.

There remains a number of technical difficulties involved in understanding the formation and relationships of the various paranoid ideas. Waelder finds that earlier theories (delusions resulting from a withdrawal of libido from the outer world and being concentrated on the narcissistic ego; delusions as products of projection; delusions as denial; delusions as attempted restitution; delusions as containing a historical truth and with those representing the return of the repressed) offer the possibility of an integrated theory.

There are three possible solutions to the conflicts between individual instinctual equipment and reality; an equilibrium can be established by changing reality (alloplasticism) or by changing the instinct (autoplasticism) or by changing neither but denying one or the other. These methods lead, wherever successful, to various types of normality, i.e., a dominating type, a submissive type, and a type with a rich phantasy life. When unsuccessful, they provide the breeding ground for psychopathy, psychoneurosis, and paranoia respectively.

Furthermore, it is suggested that if warded-off instinctual drives make their come-back, the return has the same form as the defence mechanism had; they return, as it were, through the same door through which they were ousted (ismorphism). If the defence mechanism had the form of denial, the return must have the form of an assertion. One type of paranoid idea at least, the delusion of persecution, may be the result of an (incomplete) return of a denied instinct [132, p. 176].

Freud (51) stressed the relationship between various levels of development, such as auto-erotism (severe loss of object love), narcissism (megalomania), to the various types of psychosis. He believed dementia praecox to be more regressive than paranoia and proposed for the former group the more general name of "paraphrenia." With weakened and abandoned object relationships, the patient exhibits extreme isolation and separation from the world, which is translated into such images as "world destruction," in which the patient himself or significant persons are dead or altered in the direction of being shadows, fleeting, strange, or unreal. These images and ideas may be more or less severe, depending on the economic emotional balance of the individual, but may progress to the more severe stages of depersonalization, body sensations, and catatonic stuperous withdrawal. Hypochondriacal complaints, according to Tausk, usually precede the more severe sensations of body or organ estrangement or the somatic delusions, which may be bizarre, such as "insects under the skin" or "tigers in the stomach" (130). Most patients make periodic, intense, though short-lived, attempts to establish either erotic or hostile object relationships, but their clumsiness usually prevents a durable positive benefit.

The familiar feelings of expansiveness, power, special abilities, and grandeur are akin to manic states and spiritual exaltation. There is a recapturing of the infantile omnipotence which denies injury to the prestige of the self-system and an attempt at correction by overcompensation. Those individuals who can tolerate social isolation may defend themselves with a towering, portentous aloofness which enables the patient to retain an extraordinary opinion of himself and his mission, such as saving the world, knowing the secrets of electricity, cosmic forces, or nuclear energy. This enables many of them to maintain a façade of integrity, in contrast to the glaring regressive phenomena of hebephrenia and catatonia. In this connection the work of Shakow (111) on the nature of the deterioration in schizophrenic states will help the student grasp the difficulties inherent in the concept of deterioration.

More modulated patterns of affect withdrawal have been described as the "hollow men" or the "as if" persons, who seem on early acquaintance to be intelligent, social, and adaptive but are later found to have severe emotional handicaps (24). On the other hand, French and Kasanin (41) have reported two cases of psychosis in which unconscious learning apparently took place unobtrusively behind the mask of conspicuous and disturbing psychotic manifestations.

Psychoanalysts are also contributing to the experimentation with group therapy, but in the absence of a definitive summary, only single references can be given. Slavson (113), Powdermaker and Frank (86), Grotjahn (60), Stanton and Schwartz (123, 124, 125), and Ezriel (28) are among those who have presented theories about group dynamics according to psychoanalytic principles, but most of the work is with children and neurotics. Stanton and Schwartz have carefully observed and recorded the dynamics of a hospital ward as a social organization.

Space prevents further exposition of the dynamics of automatic obedience, echolalia, echopraxia, negativism, catatonic mutism, furor, confusion, excitement, and stereotypy, but the references given will help the student's search for their meaning (37, 62, 95, 96, 103).

In summary we can state that, by the application and extension of knowledge gained from the psychoanalytic study of dreams and neuroses, the content and behavior of schizophrenics become intelligible, even though the etiology to a great extent remains unknown. It is inferred that the reality-testing functions are defective in schizophrenics and that this makes them more vulnerable to injury. This defective ego may be caused in part by poor interpersonal relationships during the early years of life. Multiple identifications with reasonably warm, stable adults, necessary to emotional health, are lacking, so that the patterns of behavior developed to meet life's needs are fragile and uncertain. Preventive psychiatry and psychiatric therapy have the task of building up such patterns, in order that the person may achieve satisfactions in a healthy fashion. This problem involves utilizing numerous methods for helping the person through both conscious guidance and "uncovering" techniques of the unconscious conflicts to integrate more adequately his means for dealing with internal and external demands. By means of examples from daily living, the patient is shown superior means of managing his affairs. The books by Bettelheim (13), Erikson (27), Levy (75), Redl (93), and Spock (122) contain excellent expositions and examples. Various studies on the separation of mothers from their babies also furnish dramatic examples of the importance of good relationships between parents and children (18, 107–9, 115–21).

MANIC-DEPRESSIVE MECHANISMS

The psychoanalytic method of interpreting the emotional content of psychotic behavior has not produced valuable differentiations between various categories of mental disorder. This is not to deny profound differences in the clinical picture, dynamics, prognosis, or treatability among the multiple manifestations of the schizophrenics and the cyclic mood disorders or their subgroups. These differences are seen to be significant phases in a complex total organization in which the symptomatology is dependent upon the economic balance of the emotional forces at play. The classic discussion at lengthy ward rounds regarding the diagnosis of dementia praecox versus a manic-depressive disorder loses much of its meaning when the genetic-dynamic development is disclosed and the current balance of power between the destructive and the restitutive powers determined. Such discussion has even less meaning when a group of experienced analysts carefully review the world literature on manic-depressive disease in the light of their own experience in numerous detailed case reviews, only to find that manic-depressive disease is probably not a sound unitary concept. History shows that Kraepelin had shrewd critics during the years he developed his diagnostic dichotomy, but their voices were lost in loud, if premature, applause from other sources. Teachers like Pappenheim, Ernest Meyer, Korsakoff, Serbski, Sommer, Bianchi, and Adolf Meyer pointed out the fallacies in diagnosing by prognosis or by ruthlessly refusing to admit that schizophrenic patients might not be treated more effectively (138).

The papers which give the basic psychoanalytic knowledge about the cyclic mood disorders are probably Abraham's "Notes on the Psychoanalytical Investigation and Treatment of Manicdepressive Insanity and Allied Conditions" (1911) (2); "The First Pregenital Stage of the Libido" (1916) (1); "A Short Study of the Development of the Libido Viewed in the Light of Mental Disorders" (1924) (5); Freud's "Mourning and Melancholia" (1917) (48); and Radó's "The Problem of Melancholia" (1927) (89). The first two stress these points: that the psychotic has nearly equal ambivalent emotions toward himself and toward others and that this is a barrier to therapy; that the ambivalence originates early in personality development (pregenital); that oral demands and conflicts expressed directly and indirectly tend to increase; and that the hatred for the self represents a turning-inward of hostility which was formerly directed outward. Freud described the "pathognomic introjection" occasioned by the loss of a love object, causing a representation of this object to become part of the superego. The ensuing battle between the ego and the superego reproduces the former fight between the ego and the lost love object.

Abraham advanced several other theories in his 1924 paper (5), as well as substantiating Freud's views. Here is outlined the familiar developmental scale of oral and anal levels of organization, each with its own problems of integration and corresponding expression of failure to maintain equilibrium. In much greater detail he pictures the interplay between the ego and the superego and the mutual recrimination which must be worked out in the depressive process. He also elaborates on the dynamics of mania as oral hunger for objects, "increased mental metabolism," which is aided by a paralysis of the superego functions, thus enabling the patient to seek gratification without inhibition and so gain a heightened sense of well-being and prestige. Conscience values are so weakened that the instinctual forces can seek direct gratification via the ego functions, and the manic can express his self-love in an unbounded fashion in contrast to the depressive, who cannot openly admit any regard for the self. The manic somehow regains his feelings of infantile omnipotence where there were no reality barriers against pleasure and no objects to fear. Abraham also offers shrewd guesses about early life-experiences which predispose the individual to depressions, stressing the probable early depressions in childhood.

Radó (89) interprets self-accusation as a means whereby the ego placates the strict superego and its ambivalent introjected object. The refinements of his explanation of the introjection of the object in both the ego and the superego, showing the multiple functions of the ego, help one to comprehend these states.

Lewin's work on cyclic mood disorders, *The Psychoanalysis of Elation* (78), studies the defenses expressed as euphoria or hypomania. In a systematic manner he presents the beginning phases of empirical analytic thinking and practice which underlie current theories. The Freud-Abraham view of mania as a triumph and such intimately related subjects as the mourning rites of savages described by Roheim (1923) (97, 98), the Radó (1928, 1926) (88, 90) observations on drug addiction, the Alexander studies on neurotic characters (1927, 1929, 1930) (7, 8, 9), emphasizing the bribery of the superego by ego suffering, are given lucid exposition. Space does not permit more than mention of the importance of the denial mechanism (Lewin, 76, 77; Deutsch, 25); the depressive position in the first year of life (Klein, 74); anaclitic depression (Spitz, 120); disappointment in infancy (Gerö, 56, 57; Jacobson, 68, 69). Lewin's own contributions on the types of denial—diffuse denial, hypomanic neurotic characters, identifications, "technical elation" as a screen affect and as resistance—the relation of mania to the sleep system, the "blank dream," and his extensions to the theory of oral eroticism and the sense of reality are important additions to the comprehension of personality patterns.

While earlier psychiatrists described reactive or situational depressions occasioned by loss of some cherished relationship through death or separation, it remained for Freud to show that the internal psychological work done in depressions was akin to the process of mourning; for in both circumstances the person is unwilling to admit the need to give up the lost object and to reinvest, so to speak, his emotional capital in some other desirable person or enterprise. The separation process becomes more complicated when the mourner has active feelings of affection and dislike simultaneously for the lost one. In fact, the mourner may for a time hate the object of his concern for deserting him, even though the latter is not responsible. Under such circumstances the mourner does not feel free to express his mixed feelings but is compelled by his conscience to turn the aggression inward to punish himself. Often the repression of hostility is incomplete, so that the mourner may impulsively exhibit his rage in active ways: he may kill the deserter and then commit suicide in order to obliterate the object incorporated within himself. Some of the fantasy material of the depressive concerns oral incorporative destruction (devouring) of the ambivalently loved object. Since the love object is represented as a part of his personality through introjection, the depressive must needs hurt himself when he attacks the introjected object. With such attacks upon loved ones comes guilt, which, in turn, demands punishment to maintain psychic equilibrium (2, 48).

As analysts became familiar with these interpretations, it was apparent that the major cyclic mood disturbances are not always adamant reactions which run a predestined course, possibly because of a genetic, endocrine, or metabolic basis. The usual textbook curves describing the course of the disease were abstractions taken from hundreds of records; but examination and the therapeutic success of many an individual case revealed that the onset was related to a psychogenic factor and that the development of the disorder had psychological coherence. It remains for more controlled studies to show what varieties of mood disorders can be so influenced.

Some differences between psychoses and neuroses become apparent from our survey, even though both have similar historical development and dynamic defenses.

1. In the psychotic, the ego functions are severely damaged in one or more spheres, especially in the loss or diminution of object relationships. The ego cannot cope with the environment, so it falsifies or distorts the data in order to maintain mastery. The neurotic tries to work out his conflicts within himself and only secondarily "acts out" his conflict.

2. The psychotic seeks infantile pleasures of rudimentary, often undisguised, type, such as narcissistic, autoerotic, symbolic, objectless pleasure.

3. The psychotic exhibits behavior of infantile origin which may be regressive (archaic language and motility, delusions of grandeur, somatic symptoms, depersonalization, and destructive fantasies about the self, other people, or the world) or restitutive (hallucinations, delusions).

4. The psychotic expresses many emotions, especially hostility, more openly than the neurotic does. He has less need for sado-masochistic refinements or ambivalence. Projection is more commonly employed by the psychotic than repression.

5. Anxiety is not so tightly organized in the psychotic, except in delusions, as compared with the neurotic. The psychotic shows much less guilt, shame, and sensitivity about his own and other persons' performance.

6. The integrative functions of the psychotic's ego are so disorganized that he seeks the satisfaction of isolated drives, and his personality is so impaired that his life may be in danger.

7. Modulated expression of personal needs compatible with conventional practices is lacking in the psychotic, who therefore is often in danger of injury or arrest.

8. Incomplete repression often causes the psychotic to be plagued with primitive thoughts and desires which cannot be controlled. When these are allied to "magic," the distress is even more acute.

9. Under stress the psychotic may resort to gross flight and massive withdrawal rather than to defensive symptom formation, as in the case of the neurotic.

Although many psychiatrists and psychoanalysts have treated psychotic patients without the use of physical methods, this area has not had strong continuity of interest. It is instructive to know of the early work at Ward's Island, New York, and Burghölzli before 1914 and the repeated efforts, with some success, at St. Elizabeth's Hospital, the Phipps Clinic, the New York State Psychiatric Hospital, Worcester State Hospital, and others (Nunberg, Kardiner, Kempf, Oberndorff, W. A. White, Paul Federn); but more concentrated attention upon psychotherapy came with the demonstration by H. S. Sullivan (1925) that psychotherapy could be carried out more effectively if human relations, as well as physical and administrative practices, were expressly designed to meet the patient's needs. To this end he selected hospital aides and nurses who had a special capacity for understanding schizophrenic patients because they themselves were sensitive, shy, and able to feel the reality of internal conflicts. With training to regard patients as hurt human beings instead of hopeless threats, the attendants became unusually skilful in their work and had corresponding success. Even after Sullivan left the Sheppard and Enoch Pratt Hospital, the attendants were able to carry on successfully. Later, in collaboration with Frieda Fromm-Reichmann, systematic long-term treatment methods were developed which have been utilized elsewhere. The active exchange of opinions regarding many techniques for treating psychotics augurs well for the future in this difficult field. At present the enormous importance of the transference-countertransference aspect of therapy is receiving increased scrutiny, for it may be one of the crucial factors in treatment (34, 29–31, 80, 110, 112). Perhaps one will learn which kinds of therapists can work with the various reaction types and then train these persons painstakingly in the arduous task of convincing the withdrawn, frightened person that ordinary living can be gratifying and worth while.

The reports by J. N. Rosen (100–102) that vigorous, direct interpretations of unconscious material carried on intensively enabled patients to improve more quickly has also stimulated wider experimentation. Until the case studies treated in this manner are brought under more rigorous control, however, it is not possible to evaluate either the methods used or the results (26, 135).

Most workers follow the methods of Federn, Sullivan, and Fromm-Reichmann.

We can hope that intensive work in many places will establish better treatment methods (135). It is certain that such studies will also make possible better collaboration with experimental psychologists, neurophysiologists, biochemists, and endocrinologists, who will reveal new aspects of the functions of the central nervous system when under stress.

BIBLIOGRAPHY

1. ABRAHAM, K. "The First Pregenital Stage of the Libido (1916), in *Selected Papers* (London: Hogarth Press, 1926), pp. 248–79.
2. ABRAHAM, K. "Notes on the Psycho-analytical Investigation and Treatment of Manic-depressive Insanity and Allied Conditions (1911)," in *Selected Papers* (London: Hogarth Press, 1927), pp. 137–56.
3. ABRAHAM, K. "The Psycho-sexual Differences between Hysteria and Dementia Praecox (1908)," in *Selected Papers* (London: Hogarth Press, 1927), pp. 64–79.
4. ABRAHAM, K. *Selected Papers* (London: Hogarth Press, 1927).
5. ABRAHAM, K. "A Short Study of the Development of the Libido, Viewed in the Light of Mental Disorders (1924)," in *Selected Papers* (London: Hogarth Press, 1927), pp. 418–501.
6. ACTH CLINICAL CONFERENCE. *Proceedings of the First Conference*, ed. J. R. MOTE (New York: Blakiston Co., 1950).
7. ALEXANDER, F. "The Neurotic Character," *Internat. J. Psycho-Analysis*, 11:292, 1930.
8. ALEXANDER, F. *Psychoanalysis of the Total Personality* (New York: Nervous and Mental Disease Publishing Co., 1929).
9. ALEXANDER, F. "Zur Theorie der Zwangsneurosen und der Phobien," *Internat. Ztschr. f. Psychoanal.*, 13:20, 1927.
10. ALEXANDER, F., and FRENCH, T. M. *Psychoanalytic Therapy: Principles and Applications* (New York: Ronald Press Co., 1946).
11. BELLAK, L. *Dementia Praecox: The Past Decade's Work and Present Status, a Review and Evaluation* (New York: Grune & Stratton, 1948).
12. BELLAK, L. "A Multiple-Factor Psychosomatic Theory of Schizophrenia," *Psychiat. Quart.*, 23:738, 1949.
13. BETTELHEIM, B. *Love Is Not Enough: The Treatment of Emotionally Disturbed Children* (Glencoe, Ill.: Free Press, 1950).
14. BLEULER, E. "Autistic Thinking" and "Autistic-undisciplined Thinking," in D. RAPAPORT (ed.), *Organization and Pathology of Thought: Selected Sources* (New York: Columbia University Press, 1951), pp. 399–450.
15. BLEULER, E. "The Basic Symptoms of Schizophrenia," in D. RAPAPORT (ed.), *Organization and Pathology of Thought: Selected*

Sources (New York: Columbia University Press, 1951), pp. 581–645.

16. BLEULER, M. "Forschungen zur Schizophreniefrage," *Wien. Ztschr. f. Nervenh.*, 1:129, 1948.

17. Boss, M. "Psychopathologie des Traumes bei schizophrenen und organischen Psychosen," *Ztschr. f. d. ges. Neurol. u. Psychiat.*, 162:459, 1938.

18. BOWLBY, J. *Maternal Care and Mental Health* (Geneva: World Health Organization, 1951).

19. BREUER, J., and FREUD, S. *Studies in Hysteria* (New York: Nervous and Mental Disease Publishing Co., 1936).

20. BRILL, A. A. *Introduction in the Basic Writings of Sigmund Freud* (New York: Modern Library, 1938), pp. 3–32.

21. CLARK, L. P. "Some Practical Remarks upon the Use of Modified Psychoanalysis in the Treatment of Borderland Neuroses and Psychoses," *Psychoanalyt. Rev.*, 6:306, 1919.

22. CLARK, L. P. "The Treatment of Narcissistic Neuroses and Psychoses," *Psychoanalyt. Rev.*, 20:304, 1933.

23. DEUTSCH, H. "Homosexuality in Women," *Internat. J. Psycho-Analysis*, 14:34, 1933.

24. DEUTSCH, H. "Some Forms of Emotional Disturbances and Their Relationship to Schizophrenia," *Psychoanalyt. Quart.*, 11:301, 1942.

25. DEUTSCH, H. "Zur Psychologie der manisch-depressiven Zustände, insbesondere der chronischen Hypomanie," *Internat. Ztschr. f. Psychoanal.*, 19:358, 1933.

26. EISSLER, K. "Remarks on the Psychoanalysis of Schizophrenia," *Internat. J. Psycho-Analysis*, 31:139, 1951.

27. ERIKSON, E. *Childhood and Society* (New York: W. W. Norton & Co., 1950).

28. EZRIEL, H. "A Psycho-analytic Approach to Group Treatment," *Brit. J. M. Psychol.*, 23:59, 1950.

29. FEDERN, P. "Bibliography," available in *Internat. J. Psycho-Analysis*, 32:242, 1951.

30. FEDERN, P. "Panel Discussion on Countertransferences and Attitudes of the Analyst in the Therapeutic Process," *Bull. Am. Psychoanal. Assoc.*, 5:46, 1949.

31. FEDERN, P. "Panel Discussion on the Theory and Treatment of Schizophrenia," *Bull. Am. Psychoanal. Assoc.*, 4:15, 1948.

32. FEDERN, P. "Psychoanalysis of Psychoses: Errors and How To Avoid Them," *Psychiat. Quart.*, 17:3, 1943.

33. FEDERN, P. "Psychoanalysis of Psychoses: The Psychoanalytic Process," *Psychiat. Quart.*, 17:470, 1943.

34. FEDERN, P. "Psychoanalysis of Psychoses: Transference," *Psychiat. Quart.*, 17:246, 1943.

35. FEIGENBAUM, D. "The Paranoid Criminal: A Casuistic Study," *M. Rev. of Rev.*, 36:222, 1930.

36. FELDMANN, S. "Über Erkrankungsanlässe bei Psychosen," *Internat. Ztschr. f. Psychoanal.*, 7:203, 1921.

37. FENICHEL, O. *The Psychoanalytic Theory of Neurosis* (New York: W. W. Norton & Co., 1945).

38. FERENCZI, S. *Further Contributions to the Theory and Technique of Psychoanalysis* (London: Hogarth Press, 1926).

39. FERENCZI, S. *Sex in Psychoanalysis* (Boston: Gorham Press, 1916).

40. FERENCZI, S. "Stages in the Development of the Sense of Reality," in *Sex in Psychoanalysis: Contributions to Psychoanalysis* (New York: Brunner, 1950), pp. 213–39).

41. FRENCH, T. M., and KASANIN, J. "A Psychodynamic Study of the Recovery of Two Schizophrenic Cases," *Psychoanalyt. Quart.*, 10:1, 1941.

42. FREUD, A. *The Ego and the Mechanisms of Defence* (New York: International Universities Press, 1946).

43. FREUD, S. "Analysis of a Phobia in a Five-Year-Old Boy (1909)," in *Collected Papers*, 3 (London: Hogarth Press, 1946), 149–289.

44. FREUD, S. "A Case of Paranoia Running Counter to the Psycho-analytical Theory of the Disease (1915)," in *Collected Papers*, 2 (London: Hogarth Press, 1946), 150–61.

45. FREUD, S. "Further Remarks on the Defence Neuro-psychoses (1896)," in *Collected Papers*, 1 (London: Hogarth Press, 1946), 155–82.

46. FREUD, S. *The Interpretations of Dreams* (New York: Macmillan Co., 1942).

47. FREUD, S. "The Loss of Reality in Neurosis and Psychosis (1924)," in *Collected Papers*, 2 (London: Hogarth Press, 1946), 277–82.

48. FREUD, S. "Mourning and Melancholia (1917)," in *Collected Papers*, 4 (London: Hogarth Press, 1946), 152–70.

49. FREUD, S. "On Narcissism: An Introduction," in *Collected Papers*, 4 (London: Hogarth Press, 1946), 30–59.

50. FREUD, S. "Neurosis and Psychosis (1924)," in *Collected Papers*, 2 (London: Hogarth Press, 1946), 250–54.

51. FREUD, S. "Psycho-analytic Notes upon an Autobiographical Account of a Case of Paranoia (Dementia Paranoides) (1911)," in *Collected Papers*, 3 (London: Hogarth Press, 1946), 387–470.

52. FREUD, S. *Three Contributions to the Theory of Sex* (4th ed.; New York: Nervous and Mental Disease Publishing Co., 1930).

53. FROMM-REICHMANN, F. *Principles of Intensive Psychotherapy* (Chicago: University of Chicago Press, 1950).

54. FROMM-REICHMANN, F. "Transference Problems in Schizophrenics," *Psychoanalyt. Quart.*, 8:412, 1939.

55. GARMA, A. "Psychoanalytic Investigations in Melancholias and Other Types of Depressions," in *Yearbook of Psychoanalysis*, 3:75, 1947.

56. GERÖ, G. "Der Aufbau der Depression," *Internat. Ztschr. f. Psychoanal.*, 22:379, 1936; also "The Construction of Depression," *Internat. J. Psycho-Analysis*, 17:423, 1936.

57. GERÖ, G. "Zum Problem der oralen Fixierung," *Internat. Ztschr. f. Psychoanal. u. Imago*, 24:239, 1939.

58. GRODDECK, G. *The Book of the It: Psychoanalytic Letters to a Friend* (London: Daniel Co., 1935).

59. GRODDECK, G. *Die psychische Bedingtheit und psychoanalytische Behandlung organischer Krankheiten* (Berlin: S. Hirzel, 1917).

60. GROTJAHN, M. "The Process of Maturation in Group Psychotherapy and in the Group Therapist," *Psychiatry*, 13:63, 1950.

61. GROTJAHN, M., and FRENCH, T. M. "Akinesia after Ventriculography: A Contribution to Ego Psychology and the Problem of Sleep," *Psychoanalyt. Quart.*, 7:319, 1938.

62. HENDRICK, I. "Contributions of Psychoanalysis to Study of Psychosis," *J.A.M.A.*, 113:918, 1939.

63. HENDRICK, I. "Ego Development and Certain Character Problems," *Psychoanalyt. Quart.*, 5:320, 1936.

64. HENDRICK, I. "The Ego and the Defense Mechanisms: A Review and Discussion," *Psychoanalyt. Rev.*, 25:476, 1938.

65. HINSIE, L. E. "Schizophrenias," in S. LORAND (ed.), *Psycho-analysis Today* (New York: International Universities Press, 1944), pp. 274-86.

66. HOCH, A. "The Psychogenic Factors in Some Paranoic Conditions, with Suggestions for Prophylaxis and Treatment," *J. Nerv. & Ment. Dis.*, 34:668, 1907.

67. HOLLOS, S. *Hinter der gelben Mauer* (Stuttgart: Hippokrates, 1928).

68. JACOBSON, E. "Depression: The Oedipus Complex in the Development of Depressive Mechanisms," *Psychoanalyt. Quart.*, 12:541, 1943.

69. JACOBSON, E. "The Effect of Disappointment on Ego and Super-ego Formation in Normal and Depressive Development," *Psychoanalyt. Rev.*, 33:129, 1946.

70. JUNG, C. G. *The Psychology of Dementia Praecox* (New York: Nervous and Mental Disease Publishing Co., 1936).

71. KATAN, M. "Schreber's Delusion of the End of the World," *Psychoanalyt. Quart.*, 18:60, 1949.

72. KATAN, M. "Schreber's Hallucinations about the 'Little Men,'" *Internat. J. Psycho-Analysis*, 31:32, 1950.

73. KIMURA, H. "Psychoanalytic Investigations of Delusions in Paranoia; Delusions of Grandeur," *Beitr. z. Psychoanal. (u. Sendai Japan)*, Vol. 1, No. 2, 1932.

74. KLEIN, M. "Contribution to Psychogenesis of Manic-depressive States," *Internat. J. Psycho-Analysis*, 16:145, 1935.

74a. KLEIN, M. "Zur Psychogenese der manischdepressiven Zustände," *Internat. Ztschr. f. Psychoanal.*, 23:275, 1937.

75. LEVY, D. M. *Maternal Overprotection* (New York: Columbia University Press, 1943).

76. LEWIN, B. D. "Anal Eroticism and Mechanism of Undoing," *Psychoanalyt. Quart.*, 1:343, 1932.

77. LEWIN, B. D. "Analysis and Structure of a Transient Hypomania," *Psychoanalyt. Quart.*, 1:43, 1932.

78. LEWIN, B. D. *The Psychoanalysis of Elation* (New York: W. W. Norton & Co., 1950).

79. LEWIS, N. D. C. *Research in Dementia Praecox (Past Attainments, Present Trends, and Future Possibilities)* (New York: National Committee on Mental Hygiene, 1936).

80. Mann, J.; Menzer, D.; *et al.* "Psychotherapy of Psychoses: Some Attitudes in the Therapist Influencing the Course of Treatment," *Psychiatry*, 13:432, 1950.

81. Mullahy, P. (ed.). *A Study of Interpersonal Relations: New Contributions to Psychiatry* (New York: Hermitage House, 1949).

82. Nunberg, H. "On the Catatonic Episode," *Internat. Ztschr. f. Psychoanal.*, 6:25, 1920.

83. Nunberg, H. "Die synthetische Funktion des Ich," *Internat. Ztschr. f. Psychoanal.*, 16:301, 1930; also, *Internat. J. Psycho-Analysis*, 12:123, 1931.

84. Nunberg, H. "Über Depersonalizationszustände im Lichte der Libidotheorie," *Internat. Ztschr. f. Psychoanal.*, 10:17, 1924.

85. Piaget, J. *The Language and Thought of the Child* (New York: Harcourt, Brace & Co., 1926).

86. Powdermaker, F., and Frank, J. D. "Group Psychotherapy with Neurotics," *Am. J. Psychiat.*, 105:449, 1948.

87. Radó, S. "An Anxious Mother: A Contribution to the Analysis of the Ego," *Internat. J. Psycho-Analysis*, 9:219, 1928.

88. Radó, S. "The Physical Effects of Intoxication: Attempt at a Psychoanalytical Theory of Drug-Addiction," *Internat. J. Psycho-Analysis*, 9:301, 1928.

89. Radó, S. "The Problem of Melancholia," *Internat. J. Psycho-Analysis*, 9:420, 1928.

90. Radó, S. "The Psychic Effects of Intoxicants: An Attempt To Evolve a Psycho-analytical Theory of Morbid Cravings," *Internat. J. Psycho-Analysis*, 7:396, 1926.

91. Rapaport, D. (ed.). *Organization and Pathology of Thought: Selected Sources* (New York: Columbia University Press, 1951), p. 401.

92. Rapaport, D. "On the Psychoanalytic Theory of Thinking," *Internat. J. Psycho-Analysis*, 31:161, 1950.

93. Redl, F. *Mental Hygiene in Teaching* (New York: Harcourt, Brace & Co., 1951).

94. Rickman, J. "The Application of Psychoanalytical Principles to Hospital In-patients," *J. Ment. Sc.*, 94:764, 1948.

95. Rickman, J. "Development of Psycho-analytical Theory of Psychoses, 1894–1926," *Internat. J. Psycho-Analysis*, Suppl. No. 2, pp. 1–106, 1928.

96. Rickman, J. *Index Psychoanalyticus, 1893–1926* (London: Hogarth Press, 1928).

97. Roheim, G. "Heiliges Geld in Melanesien," *Internat. Ztschr. f. Psychoanal.*, 9:384, 1923.

98. Roheim, G. "Nach dem Tode des Urvaters" (Abstract), *Internat. J. Psycho-Analysis*, 4:368, 1923.

99. Rorschach, H. *Psychodiagnostics* (Bern: H. Huber, 1942).

100. Rosen, J. N. "A Method of Resolving Acute Catatonic Excitement," *Psychiat. Quart.*, 20:183, 1946.

101. Rosen, J. N. "The Survival Function of Schizophrenia," *Bull. Menninger Clin.*, 14:81, 1950.

102. Rosen, J. N. "The Treatment of Schizophrenic Psychosis by Direct Analytic Therapy," *Psychiat. Quart.*, 21:3, 1947.

103. Rosenfeld, H. "A Note on the Psychopathology of Confusional States in Chronic Schizophrenics," *Internat. J. Psycho-Analysis*, 31:132, 1950.

104. Schilder, P. *Introduction to a Psychoanalytic Psychiatry* (New York: Nervous and Mental Disease Publishing Co., 1928).

105. Schilder, P. "Neuroses and Psychoses," in S. Lorand (ed.), *Psychoanalysis Today* (New York: International Universities Press, 1944), pp. 249–60.

106. Schilder, P. *Psychotherapy* (New York: W. W. Norton & Co., 1951).

107. Scott, J. P. "Genetic Differences in Social Behavior of Dogs," *Am. Psychologist*, 5:261, 1950.

108. Scott, J. P. "Genetics as a Tool in Experimental Psychological Research," *Am. Psychologist*, 4:526, 1949.

109. Scott, J. P. "Studies on the Early Development of Social Behavior in Puppies," *Am. Psychologist*, 3:239, 1948.

110. Segal, H. "Some Aspects of the Analysis of a Schizophrenic," *Internat. J. Psycho-Analysis*, 31:268, 1950.

111. Shakow, D. *The Nature of Deterioration in Schizophrenic Conditions* (New York: Nervous and Mental Disease Publishing Co., 1946).

112. Silverberg, W. V. "The Concept of Transference," *Psychoanalyt. Quart.*, 17:303, 1948.

113. Slavson, S. R. *Analytic Group Psychotherapy with Children, Adolescents, and Adults* (New York: Columbia University Press, 1950).

114. Solomon, H. D. "Newer Developments in Psychiatry," *Digest Neurol. & Psychiat.*, 18:58, 1950.

115. Spitz, R. A. "Emotional Growth in the First Year," *Child Study*, spring, 1947, p. 68.

116. Spitz, R. A. "Hospitalism: A Follow-Up Report on Investigation Described in Volume I, 1945," in *The Psychoanalytic Study of the Child*, 2 (New York: International Universities Press, 1946), 113–17.

117. Spitz, R. A. "Hospitalism: An Inquiry into the Genesis of Psychiatric Conditions in Early Childhood," in *The Psychoanalytic Study of the Child*, 1 (New York: International Universities Press, 1945), 53–74.

118. Spitz, R. A. "The Importance of Mother-Child Relationship during the First Year of Life," *Ment. Health Today*, 1948.

119. Spitz, R. A. "The Smiling Response: A Contribution to the Otogenesis of Social Relations," *Genet. Psychol. Monogr.*, 34:57, 1946.

120. Spitz, R. A., and Wolf, K. M. "Anaclitic Depression: An Inquiry into the Genesis of Psychiatric Conditions in Early Childhood," in *The Psychoanalytic Study of the Child*, 2 (New York: International Universities Press, 1946), 313–42.

121. Spitz, R. A., and Wolf, K. M. "The Role of Ecological Factors in Emotional Development in Infancy," *Child Development*, 1949.

122. SPOCK, B. *The Pocket Book of Baby and Child Care* (New York: Pocket Books, 1946).

123. STANTON, A. H., and SCHWARTZ, M. S. "The Management of a Type of Institutional Participation in Mental Illness," *Psychiatry*, 12:13, 1949.

124. STANTON, A. H., and SCHWARTZ, M. S. "Medical Opinion and the Social Context in the Mental Hospital," *Psychiatry*, 12:243, 1949.

125. STANTON, A. H., and SCHWARTZ, M. S. "Observations on Dissociation as Social Participation," *Psychiatry*, 12:339, 1949.

126. STÄRCKE, A. "The Reversal of the Libido-Sign in Delusions of Persecution," *Internat. J. Psycho-Analysis*, 1:231, 1920.

127. STENGEL, E. "The Application of Psychoanalytical Principles to the Hospital In-patient," *J. Ment. Sc.*, 94:773, 1948.

128. STORCH, A. *The Primitive Archaic Forms of Inner Experiences and Thought in Schizophrenia: A Genetic and Clinical Study of Schizophrenia* (New York: Nervous and Mental Disease Publishing Co., 1924).

129. SULLIVAN, H. S. "Conceptions of Modern Psychiatry," *Psychiatry*, 3:1, 1940.

130. TAUSK, V. "On the Origin of the 'Influencing Machine' in Schizophrenia," *Psychoanalyt. Quart.*, 3:137, 1934.

131. THOMPSON, C. *Psychoanalysis: Evolution and Development* (New York: Hermitage House, 1950).

132. WAELDER, R. "The Structure of Paranoid Ideas: A Critical Survey of Various Theories," *Internat. J. Psycho-Analysis*, 32:167, 1951.

133. WAELDER, R. "The Principle of Multiple Function: Observations on Over-determination," *Psychoanalyt. Quart.*, 5:45, 1936.

134. WEISS, EDOARDO. *Principles of Psychodynamics* (New York: Grune & Stratton, 1950).

135. WHITEHORN, J. C. "Psychotherapy," in N. G. HARRIS (ed.), *Modern Trends in Psychological Medicine* (New York: Paul B. Hoeber, Inc., 1948), pp. 219–36.

136. WHOLEY, C. C. "A Psychosis Presenting Schizophrenic and Freudian Mechanisms, with Schematic Clearness," *Am. J. Psychiat.*, 73:583, 1917.

137. WILSON, C. P., and CORMEN, H. H. "A Preliminary Study of the Hypnotizability of Psychotic Patients," *Psychiat. Quart.*, 23:657, 1949.

138. ZILBOORG, G. *A History of Medical Psychology* (New York: W. W. Norton & Co., 1941).

139. ZILBOORG, G. "Manic-depressive Psychoses," in S. LORAND (ed.), *Psycho-analysis Today* (New York: International Universities Press, 1944), pp. 261–73.

VII

PRINCIPLES OF PSYCHIATRIC TREATMENT

Maurice Levine, M.D.

A DISCUSSION of psychiatric treatment can have as its starting point some of the well-established principles of all medical practice. One precept has stood the test of time above all others. It can be phrased in this way: treatment which is based on adequate diagnosis is superior to treatment which is focused simply on the relief of symptoms.

The clearest demonstration of the value of this principle is to be seen in the treatment of a patient who has abdominal pain. In such a case it surely is not good practice to be satisfied merely with the giving of medicine to alleviate the pain. It is imperative that the treatment of such a patient be based, whenever possible, on a definite diagnosis. For example, the diagnostic conclusion that the symptom of abdominal pain of a particular patient is part of an acute salpingitis leads to treatment which is much more likely to be specific and safe and effective.

In a similar fashion the treatment of a patient who has edema is more likely to be effective if the treatment is based on a diagnosis of cardiac decompensation than if the treatment is directed merely toward the elimination of fluid. And, again, the treatment of a patient who has insomnia can be more specific and safe and effective if, in a particular case, the insomnia is recognized as one aspect of a depression. The treatment then can be based on the implications of the diagnosis of depression rather than based merely on the relief of the symptom of insomnia.

The second principle of good medical practice is, in a sense, a corollary of the first. It is that diagnostic understanding should, whenever possible, include an understanding of etiologic factors. It is not enough to make a diagnosis of salpingitis or of cardiac decompensation or of depression. It is of greater value to establish the fact that the salpingitis is due to gonorrhea, that the cardiac decompensation is based on beriberi, and that the depression is based on emotional conflict centering around feelings of guilt.

Such etiologic understanding adds still greater specificity and safety and effectiveness to the therapeutic procedures.

This emphasis on the role of diagnostic and etiologic understanding as the basis of treatment permits the comment that many of the preceding chapters of this book, which discuss various problems of diagnosis and etiology, are in a broader sense chapters on treatment as well.

But a note of warning must be sounded at this point. This emphasis on the superiority of treatment which is based on diagnostic understanding over treatment which is focused on direct dealing with symptoms should not be construed as a recommendation for a coldly scientific approach. In all fields of medical practice it is essential that the physician be interested in his patient as a person, that he somehow transmit to his patient the fact that his primary goal is to be helpful, and that his interest is not limited to the abstract intellectual process of making a diagnosis or of discovering etiologic factors. In such a therapeutic attitude he must be deeply interested in the patient's symptoms, must want them to be gone, must be able, within limits, to feel with the patient, in his discomfort, pain, and unhappiness. But his warm human interest in alleviating the patient's symptoms is not enough. It is characteristic of the work of the physician that he has a double orientation, often difficult to achieve, of having not only a therapeutic attitude of human helpfulness but also a concomitant attitude of working beyond the symptoms to an understanding of diagnosis and etiology, which then can be used for a more effective therapy.

A third principle of good medical practice is that treatment should be individualized, be adapted to and governed by the specific needs of the particular patient. Such an approach makes medical practice difficult and time-consuming, but there can be no doubt that it adds immeasurably to therapeutic effectiveness. In medicine and surgery some routinization of treatment procedures is possible and time-saving. Many broken arms can be treated in a similar fashion. Routine dosages of medication may be used in similar infections. But better medical and surgical practice takes into consideration such individually variable factors as drug-sensitivity, resistance, immunity, and recuperative strength. And the best medical and surgical practice recognizes the individual personality variables, factors such as patterns of reaction to pain and suffering, attitudes toward the physician, anxiety about sickness, and neurotic patterns which might interfere with co-operativeness in medical procedures, such as the wearing of a cast.

In psychiatry, routine procedures have little value. Human beings, in their emotions, in their interpersonal relations, in their patterns and trends, differ from one another more than one broken bone differs from another. Consequently, in psychiatry, individualization in treatment is even more urgent than in the other fields of medical practice.

It follows from the above discussion that therapy in medical practice, and especially therapy in psychiatry, must be based on a clear understanding of the problems of the patient under treatment and that, to an extraordinary degree, the prescription for treatment is written by the understanding of the problem rather than by a set of therapeutic rules. It follows, further, that a chapter on psychiatric treatment must pay more attention to the interdependence of understanding and therapy than to a description of therapeutic techniques. Consequently, a discussion of specific methods of treatment will be deferred to the end of the chapter.

To clarify further the logic of the rather unusual sequence of topics in this chapter, a parallel may be drawn with the teaching of surgical treatment. In surgery a description of the techniques of various breast operations can become much more meaningful when the student first has been given a clear conception of the ways in which various specific pathologic processes and physiologic patterns (e.g., lymphatic drainage) determine the operative procedures.

Such a formulation of the principles of treatment is not so easy to teach or to learn as one which would emphasize simple rules and routine and technical procedures. Therefore, it is of high value to have a frame of reference to use in this approach to the treatment of psychiatric patients, an approach that emphasizes diagnostic and etiologic understanding, individualization, and the basic dependence of therapy on understanding the patient as a person. One frame of reference that has proved to be of value is that of basing therapy on the following six considerations:

A. Clinical diagnosis
B. Dynamic diagnosis
C. Genetic diagnosis
D. Transference
E. Countertransference
F. Treatment possibilities

Such a frame of reference is useful in actual work with an individual patient. It provides an architecture for the formulation of the data about the patient that will permit the psychiatrist to have a broad and solid basis for his therapeutic work. And such a listing can provide the architecture for the general discussion of the problems of psychiatric treatment in this chapter. With such a framework, the discussion can be related intimately to the material of the previous chapters, rearranged and rephrased in such a fashion as to indicate its immediate pertinence to therapy.

A. Clinical Diagnosis

By "clinical diagnosis" is meant the shorthand formulation of the broad general category in which the patient's reaction belongs, such as paresis, schizophrenia, delirium, hysteria, neurotic character.

In all medicine the concept of clinical diagnosis is a complex one, with many inconsistencies in the classification systems of clinical diagnosis. Some clinical diagnostic terms are essentially descriptive, e.g., petit mal; some refer to pathology, e.g., appendicitis; and some to etiology, e.g., syphilis. In psychiatry the usage of clinical diagnosis is even more problematic. Not only is there a comparable inconsistency in the criteria of classification, but also there is an even greater variation of cases within any diagnostic category, and the points of greatest diagnostic and therapeutic importance lie in the dynamic interplay of environmental forces and personal reactions in the individual patient. In psychiatry, perhaps even more than in medicine in general, systematic diagnostic terminology is in a transitional state.

But, even with the present unsatisfactory state of clinical diagnostic formulations and the dominant importance in present-day psychiatric treatment of dynamic and genetic considerations (to be outlined below), there remains some value in a partial preservation of attempts at clinical diagnosis. A total elimination of clinical diagnosis ignores the value of reliable or partly reliable generalizations that have precipitated out of centuries of experience. Without such clinical evaluation, treatment is less soundly based and runs the risk of serious error.

The dependence of therapy on clinical diagnosis can be seen from the following examples: Depressed patients will be treated differently if their depression is part of paresis or of a deep-going depression that may be called "manic-depressive" or of a neurotic depression. The treatment of patients with manifest anxiety will in part depend on whether the anxiety is part of a typical anxiety neurosis, or is part of a traumatic neurosis, or is part of the picture of the breakdown of previous defenses during the development of a psychosis. Asthma with important emotional factors in its etiology must be treated in one way if the patient is schizophrenic and in another if the patient is a compulsive character. Psychotherapy of psychogenic headache must depend on a consideration of whether the headache is part of the general picture of conversion hysteria, of hypochondriasis, of migraine, or of anxiety neurosis.

Under this category, of clinical diagnosis, is included the diagnosis of any specific physical disorder to be found by the general practitioner or specialist with whom the psychiatrist is collaborating in the study of the patient. Such a diagnosis must be based on adequate medical history-taking, physical examination, and laboratory studies. Treatment that is soundly based must include both somatic and psychologic investigations, since errors may arise in both directions. A disorder predominantly emotional in origin may give the impression of being a disorder primarily anatomic or physiologic in origin, e.g., abdominal pain which is a hysteric conversion symptom may simulate appendicitis. In the other direction, primarily structural and physiologic disorders may simulate those primarily emotional; e.g., a brain tumor may have compulsive manifestations as presenting symptoms; a pancreatic tumor may give the clinical picture of an anxiety neurosis. Further, when both psychologic and somatic etiologic factors are of importance, psychotherapy may have to be associated with simultaneous treatment of a somatic nature. A patient who has coronary artery disease, whose attacks of pain are precipitated by conflict and anxiety, should be treated simultaneously by psychotherapeutic and somato-therapeutic measures.

In general, it is best that the relevant physical studies be made before treatment is begun or during the exploratory period. In this fashion, if the disorder is primarily psychogenic, the therapist can feel confident of his orientation and can withstand the pressure of many patients during treatment to return again and again to the defense of attributing their problems to physical disease.

Further, it must be mentioned that the psychiatrist can play a role in the evaluation of the patient's physical status. The internist must make a diagnosis of "neurosis" largely by a process of exclusion; if he finds no adequate somatic cause for the symptoms, he concludes that the disorder must be largely psychogenic. But diagnosis by exclusion is not adequate; the psychiatrist (or the psychiatrically oriented internist) must attempt to find pertinent positive factors in the psychologic sphere to account for the disorder. For example, in a case of a gross tremor of one hand, negative physical studies may, by exclusion, lead to a probable diagnosis of conversion hysteria. But a convincing diagnosis of conversion hysteria can be achieved only by the discovery of life-experiences, conflicts, anxiety, purposes, or motives which seem to have etiologic significance and can be linked with the tremor in terms of the "logic of the emotions."

Parenthetically, in connection with the problem of finding pertinent positive factors, it must be mentioned that many psychogenic manifestations are not of themselves directly meaningful. Some are; for instance, hysteric blindness may be directly understandable as a defense against unacceptable peeping tendencies. Some are not; for example, a diarrhea at times may not have psychologic meaning of itself, but may be the physiologic concomitant of anxiety, which is meaningful; a hypertension of itself is not symbolic or defensive, but the physiologic concomitant of suppressed rage, which is meaningful.

To return to the relevance of clinical diagnosis to therapy, the generalization can be made that the clinical diagnosis may serve to prevent mistakes and may give leads as to the variety and depth of treatment. When it is probable that the patient's reaction is largely schizophrenic, psychotherapy should avoid direct interpretations productive of anxiety, although this statement may have to be modified if the recent work of Rosen (39) and others is found to be generally applicable. Further, if the clinical diagnosis is that of a panic state, the psychotherapy may have to be much more emphatically supportive than if the clinical diagnosis is that of a somewhat similar anxiety state. If the clinical diagnosis is that of hypertension with episodes of hypertensive encephalopathy, the psychotherapy must be different from that of a patient with hypertension without encephalopathy. If the clinical diagnosis is of hypochondriasis, psychotherapeutic attempts must be far more cautious and circumspect than if the clinical diagnosis is of hysteria.

B. Dynamic Diagnosis

Therapeutic attitudes, responses, maneuvers, and techniques are dependent not only on the clinical diagnosis, as indicated above, but even more so on the dynamic diagnosis. This term refers to the understanding of the forces that currently are operative in the production of the patient's difficulty, the environmental pressures and internal pressures (drives, purposes, motives, anxiety) that account for symptoms, for character problems, and for disturbed interpersonal relations. For the sake of clarity, the term "dynamic diagnosis" is contrasted with "genetic diagnosis," which refers to the understanding of the genesis and origin and development of those forces which currently are at work. In a broad sense such genetic factors are "dynamic" also, as forces and stresses which molded the personality; but it is of practical value to consider the two groups of forces separately.

In the category of dynamic diagnosis are included (a) the environmental forces which are of importance either in precipitating the reaction or in keeping it active, such factors as the loss of love objects, the danger of death and mutilation (as in combat reactions), and the effect of current neurotic attitudes of a parent on a child; (b) the internal restrictive, permissive, punitive, and standard-setting forces of the personality, which go by the shorthand term of the "superego"; (c) the instinct derivatives, the drives, impulses, unacceptable attitudes, and fantasies of the patient, which are spoken of as the "id" (including sexual, hostile, narcissistic, passive, and other drives); and (d) the integrating, synthesizing, compromising, solution-forming, defense-creating aspects of the personality, called the "ego," which is in contact with the environment (through external perception and control of motility) and in contact with id and superego through a kind of internal perception and influence. In a sense, the ego serves three masters—id, superego, and external world—and at the same time attempts to be their master. As indicated in other chapters of this book, most of the forces involved in such psychodynamics are unconscious.

It must be stated, with emphasis, that such a formulation of dynamic forces in terms of id, superego, and ego is not to be understood as indicating that there are three separate and distinct compartments, or three little men fighting for control. The terminology is used only as a convenient shorthand, as a way of indicating that there are three sets of forces and functions, blending and interacting, each one being many-sided and complex, partly organized and partly unorganized. Understood in this fashion, this terminology provides a useful tool for clear thinking.

Essentially, the dynamic diagnosis in an individual case is the understanding of the forces of the above four groups (id, ego, superego, and external world) as they operate and interact in the specific person and situation under consideration. It is the formulation of the ways in which certain environmental and internal (id and superego) forces in conflict produce anxiety, which, in turn, leads to specific defensive attempts by the ego to lessen the anxiety and to provide some solution of the conflict.

Unfortunately, it is difficult to outline such a condensed formulation of the essence of psychodynamic thinking without seducing many students into using a too theoretical formulation of the problems of individual patients and a too theoretical approach in therapy. Perhaps such a tendency can be counterbalanced by emphasizing the fact that it is far more important for the student to observe or to sense correctly one single dynamic force, e.g., that the patient, underneath his amiable attitude, really hates his boss, than for the student to be able abstractly and without immediate feeling to write a five-page theoretical discussion of id and superego. The student should use theoretical learning only as a way of general orientation to the field and later as a way of cross-checking his thinking about a specific patient against known theoretical concepts. While he is in the interview room with the patient, he need not try deliberately to think of general or theoretical constructs. In such an exploratory or psychotherapeutic interview he should essentially be an understanding, thinking, feeling, responding sample of humanity in direct contact with another sample of humanity in trouble.

The above comment, on the attitude of the therapist during interviews, leads to another, on the processes occurring in the therapist in his interviews with patients. Essentially, two processes occur, as part of the therapist's attempts to understand the forces operative in the patient and to understand the ways in which the patient might be helped. They are: (a) the "intellectual" process and (b) the "empathic" process. (Again, such terminology is not to be taken too literally or rigidly. It is quite possible that the intellectual approach is, in the last analysis, based on empathic processes involved in any process of perception. The terminol-

ogy is used simply to characterize the two rather different processes by which one human being comes to understand another.)

The intellectual process involved is that the therapist uses
his perception and logic and reason to figure out what is
wrong with the patient and what forces are at work. He collects
pertinent evidence and correlates it. He puts together past history and significant recent events, notices chronologic sequences,
observes discrepancies. For example, he notices that a patient becomes flushed and tense when he mentions his boss, even though
the patient says that the relationship is all that it should be. The
therapist's reason tells him that such a discrepancy must mean
that conflicting forces are active. Or the therapist notices that the
patient talks a great deal about his father, his siblings, and his
associates but never mentions his mother, even though the patient
might be expected spontaneously to make some comment about
her. The therapist must suspect that such an omission may be
meaningful. Or the therapist, knowing from the relatives or referring doctor or from the patient himself about some of the
patient's demanding and controlling attitudes and observing now
that the patient is anxious and bewildered after some frustrating
experience, may intellectually construct the hypothesis (to be
verified) that the patient has a pattern of becoming anxious and
bewildered whenever he cannot succeed in dominating or controlling his environment or his problems.

The second process involved in interviewing which leads to an
understanding of the dynamic diagnosis may be called "empathic," a process essentially of limited and temporary identification with the patient. What happens in empathy may be phrased
in this way: "How would I feel under the same circumstances?"
"If I were in his shoes and behaved that way, how might I really
be feeling?" Another phrasing may be used, which in part involves empathic and in part intellectual processes: "How would
a child feel under the circumstances?" The latter phrasing occasionally is very effective in giving the therapist some conception
of the patient's hidden reactions, since a child under the same
circumstances would be less likely to keep his feelings hidden
from others or from himself and would be less likely to have
complicated his direct feelings by evasions, subtleties, and complex patterns. As an example: Suppose that a patient, who has
always been very independent and self-sufficient, tells, without
appealing for pity or sympathy, of the many jobs he now has to

do and at the point of going on to some other comments sighs fairly deeply without noticing it and has a momentary slump in his body attitude. The therapist at that moment, out of his "free-floating attention" and "unconscious speaking to unconscious," identifies himself with the patient momentarily and then says to himself: "Under those circumstances I'd certainly want to sigh many times; I'd feel very tired; I'd like someone to help me out while I relax; a child in such circumstances might feel over-whelmed and very eager for someone to take over and help and protect; I wonder if this man doesn't have some dependency needs that he is unable to express or to satisfy."

The process of empathy is, of course, facilitated if the therapist has had comparable experiences. One internist, after a discussion of the material of the preceding paragraphs, remarked that his understanding of the problems of his patients during the experience of illness was tremendously improved after he, for the first time, had had a serious illness. Another stated that he had had no tolerance for the complaints of patients with backache until he himself had a slipped intervertebral disk. It is to be hoped that neither became too sympathetic!

But empathy is possible without actual comparable experience. All human beings have similar impulses, conflicts, and anxieties; and usually an inner awareness of the therapist's own human problems, combined with an ability to feel for and with others, provides an adequate basis for the necessary understanding of the experiences or feelings of the patient.

Parenthetically, the danger of excessive identification must be mentioned, as leading to too great an agreement with the patient's rationalizations, to too much sympathy with the patient's attempts to "blame" others, to too great participation in the patient's anxiety, to too little expectation of better adjustment, to too strong an attitude of permissiveness for the satisfaction of neurotic needs, to the loss of the independent leadership necessary for a good therapeutic relationship. But, with all its dangers, the process of identification is crucial in psychodynamic understanding and therapeutic progress. If it is handled correctly, it can lead to a type of immediate comprehension of the patient's problems that in many ways is superior to the intellectual variety of understanding. The insight gained through empathy is, of course, to be checked intellectually, with the added accumulation and correlation of pertinent evidence.

From the above comments on the empathic and intellectual processes in interviewing, it should be obvious that a question-and-answer type of interview is far less likely to produce valid and pertinent information than an interview in which spontaneity, free flow of thinking and feeling, relaxation, and undirected recounting of events and ideas and feelings are fostered.

Out of such intellectual and empathic processes the therapist comes to have an understanding of some of the forces at work in specific cases, to arrive at some of the elements of the dynamic diagnosis. For example, he might conclude that basic in some cases of prolonged convalescence is such a motivation as a desire for attention, for protection, or for control of the situation; that basic in some cases of constipation is the force of fear of a loss of security and possessions; and that in some cases of handwashing compulsion the basic force is guilt over masturbation and masturbation fantasies.

And through such intellectual and empathic processes the therapist comes to understand the interrelation between current situational or precipitating forces and the internal drives which are mobilized. For example, in one case he may conclude that a child's overeating and obesity are based on the child's attempt to compensate for his rejection by his mother. In another case the therapist may come to recognize that a certain patient's emotional upheaval is based on the fact that the marriage of his motherly older sister put an end to their usual relationship and mobilized in him intense ungratified needs for dependence and security.

The interrelation of understanding and therapy—the guiding concept of this chapter—is most evident in connection with the material of this section on dynamic diagnosis. The therapeutic work of the psychiatrist in any particular case is pre-eminently based on his dynamic diagnosis; and the chief purpose of supervised training in psychotherapy is to increase the student's ability to understand the dynamic problems of his patients and to base his therapy on dynamic understanding.

As a sample of the close dependence of psychotherapy on dynamic understanding, the following may be cited: The study of the psychodynamics of a number of patients with duodenal ulcer indicates that the ulcers are primarily the end-result of physiologic patterns set up by strong dependency needs which could never be expressed or satisfied because of the force of the patients' internal condemnation of their dependent wishes, a condemnation based on the narcissistic attitude that to be dependent is to be inferior, second-best, infantile, or feminine. In any specific patient whose patterns may approximate this formulation, psychotherapy must, first of all, be based on the decision that, qualitatively, these two forces—his dependency drives and his narcissistic drives—are actually the important ones in his personality problems. Further, the psychotherapy must be based on a quantitative estimate of the force of these drives. As one component of the therapy based on such evaluations, the patient must be given some satisfaction of his dependency needs. If they are not too great, the gratification provided by the therapeutic relationship may lead to a diminution of gastric symptoms. If his narcissism is very strong, however, the satisfaction of the dependency needs cannot be direct and open (until later in treatment) and must be presented as a medical necessity, e.g., the need for close nursing care, frequent feedings, and medication. If a workable therapeutic relationship is developed, incidental comments can then be made which indicate that even mature adults can have strong dependent wishes and legitimate dependent satisfactions, without considering themselves weak, and without hurt pride. Further, the patient can be given the living experience that in the relationship with the therapist he can have a moderately dependent role, without having the experience of being treated as second-best or inferior. In some cases more extensive "insight" into the interplay of dependency needs and pride may be given. From these comments, which indicate some of the possible therapeutic procedures, it is clear that in such a case psychotherapy must include specific attitudes, specific actions, and specific comments on the part of the therapist which are related directly to an understanding of the dynamic diagnosis. (The foregoing is by no means a complete statement of the psychotherapeutic possibilities in such cases; therapy may include responses to genetic factors as well, i.e., to the sources of the dependency and narcissism.)

A second example of the dependence of therapy on dynamic diagnosis: if a patient gives evidence of having a "hypertrophied" superego, of internal restrictions and prohibitions that are excessive and rigid and overly strict (e.g., if it is obvious that he can permit himself no pleasure without great guilt; that he must overwork to satisfy his conscience; that he cannot even have a hostile or sexual or imperfect thought), the therapist must respond with a permissive attitude and must attempt, by his attitude and comments, to indicate that normal adults may permit far more than the patient permits himself and that he can identify with someone who has a more tolerant attitude toward himself. Involved in this is the fact that in therapy the patient may come to see that he may have impulses toward the therapist of a sort which he previously had regarded as intolerable but which the therapist obviously now regards as unimportant. The end-result may be that the patient may come to be less self-critical and self-punitive and may eventually integrate some of the therapist's attitudes into his own superego.

If the therapist has come to understand that the patient's strictness toward himself was based on his fear that, without such excessive internal prohibitions, he might become uncontrolled and unlimited in his drives toward satisfaction, it is part of the therapist's function to indicate by attitude, comment, and living experience the fact that new and strong limits can be set which are healthier and more mature, in the therapeutic relationship and in life.

In another case the therapist may come to see that the patient has never developed adequate internal limiting forces—that, in contrast to the previously mentioned patients, this one has developed proficient techniques of bribing or cajoling or side-stepping his too permissive conscience. In such a situation the therapeutic responses may have to be much more in the direction of the setting of limits, of a clarification of the ways in which undue permissiveness toward one's self may actually block an intelligent self-interest, of providing a new parent-figure (the therapist) who combines realistic permissiveness with a realistic acceptance of limitations.

The dependence of therapy on dynamics is even more apparent when it is recognized that one of the general functions of psychotherapy (in many cases) consists in the giving of insight, the development of a conscious awareness and understanding of previously unrecognized trends, impulses, and fantasies. The therapist cannot use the technique of insight unless he previously has made a diagnosis of the existence of specific pathogenic forces, which he now will attempt to clarify.

Further, the dependence of therapy on dynamic diagnosis is shown in the fact that the therapist (in many cases) hopes to point out to the patient the differences between his distorted expectations in human relations, now clearly reflected in his attitudes toward the therapist (expectations based on his dynamic patterns and his unfortunate previous experiences or fantasies), and the actualities of his relationship with the therapist. Such a contrast, clearly explained by the therapist, may have great value in bringing home to the patient a real awareness of his patterns of distorted expectations in human relations, which may have played a role of high importance in his symptom formation and life-problems. The patient may thereby develop a profound conviction that human beings actually are far different from his expectations, and on that basis his own patterns and anxieties may diminish. This process has been called the "corrective emotional experience" (3). To be able to point out such a contrast between the patient's expectations and the realities of the therapist's attitude, the therapist must previously have come to a diagnostic understanding of the patient's relationship with others and the part which the patient's distortions played in disturbing those relationships.

A final example of the dependence of therapy on dynamic diagnosis is evident in the rational use of environmental manipulation. For example, if adequate study of the problems of an overly aggressive, "predelinquent" boy indicates that the neurotic pressures emanating from his parents are predominant, one essential therapeutic move may consist in the removal of the boy from his home environment.

The above discussion of the ways in which therapeutic maneuvers or responses are prescribed by the dynamics of the person or of the situation to be treated is focused on the correlation of specific psychotherapeutic responses with specific dynamic configurations. There is, however, a more fundamental issue which must be presented in this section on the interrelationship of dynamics and therapy.

This basic issue can be formulated in this way: that fundamental to all therapy is a sound "therapeutic attitude," to which various specific types of therapeutic activity may be added. Essentially, the sound therapeutic attitude is simply one of human decency and respect for other human beings, of helpfulness and understanding. Such an attitude sounds simple and easy to achieve and to maintain, but it is not. Patients often present a surface that is unpleasant and illogical and provocative, and the therapist often has immature tendencies of his own, ready to be called into action in a way that would be at variance with a therapeutic attitude.

The most effective way of achieving a persistent therapeutic attitude is by having extensive psychotherapeutic experience, under adequate supervision, with a stringent scrutiny and discussion of the student's deviations from a therapeutic attitude. Such supervision and self-scrutiny (and, in some instances, psychotherapy) offer a far-reaching stabilization of therapeutic attitude. No study of textbooks can substitute for such experience, and the following paragraphs are not intended as a substitute. Rather they are an attempt to clarify the basic meaning and purpose of a correct therapeutic attitude. To do this, some of the material on dynamic diagnosis given above can be reformulated and simplified. If one wants to have a label, the following paragraphs may be entitled the "three-layer approach" to dynamic understanding and psychotherapy.

The starting point for such an approach is the fairly well-established central fact that a large part of human problems may be understood in terms of the simple concept of anxiety and defenses against anxiety. (This excludes those difficulties which are the direct result of hereditary factors, e.g., some types of feeble-mindedness; or which are the direct result of brain damage, e.g., the memory defects in organic psychoses; or which are the direct result of intoxication, e.g., the disorientation in a bromide psychosis. But even in some of these conditions, basically not to be understood as defensive reactions against anxiety, the anxiety-defense concept is of value. In a bromide delirium, for example, the brain malfunction may lead to a loss of the usual activity of the forces of repression, and auditory hallucinations may appear, e.g., hallucinated voices which speak of the death of a relative toward whom the patient for some time had had obvious but repressed death wishes. With the breakdown of the usual defense of repression, anxiety appears, and a different defense is called into play in the emergency—the defense of projection, which permits the patient again to "disown" the hostility by having its content attributed to a source, a voice, outside himself.)

The concept of defenses against anxiety is a fundamentally simple one, as simple and as clarifying as the concept of homeostasis in the field of physiology. In fact, the defense-against-anxiety concept can be considered as an extension into the field of personality reactions of the physiologic principle of homeostasis. Essentially, the concept of homeostasis is that the organism must adapt not only to the environment in which it lives, to its external milieu, but also to an internal milieu, to the changes within itself. In this adaptation, patterns of response have been developed, some healthy and some not, to meet the changes in the internal milieu and to avoid the internal danger that would arise if the threatening forces, e.g., an excessive retention of water, were not stabilized or balanced or brought into equilibrium.

In the field of personality problems such a concept stresses the fact that there are internal as well as external personal dangers which threaten the organism. External dangers (fire, wild animals, robbers, etc.) produce the danger signal of fear, to which the individual responds with defenses, such as flight or fight or calling for the fire department or the police. Internal dangers (unacceptable impulses, severe pangs of conscience, etc.) produce a type of fear also, which usually goes by the term of "anxiety." Against such internal dangers, defenses are developed as well, defenses which appear as adequate adaptations, as psychiatric symptoms, as character traits, and as disturbed human relations.

Examples could be given that would cover an enormous part of the field of human psychology and psychiatry. A few will suffice to indicate the extraordinarily clarifying value of this concept which stems largely from Freud. A boy in the throes of a masturbation conflict, who believes that masturbation is making him into a weakling and that he will become psychotic or impotent, develops severe anxiety and responds to that anxiety with the defense of trying to show his great strength, of becoming aggressive and domineering, defiant, afraid of nothing, sneering, contemptuous, and bullying toward smaller children. A mother, unconsciously having antagonistic rejecting impulses toward her child, develops anxiety and becomes oversolicitous and overprotective and prevents the child from having those pleasures which entail average risks. A man has a coronary occlusion, develops anxiety of desperate intensity, and tries to protect himself against the anxiety by an emergency defense of using those techniques which in his childhood were effective in alleviating what seemed overwhelming anxiety, such techniques as feeling and behaving in a helpless fashion, making excessive demands, becoming whining and domineering. A patient developing a Korsakoff psychosis, unable to remember events of the immediate past, develops anxiety about disintegration, loss of ability to deal with life, loss of one of man's most prized functions, his memory; and then develops the second Korsakoff symptom, confabulation, which acts as an effective defense against his anxiety, by a total concealment, from himself, of his defective functioning. A child who has had repeated convulsions in school, who thereby has aroused anxiety in the other children which has led them to reject and stigmatize him, develops anxiety and then defends himself by the development of patterns which play a part in what at times is called the "epileptic personality": patterns of egocentricity (of self-aggrandizement, as a defense against this anxiety of feeling rejected), of suspiciousness (an exaggerated defensive alertness against the possibility of further slights or hurts), and of unpleasant aggressiveness (based on the attitude that attack is the best defense).

In some instances the anxiety is so great or the defensive capacity so diminished that the anxiety appears on the surface, either in acute anxiety attacks or in chronic psychologic or physiologic expressions of anxiety.

It is to be noted that in the above examples many of the defenses were unpleasant, e.g., demanding attitudes, suspiciousness, overprotectiveness, bullying. In the face of such defenses, a therapeutic attitude is not always easy to maintain.

The concept of defenses against anxiety can be formulated schematically, as involving two layers—the outermost layer, the defenses; and an immediately subjacent layer, the anxiety. Here one must add that anxiety and defenses do not occur in a vacuum; that there is a third, a deeper, portion (or layer) of the personality, which, for simplicity, can be called the "basic layer." And to this must be added the fact that experience with human beings points strongly to the conclusion that the unpleasant aspects of their personalities inhere essentially in the first layer—the defenses—and that the third layer often includes many unexpected assets of warm humanity, of decency and worth-whileness. Psychiatric experience indicates that, fundamentally, human beings have many potentialities and positive qualities, when one looks beyond and beneath the defenses forced upon them by their anxiety.

Again a note of warning must be sounded about the possible misuse of such a schematic mode of phrasing. This "three-layer" formulation is intended again as shorthand, as a clear way of expressing some simple and vital relations of groups of forces and functions. It is not to be regarded in the same manner as a geographic or geologic description or an anatomic dissection. At times many sequences are involved, all of which could be called "layers." Some defenses lead to further anxiety and thus to further defenses. For example, the defense of becoming unaggressive and noncompetitive may lead to the anxiety of being beaten and hurt; this, in turn, may lead to a defensive urge to show strength by fighting; this, in turn, to anxiety; and this to a defense of being obsequious and sycophantish. The concept of three layers is one of the useful concepts in which the designation is far from exact; there often are many more layers than three, and actually there are no layers at all in the dictionary sense.

This three-layer concept of defenses against anxiety helps to clarify the problems of psychodynamics, but more important is the fact that it also clarifies the problem of therapeutic attitude and atmosphere. An adequate therapeutic attitude must be based on the needs of each of the three layers. The very existence of defenses, of anxiety, and of the basic layer of personality calls for a therapeutic attitude that has at least three facets.

The therapist must respond to the first layer—the defenses—with a nonjudgmental, noncondemning attitude, a feeling of human tolerance, and a conviction that they are merely defenses. He must have the feeling that the defenses, even though they are in part unpleasant or unacceptable, could not lead him to a rejection of the patient as a human being. Out of this must grow the recognition that an attitude of contempt or punishment is not only wrong therapeutically but also wrong in terms of fact and logic and that the response called for is a response to the total person, not just to his defenses. Fundamentally, the therapist must be guided by a full awareness of the fact that beneath the defenses are two other, more significant, layers. Perhaps this point may be underlined by such expressions as "a misbehaving child is almost always somehow a frightened child" (even the spoiled child, in large part, continues his self-centered behavior out of anxiety) and that "the irritating qualities of human beings are fundamentally the result of anxiety which the patient could not handle otherwise."

But such a tolerant, permissive, understanding attitude is not the only component in the therapeutic response to the defenses.

The tolerant attitude must be combined with a varying amount of firmness, of an expectation of better adjustment, and of setting limits to the acting-out of unacceptable defenses. A certain amount of such firmness must be pervasive in the therapeutic attitude generally, as it must be in the leadership attitude which all parents must have during the normal development of their children. And, in certain instances, firmness must be the dominant note in the therapist's attitude (although the understanding and fellow-feeling attitude must always persist strongly as well). Absolute firmness is necessary in the presence of great anxiety or of panic or when there is actual danger to the patient or to others; a depressed patient may be made to feel more guilty when tolerance and acceptance are accentuated and less guilty when strict firmness is emphasized; a dependent patient may need emphatic firmness as a prerequisite for a therapeutic relationship; a patient afraid of his own inability to control his unacceptable defenses may require great firmness as an essential aspect of the therapist's attitude.

Along with the above tolerance-and-firmness combination as the response to the layer of defenses, the therapist must respond to the layer of anxiety. Again his response must be generally the same, with individual variations in specific situations. In general, his response must be one of human friendship and warmth and reassurance, of providing a certain security and feeling of acceptance, which often acts as a force to lessen anxiety. The therapist must somehow put across to the patient the fact that he now provides a new potential source of strength. He must transmit to the patient the vital reassurance that an adult of some strength and experience will now try to help him solve some of the problems that have led to anxiety and that the therapist believes the patient to be capable of learning how to meet his conflicts and anxiety more adequately than before. When it is true, he must give the patient the feeling that the situation, external or internal, does not call for the amount of anxiety which he now has. Often the therapist, by his detachment and objectivity and by his emphasis on talking of hidden problems, creates in the patient a greater objectivity, with the feeling that the anxiety is not so threatening as it seemed to be. Still another factor in lessening the patient's anxiety is that the therapist does not join in the patient's anxiety, even when the patient has told him of a condition or situation which has evoked great anxiety in the patient himself.

In addition to such general security-giving aspects of the therapeutic attitude, the therapist tries in more specific ways, whenever he can, to lessen or undercut or eliminate the anxiety. If the therapist knows the nature of the specific anxiety which has led to the defenses, his reassurance can be more pointed, and he gives specific information or clarification or interpretation. If he knows that the aggressively hostile boy is defending himself against anxiety based on distorted ideas about the effects of masturbation, he can give emphatic reassurance. If he does not know the specific anxiety, a large part of his therapeutic work will consist of attempts to discover the dynamic conflicts which are operative in the anxiety (if such exploration is not contraindicated in the particular case); he then works directly to alleviate the anxiety by comments or explanations or attitudes which will change the dynamic picture. It is to be emphasized that in such a dynamic exploration and therapy there is implicit the fact that the therapist believes the individual patient to be strong enough to use the insight—a fact which in itself tends to alleviate anxiety. In summary, the therapeutic attitude toward the second layer—the anxiety—consists of offering a certain general security and affection and help and reassurance, and a specific reassurance when specific anxieties are evident or uncovered.

Along with the response to the "upper" two layers, the therapist must have a healthy positive attitude toward the third layer—the basic personality. This is not difficult with patients whose anxiety and defenses have not prevented the obvious development of many trends toward maturity and strength and achievement. But, even with other, less fortunate patients, he must somehow sense, with conviction, that, underneath the defenses and the anxiety which are so disturbing to the patients or to others, there exist important aspects of the personality which are worthy of respect. The therapist must know that with many of his most neurotic patients he is dealing with persons who fundamentally are likable and worth while and who have potentialities for self-development which have been blocked by unfortunate external or internal forces. With some of his patients, in whom he finds layer after layer of defensive distortions, he must know that beneath all these distortions is the inborn capacity for healthy development. He must have a genuine regard for his patients as human beings and know that they are, or could be, worthy of warmth, of respect, and of acceptance. If the therapist has such a conviction of his patients' fundamental acceptability, the patients will know it, even though it remains unspoken. And it is probable that no psychotherapy of lasting value can be done unless the therapeutic atmosphere includes such a response to the basic personality.

In connection with the above material about the three-layer concept as it relates to therapeutic attitude, the following should be added: Mistakes in psychotherapy are often based on an overemphasis on one or another of the three layers. An overemphasis on the anxiety layer may lead the therapist to have too sympathetic and permissive an attitude, which can have a noxious, rather than a therapeutic, effect. A strongly permissive attitude should be the result of the fact that the patient requires such an attitude for therapeutic reasons (e.g., because his parents were too punitive and prohibiting); a strongly permissive attitude should not be the result of the therapist's being too impressed by the patient's anxiety. Further, an overemphasis on the layer of defenses may lead to an underestimation of the need to respond to the other two layers as well, so that the therapist's approach becomes superficial and often punishing or rejecting or controlling. The essential point is that the therapeutic attitude must include responses to all three layers of the patient's personality and that the modifications in therapeutic emphasis must be based on the dynamics of the problem at hand, not on an inadequate orientation to the general problem of therapy or on the countertransference problems of the therapist.

C. GENETIC DIAGNOSIS

Whenever possible, psychiatric therapy should be based not only on clinical and dynamic diagnoses but also on genetic diagnosis. This last term refers to an understanding of the origin and development of the patient's personality and current conflicts and to an appraisal of the situations, experiences, and reactions which led to the development of the current dynamic constellation.

A passing comment on terminology must be made. Students trained in biology occasionally infer that the term "genetic diagnosis" connotes heredity or constitution, since in biology the term "genetic" is the adjective referring to the genes and chromosomes. In psychiatry the term "genetic diagnosis" refers to the totality of those forces involved in the genesis and origin of current forces; such genetic forces are hereditary or constitutional in small part but are predominantly a matter of early life-experience and individual reactions.

As typical examples of the genetic factors which are to be considered in individual cases seen in psychotherapy, the following can be cited: prolonged contact of the patient as a child with an adult whose personality or behavior provided material for unhealthy identification; cruelty, deprivation, overindulgence, overstimulation, excessive gratification, intimidation, or inconsistency, in infancy; problems of weaning and toilet training; problems of infantile sexuality; development of attitudes of fear and envy and feelings of inadequacy in connection with sexuality (e.g., the little girl's envy of the penis and the little boy's anxiety about castration); a pervasive disturbing atmosphere in childhood (e.g., emanating from a sadistic father) which was productive of early anxiety; specific traumatic experiences, e.g., a circumcision for which the child was not prepared, at a time when he expected drastic punishment for his activity or wishes; only-child or oldest-child or youngest-child or middle-child experiences. These and a host of other life-experiences which, occurring with undue intensity or at a vulnerable period in the life of the child or in a particular sequence or configuration, may have led to the development of the unhealthy aspects of the child's personality, to those forces which currently are operative in producing the patient's disorder.

The genetic factors leading to strength (such as identification with an emotionally healthy older sibling) must also be included in the evaluation, since the sources of relative maturity provide therapeutic leads, as do the sources of unhealthy development.

It must be stressed that genetic diagnosis must include an understanding not only of the environmental forces which impinged on the patient earlier in life, for better or for worse, but also the patient's reactions to those forces, his impulse stirrings, his anxiety, his defenses, and his fantasy distortions of the environment, either at the time or in retrospect.

To illustrate the content of a genetic diagnosis, the group of patients with peptic ulcer referred to above may be considered again. The predominant elements in the dynamic diagnosis were their strong unconscious dependent trends and their narcissistic rejection of dependency as weakness. The genetic diagnosis would then be the statement of the origin of both the dependency pattern and the excessively high standards. For example, the genetic diagnosis might include the fact that in childhood such a patient was seriously unwanted, unloved, and rejected, leading, on the one hand, to a lifelong hunger for love and protective care, i.e., for dependent satisfactions, and, on the other hand, to the attitude that never again will he permit himself to be in a position of weak dependency when he might be hurt or humiliated. Or in another case the dependent attitude might have had its origin as a regression, as a flight from the fears connected with genital sexuality, and the excessive rejection of dependent roles might be based on a fantasy of the bodily dangers related to passive dependent homosexual impulses.

Therapeutic decisions and procedures are, in various ways, based on an understanding of such genetic factors. If dependency trends and excessively high standards have their genesis in the childhood experience of serious rejection, the therapist must know that the therapy will involve a long period of the patient's testing him out to see if the therapist will reject him. He will know that he must have unending patience and acceptance and must refuse to be provoked into a rejecting attitude. But he must set realistic limits (e.g., not permit the patient to phone him at all hours), even though the patient may construe the setting of limits as a rejection. If such limits are not set, the patient may develop a too dependent attitude. And, more important, if such realistic limits are not in force, the patient may fail to have the necessary living experience that there can be patterns of adjustment other than his usual dichotomy of either being totally dependent or being rejected.

In the above example it is apparent that the genetic diagnosis determines some of the therapist's attitudes and behavior. If, in addition, insight therapy along genetic lines is to be used, it is obvious that the interpretive comments made to the patient must be based on an understanding of the genetic diagnosis.

One essential aspect of genetic diagnosis in relation to therapy is the attempt to establish the relative importance of fixation and of regression. In an impotent man it is of importance to know whether his impotence is essentially based on regressive patterns—i.e., is based on childhood experiences and reactions which led him to have and to retain a fear of masculine sexuality and its supposed dangers—and whether such experiences then led him to regress to the attitude of wanting to be a protected baby instead of a man. In such a case the impotence then would have at least two sources: his fear of sexual activity itself (and what it symbolizes) and, second, his fear that sexual activity, as a sign of being a man, would jeopardize his hoped-for role of being a protected baby. In another patient the impotence may be much more a product of fixation. Then the impotence would not be related to childhood experiences that led to fear of masculine sexuality or to a regression to the role of being protected but, instead, would be based primarily on experiences that led to fixation at a level before the development of strong masculine impulses or fantasies. Overindulgence or its opposite, severe rejection, in the first two years of life is an example of the type of experience which can lead to an enormous accentuation of the need passively to be loved, to be protected, to be treated as a baby. In such a case the later impotence would not be the expression of a fear of masculinity or of the loss of the dependent position assumed in flight but fundamentally would be the direct continuation of a very early pattern, that nothing must be allowed to jeopardize the possibility of receiving a baby's type of love. There the impotence would be the result of a fixation on oral dependency, and masculine potency is to be avoided as representing maturity, responsibility, and a giving attitude, which would be at variance with the lifelong orientation toward passivity. Further, such an oral fixation may lead to marked feelings of inadequacy and inferiority, since the patient comes to feel weak and childlike. In the face of adult situations to be met, the patient may feel totally inadequate and afraid, emotions which, in turn, can interfere with his masculine performance. (Again, a warning against regarding such a teaching formulation as complete, e.g., most patients with impotence also have serious problems in the area of hostile aggressiveness.)

The pertinence to therapy of genetic formulations which include the problem of "regression versus fixation" can be phrased in this way (and usually it is not an "either-or" decision but one of relative emphasis): If the emphasis, genetically, is on regression, it must be recognized that the patient had previously made some strong developmental thrusts toward maturity, which may be repeated in the treatment with greater chance of success, and hence the prognosis is better. Often, if the emphasis is on regression, the patient has greater ego strength, is more able to make use of the therapist's help and more able to go along with a more rapid therapy. If the emphasis is on regression from anxiety about something (e.g., masculine sexuality) which is fundamentally acceptable to the adult ego, the efforts of the therapist receive assistance from the adult strivings of the patient and from the added increment of pleasure which the patient knows improvement will bring. If the emphasis is on fixation, however, the therapist is in a sense asking the patient to give up a pleasure, or a hoped-for pleasure (dependency), around which his whole life has been oriented and to substitute for it a pleasure toward which he has developed little or no drive, which is for him rather hypothetical. More directly, the implications for therapy in this problem are these: Emphasis on regression permits more active therapy, emphasis on fixation calls for slower, more cautiously dosed attempts at therapy. Emphasis on regression permits a greater implication of the need to face and conquer anxiety and a greater chance that, in the setting of the therapeutic situation, life can be met more directly and effectively, and successful life-experiences can add their curative value. Emphasis on fixation calls for the expectation of a much more protracted therapy (if it can be done at all), in which a prolonged process of gradual identification with the therapist may be the most effective tool of modification. In addition, in the patients in whom fixation is more important than regression the therapist must concentrate his attention, his attitudes, and his comments on the pregenital problems, in the hope that through the patient-physician experience and through insight some resolution of the fixation may take place; in the patients in whom regression is more important the therapist may concentrate his attention on the patient's hidden anxiety about masculinity and maturity, anxiety toward the therapist, toward current situations in the patient's life, and toward the important figures of his childhood.

Another aspect of the relevance of genetic understanding to therapy: If the therapist becomes convinced that the patient's childhood was permanently and basically disfiguring to his personality, he may decide that little can be done and that he must limit his therapy to superficial techniques, such as environmental manipulation or some supportive contact. Even in such superficial psychotherapy, genetic understanding is of value; if the therapist recognizes that the patient, in childhood, had a good relationship only with an elderly aunt, he may try to arrange for a therapeutic contact with a social case worker who is older than the patient.

The last statement—on the choice of a woman therapist—deserves some amplification, since the whole problem of the choice of a therapist offers a good example of the use of genetic data in therapeutic work. If, for example, it is clear that in childhood a man patient had an extremely conflictful relation with his father and other men figures but fairly good relations with his mother and sisters, it probably would be best to arrange for a woman therapist; otherwise, the transference distortions with a man therapist may be too great to permit perspective and the growth of insight. If the patient then matures in therapy, a period of therapeutic work with a man therapist may be advisable. On the other hand, the opposite decision as to male or female therapist may be made in another case if the childhood conflict was not quite so intense and the patient is more mature and evinces greater strength. If, for example, a male patient, with a relatively strong adjustment capacity, had a childhood characterized by slight problems with his mother and moderate problems with his father, the decision might well be to have him treated from the beginning by a male therapist. Usually such a patient will not develop too great distortions in his transference attitudes. Further, it will be of high value in the therapy to have him confronted with the need for an adjustment with a new father-figure, to have his problems with fathers mobilized by the situation, to have the corrective emotional experience of a good relationship with a father-figure, and (if insight therapy is used) to develop insight into his own problems in relation to authoritative male figures.

The above type of application of genetic understanding to therapeutic work has its greatest sphere of usefulness in psychoanalytic therapy. But it is applicable in less deep-going contacts. A man internist may decide to treat a patient himself or refer the patient to a woman internist or psychiatric case worker (granting that all are qualified for the type of therapy they are attempting) on the basis of genetic considerations such as those given above.

D. Transference

It will be apparent that a good part of the material of the following two sections (on transference and countertransference) could logically be included as part of the preceding sections. But an emphasis on transference and countertransference is so vital to the student's orientation and understanding and so important in work with individual patients that it seems best to present them as independent topics.

Until the development of psychoanalytic therapy by Freud, little attention was paid to the physician-patient relationship, other than to make use of the passive dependent attitudes of patients for the purpose of authoritarian orders or suggestions. Other attitudes of patients were taken personally and were regarded as lack of co-operation, as stubbornness, as disturbing attachments, as situations to escape, or as adulation which was pleasing to the physician's pride and competitive strivings. Fortunately, Freud's use of the technique of relaxed free association and his close attention to the nuances of meaning of the patients' talk and attitudes and behavior led him to see the essential importance of the patient-physician relationship, which now plays a crucial role in dynamic psychotherapy.

Freud saw that patients often reacted to the therapist in many ways that were not logical or appropriate to the actual situation of patient and doctor. With no provocation on the part of the physician, patients may develop fear, hostility, suspicion, resentment, defiance, undue dependence, excessive compliance, love, idolatry, contempt, etc. For these spontaneous, excessive, illogical, and inappropriate reactions he suggested the term "transference," to indicate that the dynamic meaning of such responses was that the patient was reacting to the therapist not in terms of reality but in terms of transferring to the therapist feelings and reactions which he had had to other important figures in his life, particularly his parents.

The term "transference" actually has a somewhat broader meaning than is indicated by the concept of "transferring" from one to another. It refers to all the patient's illogical reactions to the therapist, including his stereotyped and patterned responses applied when they are not appropriate, his various automatically applied defenses, his attempts to satisfy ungratified wishes, and his projection of his own conscience attitudes.

Such transference reactions exist alongside the more appropriate reactions to the physician, of a realistic acceptance of him as someone who is trying to help and to cure, as an experienced, trained person in whom the patient can have a reasonable trust and confidence.

In psychotherapy, the attitudes of the patient to the therapist must be of profound importance, since psychotherapy consists largely of the transmission from patient to therapist and from therapist to patient of words, of attitudes, of interpersonal contacts. The tools of interpersonal communication (and so of psychotherapy) are language, intonation, gestures, facial expressions, and behavior. Such communication between therapist and patient is dependent on the development of a workable relationship. The transference distortions of the patient may seriously interfere with such communication and therefore with the therapeutic process. Consequently, one of the basic problems of some aspects of psychotherapy is to by-pass or to minimize or to eliminate the transference distortions.

In other aspects of psychotherapy, however, the therapist, instead of trying to by-pass the transference problems, puts them in the foreground as the focus of therapy. The rationale of such a procedure can be phrased in this fashion: Emotional problems are largely based on interpersonal difficulties and frequently are expressed as interpersonal difficulties. Consequently, it is of value to have such problems under direct observation in a controlled interpersonal situation. The contact of therapist and patient offers, in a sense, a laboratory setting of a standardized procedure. If the therapist's reactions are not distorted, the distortions which arise may clearly be understood as originating from the patient. His reactions then become significant samples of his behavior and motivation, and the therapy can work directly with the transference manifestations as a reliable sampling of the patient's personality problems. The hope then is that modification of the patient's patterns in this significant situation will lead to a modification of patterns in other aspects of his life-adjustment.

From this it is clear that transference attitudes must be of great pertinence to therapy. In documenting this pertinence, one simple but fundamental point should first be made, viz., that good therapy must be based on a knowledge of the inevitability of transference manifestations. A good therapeutic attitude cannot be based on the naïve assumption that all patients will be logically co-operative, eminently reasonable, properly grateful, and so considerate that they will have illogical reactions to others but not to the therapist. If the therapist expects transference problems, he is not shocked or surprised or taken in when they appear, and he may then preserve a good therapeutic relationship. For example, if a therapist has done a good job and yet the patient becomes openly hostile and critical toward him, the therapist can recognize such a reaction as transference and deal with it objectively, without regarding the patient as an ungrateful wretch. He can avoid being angry and can thus prevent a situation in which his own resentment would block his usefulness to the patient. Or, for example, if a patient is high in his praise of the therapist and regards him as the embodiment of perfection, the therapist must avoid the temptation to be flattered and must recognize the patient's attitude as a transference distortion.

In a variety of ways specific therapeutic decisions and responses should be based on observation of the transference. In the exploratory period the transference reactions of the patient give important clues in the three categories of diagnostic thinking listed above, and so are helpful in determining the type of therapy to be used. For example, an atmosphere of coldness, of withdrawn separateness, in the attitude of the patient to the therapist may help in the making of a clinical diagnosis of schizophrenia, with the therapeutic implications of that diagnosis. If, in the introductory interviews, a depressed patient is unable to make a workable positive contact with the physician and has a transference attitude of exclusion and impenetrable self-absorption, the advisability of shock therapy concomitant with, or followed by, psychotherapy is suggested; if a depressed patient turns more rationally for help or has a transference attitude of seeking dependence and forgiveness, the possibility of further attempts at psychotherapy is suggested.

With regard to dynamic diagnosis, the transference attitudes are even more important and significant for therapy. Transference attitudes often are indicative of the patient's predominant trends, the defenses and current forces at work which are the most important to deal with in treatment. Often a patient presents a psychodynamic picture that is complicated and even chaotic; he may show, in his life-patterns and relations, various problems of dependence, aggression, sexuality, narcissism, guilt, and a variety of defenses, all apparently of significance. A rather reliable guide in estimating the immediate importance of a trend is the transference; if narcissistic attitudes toward the therapist appear with some frequency or intensity, he can be certain that such attitudes are a vital part of the current dynamic problems of the patient. As a corollary, in therapy it may be difficult to decide where "the abscess is pointing," where therapeutic work is most promising, if one relies solely on dynamic study of the patient's reactions in life. In such a case it may be extremely helpful to center the therapy about those problems which appear in the transference.

Another angle of the value of transference manifestations in dynamic diagnosis should be mentioned. If the dynamic diagnosis is based on data about the patient's relations with his family and friends, the diagnosis may at times be uncertain. The relatives or friends often have their own distortions. It may be difficult to decide whether the patient's reaction is distorted and, if so, to what degree. For example, if a woman complains repeatedly of mistreatment by her husband, one may conclude, on the basis of what she says and how she says it and on the basis of similar attitudes in the past, that she is masochistic and is exaggerating the mistreatment by her husband, or perhaps provoking it. But in some cases the conclusion will still be under question. If, then, she attempts to provoke the therapist or if she interprets his objectivity as coldness and his comments as attempts to hurt her and insult her, the doubt of the dynamic diagnosis disappears completely. In such fashion, diagnostic thinking becomes certain, and therapy more soundly based. The therapist then knows that he must avoid being provoked and must maintain a steady, firm leadership. Still further, if insight therapy is to be used, he then will have incontrovertible data for interpretation. If he were able to interpret her masochism only by referring to her relations with her husband, she might be unconvinced, saying that the therapist would agree with her if he knew her husband. If, however, he can interpret her masochism on the basis of her attitudes toward himself, he can be much more convincing.

With regard to genetic diagnosis, the transference manifestations are of high value and again give leads for treatment. If a patient regards the therapist as a father-figure and constantly seems to expect rejection, the conjecture is called for that the patient was rejected by his father, or felt rejected by his father, or had impulses toward the father (and now toward the therapist) which made him feel, out of guilt or anxiety, that he should be rejected by his father.

In such fashion, transference manifestations contribute to diagnostic decisions, clinical, dynamic, and genetic, which have therapeutic pertinence of the type described in previous portions of this chapter.

To illustrate the value of transference manifestations in dynamic understanding and therapy, a portion of the treatment of a specific case of essential hypertension can be given. In some such cases the clue to the understanding of the chronic elevation of blood pressure may be found in the transference. The patient in question was one whose life, as far as could be seen, was free of emotional conflict and problems. So far as he and his family could tell, he got along well with everyone, was liked by everyone, let nothing disturb his equilibrium. At first glance, there was nothing to suggest that there were emotional tensions in his life that might be causing a high tension in his blood pressure. In his relation with the psychiatrist he was cordial and agreeable, and it soon was obvious that he was much too amiable, too agreeable, too pleasant, too submissive. Shakespeare, long before Freud, might have said, "methinks the gentleman doth protest too much." Shakespeare, like Freud, would have been benevolently skeptical about this patient's degree of amiability and imperturbable docility. If the telephone bell interrupted an interview, he would be obviously tense and flushed, as if in anger; but he denied being angry and said that the interruptions were of no consequence, that the psychiatrist was a very busy man who must take his calls, and that he, the patient, did not mind it in the least. From many sequences such as this in his behavior with the psychiatrist, the inference became highly probable that beneath his calm exterior there existed intense reactions of anger, which are known to be associated with a rise of blood pressure. This dynamic diagnosis of an underlying unexpressed hostility was verified when, during treatment, he repeatedly had dreams of obvious hostility, such as shooting an enormous fountain-pen-full of muddy black ink over the face of a man he did not recognize, who had a small mustache, who was partly bald, who wore steel-rimmed glasses, and whose business seemed to consist of trying to look through a skull with X-ray eyes. The patient did not recognize his victim in the dream, but from the description it was obvious that it was the therapist, whose work as a psychiatrist might be lampooned as an attempt to look into heads with X-ray eyes. In essence, a study of the patient's transference revealed the dynamic picture of a façade of excessive amiability concealing intense unexpressed hostility, which may have been associated with his hypertension.

Such dynamic understanding, of which the transference data

are an essential part, has clear-cut implications for therapy. In such a case the therapist must not be too appreciative of the patient's considerateness and amiability and docility. He will know that the patient will agree with any interpretation that the therapist makes, in order to be agreeable and friendly, even if he is unconvinced or if he disagrees. The therapist must know that hostility which is so denied and so concealed by totally opposite behavior must provoke serious anxiety in the patient and, consequently, that "bull-in-the-china-shop" early interpretations must be avoided. The therapist must work for the creation and development of a relationship in which the patient will feel safe enough to have some hostility, to express it slightly, and eventually to recognize and not be concerned about the fact that he has certain hostile tendencies. Then, if genetic material is to be worked through in a psychoanalysis, the patient can eventually come to understand and to modify some of the sources of his excessive hostility or of his superego strictness which would not countenance even a trace of hostility.

Another point to indicate the importance of transference in therapeutic procedures is this: By emphasizing transference problems, the therapist is dealing with actual current living experiences which are vividly meaningful to the patient, and the therapy may have an immediacy and aliveness that otherwise may be difficult to achieve. Interpretation of past events and reactions often has a distant and unconvincing quality that may disappear completely when they are seen from a fresh point of view, arising out of an understanding of the immediate living relationship with the therapist.

Further, in psychotherapy a lessening of transference problems may clear the way for acceptance of insight along other lines; if the patient has an unresolved attitude of being mistreated by the therapist, it will be difficult for him to accept as helpful any comments made by the therapist about the other aspects of his life-adjustment. Consequently, in psychotherapy with some patients (particularly those who are likely to develop negative transference attitudes) a clarification of transference distortions becomes the first essential of the therapy.

Another item: for various reasons, the patient often resists the efforts of the therapist to help him. The whole problem of such "resistance" in psychotherapy often can best be handled through the transference, since many types of resistance tend to focus on the relationship between patient and therapist. The resistance based on anxiety over becoming aware of unconscious trends, the resistance based on the urge to avoid the narcissistic blows of having to admit mistakes or of being helped by someone else, the resistance based on fear of being dominated by another person, the resistance based on the urge not to give up infantile pleasures, all lead to defenses directed toward the therapist and can best be dealt with by attention to transference problems.

In essence, then, treatment which is based on adequate understanding of transference manifestations has many advantages: clinical, dynamic, and genetic diagnoses are made more clear and reliable; leads become apparent for the focusing of attempts at therapy; and insight and corrective emotional experiences are made far more productive.

E. COUNTERTRANSFERENCE

It seems probable, although there is no statistical evidence to support the conclusion, that countertransference accounts for a large percentage of mistakes and failures in psychiatric treatment. For example, shock treatment may be used inappropriately because the psychiatrist is unwilling to use more time-consuming methods or because he is unduly aggressive or because he is unable to withstand the family's urging that he do something drastic immediately. Another example: Psychotherapy, in a modifiable patient, may fail because the therapist is unable to resist being hostile and rejecting when the patient is provocative. Consequently, it is urgent that all therapists have a vivid understanding of countertransference problems and of their implication for therapy.

In the previous section, the debt of psychiatry to Freud for the concept of transference was indicated. But Freud did not stop with the understanding of the transference. He realized that all human relations are two-way streets, that the patient is not the only fallible human being in the interaction of patient and physician. In fact, in all of the contacts of two human beings, it must be recognized that both may be responding illogically as well as logically. When a husband complains that his wife is behaving irrationally toward him, the psychiatrist who hears the story must wonder if the husband also does not behave irrationally toward his wife and perhaps provoke some of her illogical behavior. When a mother complains that her child reacts with defiance and antagonism to her, the psychiatrist must wonder if the mother also is not reacting illogically to the child. And so Freud put the question, What of the medical two-way street, what of the physician's reactions to the patient? And, observing himself, with his customary courage and honesty, Freud discovered certain tendencies in himself that were inappropriate and tended to interfere with his successful work with patients. Subsequently, he made the same observation in supervising the work of the physicians he was training in the use of his new techniques. For this phenomenon—the distorted reactions of physicians to patients—Freud suggested the technical term of "countertransference."

Some examples, taken from the general practice of medicine, can be given to indicate typical mistakes based on countertransference. A physician who is too sympathetic with sick people may pamper his patients, may make them realize too vividly that sickness has its pleasures, and so prolong his patients' convalescence. On the other hand, a physician who is overdemanding that his patients be strong and mature and self-reliant may do injury by holding up to his patients an impossible ideal. Patients of such a physician may become excessively critical of their own human limitations, may ignore their actual need for rest, for leisure, and for recuperation, and may struggle too strenuously to be as strong as the physician expects them to be.

Every physician must resist the importunities of some of his patients for more and more medicine. If the physician has the personality characteristic of being unable to say "No," of being too amiable and agreeable, he is very likely to give too much medicine to demanding patients or to patients who play on his sympathy. And, of course, the excessive use of medicine has its dangers, of drug addiction or of undue dependence on medicine or of some accumulated physical effects of the medicine itself.

Another type of mistake is based on what can be called excessive therapeutic ambition. All physicians must have some therapeutic ambition, must want to help their patients, must try in part to build their security and prestige by being successful, by curing their patients as quickly as possible. Such therapeutic ambition is of real value to the doctor and to the patient. But therapeutic ambition may be excessive and defeat its own ends. If the physician is very insecure and has too great a need for fame and fortune, he may then have too great a need for cured cases, for the kind of case he can boast about or expect others to boast about for him. He may then become impatient with those who do not respond or may, in an open or concealed fashion, be angry and resentful toward them. Some medical problems are complicated and difficult to solve, requiring patient consideration of a number of diagnostic possibilities and the use of one after another of therapeutic attempts until the problem is solved. The emotions of anger and resentment that arise in the doctor when excessive therapeutic ambition is thwarted are not conducive to clear thinking or to the gradual working-through of a difficult medical problem. Furthermore, a patient may sense the physician's impatience and resentment and become anxious or resentful or self-critical, so that a secondary neurotic problem is superimposed on the primary problem, which is still unsolved.

Another example of countertransference has to do with the unnecessary stimulation of anxiety in patients by a physician who likes to be totally safe in his diagnoses, who has an excessive fear that some other physician who may later examine the patient will find something that the first physician has missed. In moderate degree such concern for one's reputation is valid and appropriate and one of the safeguards of medical practice, tending to assure adequate and careful examinations. But, like all good things, such concern can be overdone. The physician who is excessively afraid of the opinions of others may try to protect himself by avoiding definite diagnoses, may try to straddle the fence so that, no matter what happens later, he cannot be said to have missed a point. If such a physician examines a patient who thinks he may have heart disease, does a thorough job plus whatever special examinations are called for, and finds absolutely nothing except an almost surely functional murmur, the physician may then be unable to give the necessary reassurance. He may damage the patient and help to produce a cardiac neurosis by remarking that the examination is essentially negative but that there is a little murmur that might be watched or that the patient's heart is in fine shape but that it might be better not to take quite so much exercise as before. Such excessively conservative statements produce anxiety which is totally unnecessary. They may protect the physician from criticism in an occasional case, but at the expense of the well-being of some of his patients.

The above examples were chosen from the general practice of medicine, to indicate that countertransference is a problem not only of psychiatry but of all attempts at human helpfulness.

The specific countertransference mistakes indicated in these examples, e.g., excessive therapeutic ambition, are, of course, problems of psychiatric therapy as well. In fact, countertransference problems are more frequent in psychiatry than in general medical practice, in part because psychotherapy makes greater use of the patient-physician relationship and in part because the psychiatric atmosphere is to some degree permissive and the patient is more likely to express feelings or attitudes that may stir counterreactions on the part of the psychiatrist. Further, countertransference problems are important in psychiatry because the psychiatrist so frequently tries to modify the patient's adjustment, an attempt that often arouses resistive defenses on the part of the patient, which, in turn, may lead to inappropriate responses on the part of the psychiatrist. If the patient uses the defense against the treatment of appealing for sympathy, the psychiatrist may become too sympathetic or may have an attitude of contempt for one who seeks sympathy. If the patient defends himself against change or against unpleasant insight by attacking the psychiatrist as a threat, the psychiatrist, in turn, may counterattack or become frightened and appeasing. Another patient may defend himself against the arousal of guilt feelings by the time-honored technique of feeling less guilty if one can make someone else feel guilty. In such a defense he may try to make the psychiatrist feel guilty over having done something, over not having done something, or over not having achieved a cure. The psychiatrist, even though he has done his best, may easily make the mistake of feeling guilty. Obviously, such countertransference reactions may give the patient momentary satisfaction, but they have no therapeutic value and may delay the patient's recovery.

In psychiatric practice, countertransference reactions may appear even when they are not mobilized by specific reactions on the part of the patient, as in the above examples. A therapist may be afraid of older women and so with older women patients may have an attitude of anxiety or of defensive aloofness or of aggressive domination. Or a man therapist may have excessive competitive attitudes toward men of his own age, and with such patients may have a need to show that he is brighter, quicker, more successful, and better adjusted. In such circumstances he unconsciously may be averse to having the patient improve and thereby become a stronger potential competitor. Or the therapist may have a lifelong defense of his own of overintellectualization, and so his contact with patients becomes a sterile intellectual game instead of an interpersonal process that includes feeling tones, warm human contact, and understanding empathy.

Countertransference problems may lead psychiatrists to an incorrect evaluation of their patients' conflicts. One psychiatrist may be unable to see some of the important problems of his patients because they are problems which he does not want to see in himself. His defense is trying to ignore the existence of such problems altogether, and so he cannot see them in his patients even when they are of central importance. Another psychiatrist may see too much instead of too little, may believe that some of his patients have certain conflicts which actually are not present or are of little consequence. His mistake is based on a defense which is different from that used by the other psychiatrist. He attempts to alleviate his anxiety over some conflict of his own by imputing that conflict to others in an even greater degree, so that his own seems unimportant by comparison. With such a defense, he may come to believe that some insignificant problems of his patients are of high importance in their psychodynamic picture.

The implications of the countertransference for therapy need hardly be detailed, since they are obvious, once the problem is stated. Some of the implications are these: The therapist need not be shocked if he has countertransference problems, since they are universal; but he must not permit himself to act out his tendencies to the detriment of the patient. If his distorted reactions are mild and under control, he need not be concerned about them. If they are intense or out of control, he needs psychotherapy for himself. If he finds that he has difficulty with one type of patient, he should refer such patients to other therapists until he has lessened his own problem.

In general, the safeguards against the interference of countertransference with therapy consist of intensive supervision over an adequate period of time with an adequate variety of patients, stringently honest self-scrutiny, and psychotherapy of the therapist.

It is apparent, then, that treatment in psychiatry has a much greater chance of success if the countertransference is minimal and undisturbing. In such circumstance, mistakes in diagnosis and therapy can be lessened, the transference reactions are more significant and more reliable tools of treatment, the patient has a far greater chance to correct his mistaken expectations in interpersonal relations, and the therapist's responses and comments are far more likely to be suited to the actual needs of the therapy.

F. Treatment Possibilities

The treatment of an individual patient is dependent on the points of understanding outlined in the preceding five sections. In addition, the following must be taken into consideration in reaching decisions about therapy: (1) the specific techniques of treatment which may be suitable; (2) the training and skill of the therapist in the use of specific techniques; and (3) the practical aspects of treatment. The remainder of this chapter will consist of an elaboration of these points.

1. TECHNIQUES OF PSYCHIATRIC TREATMENT

The following groups of therapeutic procedures for the amelioration or cure of psychiatric difficulties may be listed:

a) Procedures intended essentially for the protection, safety, and general care of the patient, his family, and society. They include hospitalization (at times commitment) of seriously disturbed patients; prevention of aggressive acting-out (suicide, antisocial behavior); custodial care of those unable to care for themselves, e.g., the feeble-minded; specific procedures of general care, e.g., feeding of patients who refuse to eat, hydrotherapy in states of excitement. In the use of such procedures, their psychotherapeutic implications must be considered as well as their more obvious purposes. For example, hospitalization may provide a valuable temporary satisfaction of dependent needs but, like all such satisfactions, runs the risk of stimulating regressive tendencies. Another example: Individuals who are near panic because of their anxiety that some unacceptable unconscious impulses may break through may find the restrictions of hospital life a welcome auxiliary source of control.

b) Procedures aimed at a correction of structural pathologic processes, e.g., surgical removal of a brain tumor or evacuation of a subdural hematoma.

c) Procedures aimed at a correction of pathophysiologic processes, e.g., medicinal and other treatment of delirium tremens and bromide delirium; medicinal and fever treatment of paresis; thyroid medication in cretinism.

d) Medicinal or surgical treatment to ameliorate some of the physiologic concomitants of emotion, e.g., the limited use of sedatives and antispasmodics in anxiety-tension states; the use of stimulants in certain depressive states; the use of hypnotics when insomnia is troublesome; vagotomy in some cases of peptic ulcer. In such circumstance, when the problem is essentially psychogenic, it is often wise to be direct with the patient about the role of the medicinal treatment and to state clearly to him that the medicine is not intended to be a cure but rather to give symptomatic relief and that some variety of more direct dealing with his personality problems is in order.

e) The use in selected cases of such physical methods of therapy as electric shock treatment and insulin coma (see also chap. x). A variety of modifications and combinations of physical methods of therapy have been developed in recent years, and the student is referred to the pertinent literature for a statement of techniques and procedures (5, 23, 24, 41). The chief current procedures are those of electro-convulsive therapy and insulin coma therapy, in which patients are in the one instance subjected to an electric current through the brain substance, with the production of a convulsion, and in the other are given enough insulin to produce a response of several hours of hypoglycemic coma. The electro-convulsive procedure is usually repeated some five to fifteen times over a period of several weeks. The insulin coma procedure is usually repeated some twenty to sixty times over a period of several months. Electro-convulsive therapy seems to have its greatest sphere of usefulness in severe depressions which usually are labeled "manic-depressive" and "involutional melancholia," and in many instances when psychotherapy is unpromising it is the treatment of choice. It may be of value in certain other cases, in bringing about an increased interpersonal contact which is basic for psychotherapy. Insulin coma therapy seems to be of value in the treatment of some cases of early schizophrenia. It seems probable that in most instances shock therapy should be combined with appropriate psychotherapy.

The rationale of these physical methods of treatment is far from established. Many physiologic explanations have been offered, but none is accepted generally. Various attempts at a psychodynamic formulation of the influence of such treatment have also been offered. It has been suggested that the treatment arouses a fear of death, which leads to a defensive attempt at a re-establishment of contact with the world of reality. It has been suggested that the treatment offers a punishment which is avidly seized on by the guilt-laden patient as a way of doing penance and receiving absolution and thus rendering unnecessary any further self-punishment, which had been the motivating force in some of his previous symptoms; this would apply particularly to the self-destructive tendencies of the depressed patient. It has also been suggested that the treatment may work especially in patients whose resistance to interpersonal influence had blocked any attempt at psychotherapy or workable personal contact but who now in shock therapy are up against overwhelming physical forces which cannot be resisted, with the end-result that the patient gives up his pattern of resistance and begins to conform.

Other physical methods of treatment are now being investigated: lobotomy, which involves a surgical interruption of pathways between frontal cortex and subcortical structures, and topectomy, which involves a surgical removal of small areas of cortical substance.

f) Psychotherapy, which may be roughly defined as the carrying-through of a planned program for modifying the emotional life and adjustment of the patient, through new life-experiences and psychologic processes which can influence the patient in the direction of health. Most often this occurs in the setting of an interpersonal relationship between one patient and one therapist.

In a textbook of dynamic psychiatry, it is this form of psychiatric treatment which should receive greatest attention. In the following pages, the most useful modes of psychotherapy are summarized.

One general comment is necessary before embarking on a discussion of the techniques of psychotherapy. In line with the persistent emphasis in this chapter on the fact that psychotherapy must be based on adequate diagnostic understanding, it is clear that any type of psychotherapeutic approach must be preceded by an exploratory period of one to ten interviews with the patient. Such an exploratory period will provide an opportunity for the accumulation of significant clinical, dynamic, and genetic material, so that decisions can be made as to the variety of psychotherapy to be considered. In such an exploratory period the explorer must have an adequate therapeutic attitude, in order to avoid doing damage. And occasionally a good therapeutic attitude during the exploratory period will lead to an amelioration of the presenting symptoms.

In this connection it must be stressed that even a single consultation interview or examination must be thought of in therapeutic as well as diagnostic terms. With such an emphasis, it is possible to avoid having the experience be traumatic or antitherapeutic. With such a therapeutic attitude, a therapeutic gain is possible even from a single contact. And if the consultation leads to the recommendation that treatment is indicated, acceptance of the recommendation will be facilitated if the consultation itself had a therapeutic orientation. In brief, a diagnostic consultation must not concentrate so intently on the eliciting of information of diagnostic value that the therapeutic implications of the consultation are forgotten.

To return for a moment to the exploratory period and the understanding which is its goal. From the preceding sections of this chapter the student may have the impression that in all cases the exploratory period must lead to a rather thorough understanding of clinical, dynamic, and genetic diagnosis, of transference and countertransference. Thoroughness is of value in many instances, but unnecessary in others. For example, in the study of a patient who may have delirium tremens, the clinical diagnosis is at first the important consideration, for the determination of the immediate treatment regime. The other facets of the study are at that time of only secondary value. Later, during the treatment of the delirium, an understanding of some of the other aspects of the case may occasionally be useful. For example, the patient's attitude to his parents and his customary modes of dealing with authority may give leads that can be of value in the management of his reactions on the ward. Still later, when the delirium is over and the question of psychotherapy in the treatment of the patient's chronic alcoholism becomes the central issue, the other aspects of psychiatric study, e.g., dynamic and genetic appraisal, become crucial. In other words, the psychiatric study must be oriented around the pertinent goals of therapy at the time that the study is made.

PSYCHOTHERAPEUTIC PROCEDURES

Psychotherapeutic procedures, rather artificially, may be subdivided in the following fashion:

a) Indirect psychotherapy.—Indirect psychotherapy consists of procedures which influence the patient indirectly through having a direct effect on his surroundings. One example is environmental manipulation, i.e., a modification of the external living conditions to lessen noxious pressures or to provide a more beneficial type of influence. A simple example of this is the placement of a child in a well-chosen foster-home. Another type of indirect psychotherapy is the treatment of a parent to produce changes in his attitudes toward the child who was the original patient. In this type of indirect psychotherapy, the emphasis is on the improvement of some key person in the child's surroundings rather than on removing the child from the environment or manipulating it in some other fashion.

At times the treatment of a parent may be concurrent with the direct treatment of the child. Usually the two are treated by different therapists, to avoid such complications as the competitive struggle for the attention of a single therapist. There is another, rather paradoxical, reason for having such a tandem arrangement. If the parent has a separate therapist, there is a greater possibility that the therapy of the parent will not be too exclusively related to the needs of the child. Even though the original recommendation for treatment of the parent was motivated by the needs of the child, it will usually be found that the parent in treatment is more likely to make progress if he or she feels that his or her interests are not being neglected and that he or she has a right to happiness and to therapy on his or her own. To have a therapy of one's own, like a "room of one's own," can satisfy deep needs and can provide a basis for improvement which then can be reflected in a more productive relationship with the child.

These comments on the parent as a patient suggest the relevance of a more general comment, that, even when the parent is not officially a patient, a therapeutic attitude toward the parent (and other relatives) is worth having. When the parent obviously is behaving in a disturbing fashion toward a child, it is easy for the child's therapist to develop hostile attitudes toward the parent in their incidental contacts. Such hostility often provokes unmanageable guilt or counterhostility in the parent, which may then be expressed toward the child. Consequently, the therapist's attitude toward the parent should, in general, be one of regarding the parent as being, in a sense, an incidental patient also and thus of having toward the parent a noncondemning, accepting attitude along with an attitude of firmness and an expectation of sincere attempts at more mature behavior. Strongly critical attitudes to relatives of patients or strongly sympathetic and forgiving attitudes are valuable only in special instances, when they happen to meet the dynamic needs of the relatives themselves. Such attitudes are to be used, not as an expression of the therapist's emotional reactions, but as a technique of helpfulness to the relatives and the patient, and only when the therapist has some conviction that they are dynamically correct.

b) *Direct psychotherapy.*—"Direct psychotherapy" is the category of procedures which influence the patient directly and which may be classified as (1) suppressive, (2) supportive, (3) relationship, and (4) expressive psychotherapy.

(1) *Suppressive psychotherapy.*—Suppressive psychotherapy employs such techniques as authoritative firmness and commands, the ignoring of symptoms and complaints, placebos used with dogmatic assurance, suggestions under hypnosis to repress symptoms, comparable waking suggestion, exhortation, and persuasion. Essentially, in this approach, the therapist acts as a dictator, as an adjunct to the forces of repression, as an omniscient and omnipotent father who expects to be obeyed.

Such an approach is aimed in part at the suppression or re-repression of unconscious material which is threatening to erupt, and at a strengthening of the usual defenses. In part, it is intended to counteract the secondary benefits of neurotic illness, such as the striving for attention and sympathy and the use of symptoms to control the environment.

It shades over into the next variety, supportive psychotherapy, and in some instances actually is a productive variety of supportive psychotherapy, if it is used in a deliberate attempt to meet a patient's need for a strong, firm, guiding, controlling hand.

In general, however, present-day psychiatry has little respect for the suppressive techniques, recognizing that they are often used without reference to the actual psychodynamic problem and that, even if they have some effect at times, they leave the problem unsolved and the patient seriously vulnerable to subsequent stresses and strains.

(2) *Supportive psychotherapy.* — Supportive psychotherapy uses such components as a warm, friendly, strong-leadership type of support and reassurance; help in the development of hobbies and outlets (e.g., in occupation and recreation); symptomatic medication; adequate rest and diversion; the removal of external strain; hospitalization; the provision of a period of necessary dependence; and guidance and advice in practical issues. Group psychotherapy also may have a valuable supportive effect.

Essentially, supportive therapy uses those techniques which will make the patient feel more secure, reassured, accepted, protected, encouraged, safe, less anxious, and less alone. In good part, even a supportive psychotherapy must be individualized and be dependent on the understanding of the specific individual. For example, in one patient symptomatic medication will have excellent supportive value; in another it may mobilize sharp anxiety about the development of a drug addiction. Its goal is a rather limited one, that of offering support during a period of illness or turmoil and at times of restoring or strengthening the defenses and integrative capacities which are temporarily impaired during the illness. It provides a period of acceptance and dependence when the patient is acutely in need of help in meeting his frustrations, his guilt, and his anxiety or the external pressures which are too great for him to handle.

Often supportive psychotherapy shades over into relationship therapy or is combined with it. And supportive psychotherapy may use a limited amount of expressive psychotherapy, such as the verbalization of unexpressed emotions. The verbal expression of emotion has the value of some relief of emotional tension. And, in a therapeutic situation, the expression of emotion and its subsequent discussion may lead to a greater objectivity in evaluating a current problem. In this fashion the patient may achieve some relief of anxiety and symptoms and get help, through superficial insight, in reaching some sort of solution of a current problem or reactive upset.

The therapist must keep in mind the fact that supportive help may foster regressive tendencies and too great a dependency. He must keep in mind the obligation to avoid the development of undue dependence and the need for a persistent weaning to a resumption of independence.

In practice, supportive psychotherapy is of value in psychiatric conditions such as these: relatively mature individuals in reactive upsets largely based on extraordinarily severe environmental pressures (e.g., some traumatic neuroses, some reactive depressions); individuals who, in general, have made a rather good adjustment and are in what seems to be only a temporary period of pressure, of turmoil, of temptation, or of indecision; individuals who have been fairly responsible and giving in their life-adjustment but who now are required to give beyond their psychologic means (e.g., a wife whose husband is behaving in a more infantile fashion than usual) and who need to be given to, so that they will have more to give; individuals who are extremely resistant to expressive psychotherapy and those who the therapist concludes are fundamentally too sick to respond to expressive psychotherapy; and, finally, patients who have no drive toward a fundamental change in their adjustment and are essentially interested in a restoration of a more comfortable previous adjustment.

In some instances a period of supportive psychotherapy may lead to the joint decision that expressive psychotherapy is the procedure of choice. And the reverse in part may be true; during an expressive psychotherapy the therapist occasionally must be flexible enough to provide a period of supportive therapy.

It must be added that in the present transitional period of a plethora of patients and a paucity of psychiatrists, supportive psychotherapy at times is used not as the procedure of choice but of practical necessity.

(3) *Relationship therapy.*—Before embarking on a description of relationship therapy, a transitional comment should be made, contrasting the types of psychotherapy with regard to one essential difference, viz., the goals of therapy. It can be said that, in contrast to the supportive type of psychotherapy (described in the preceding section), a relationship psychotherapy (described in this section) and an expressive psychotherapy (to be described in the following section) have more extensive goals. The latter two types aim not only at a restoration of the *status quo ante*, at the re-establishment of a former equilibrium, but also at a change in personality patterns and at a decrease in vulnerability to external pressures.

Then, to contrast these two, it can be said that a relationship therapy has more limited goals and techniques than does expressive psychotherapy. The differences will become apparent in the description of the two in this and the subsequent section.

The present section—an attempt at a delineation of relationship therapy—provides difficulties in presentation and clarification. The concept of a relationship therapy is fundamentally a simple one, and yet it is so much a matter of atmosphere and feeling and personal interplay that a clear phrasing of its essence in brief form is difficult to achieve.

Perhaps a relationship therapy can best be described as a fairly prolonged period of contact of patient and therapist in which the therapist can maintain, without much conscious effort, a good therapeutic attitude of the sort described in previous pages of this chapter. In response to such a therapeutic attitude, the patient behaves in various ways, and there develops an interplay of feeling, of communication, and of new experience. In such a growing relationship certain therapeutic experiences occur, which may be listed in part as follows: (*a*) the experience of being accepted as of value, or potentially so, and of not being condemned or rejected because of defensive distortions; (*b*) the growth of an identification with some of the more successful techniques and adjustments of the therapist as they may fit the individual needs of the patient; and (*c*) spontaneous corrective emotional experiences, based on the fact that the therapist does not respond in the manner expected by the patient. These points will be elaborated in subsequent paragraphs.

The essence of the technique of a relationship therapy can be phrased in this way: It consists of a series of interviews in which current and past life-problems and situations and conscious conflicts and wishes and fears are discussed but in which the therapist is less interested in the dynamics of the problems than in the fostering of a good therapeutic relationship. The cornerstone of the relationship is that during the interviews the therapist has toward the patient the sort of attitude that is characteristic of a good father or mother or of a good older brother or sister.

In such an attitude and such a relationship the element of support must play a vital role, of course; a good parent or a good older sibling does offer support. In fact, a relationship therapy may, at times, use some of the specific techniques of a supportive therapy. And, in a sense, relationship therapy can be considered a protracted variety of supportive therapy, in that the therapist may see the patient over a period of months or years (usually once a week or so) in an atmosphere of friendliness and support. And such a sustaining relationship has some value on that basis alone; it offers a limited satisfaction of some of the deep needs for acceptance and dependence which develop in many patients in an attempt to counterbalance their neurotic frustrations, their guilt, and their anxiety.

But in this technique of relationship therapy the therapist avoids being too supportive, because he hopes not only to offer sustaining help but also, through his therapeutic attitude of being nonjudgmental, noncondemning, nonsubmissive, nonanxious, noncontrolling, firm, consistent, and realistic, to have a modifying effect on the patient's personality. He knows that the constant playing of the note of supportiveness is often not enough. He knows, further, that a too emphatic or a too prolonged sounding of that note may infantilize the patient. And the therapist wants the patient to obtain more from the therapy than the security and reassurance that comes from feeling supported and sustained.

Consequently, the therapist would like his attitude to include all the attitudes that can characterize the helpful parent or older sibling. A good father is not too supporting; the therapist must not be. A good father sets limits to unacceptable behavior; so must the therapist. A good father can point out mistakes; so can the therapist. A good father is not frightened by threats; nor is the therapist. A good father can be firm without hostility; so can the therapist. A good father expects a growth in self-reliance; and so should the therapist. A good father gives respect and acceptance; so does the therapist. A good father is not always good and can make mistakes; the same goes for the therapist. A good father need not try to be the perfectly good father or completely well adjusted with his children; nor need the therapist with his patients.

A further contrast of supportive therapy and relationship therapy is this: The therapist's basic role in a relationship therapy is not that of a supporting crutch but rather that of a firm, helpful friend, who wants to help and be sustaining but expects the patient to be as self-reliant and independent as he can be. The therapist would prefer to help the patient see facts and issues and alternatives, so that he can make his own decisions, rather than to try to make the patient's decisions for him. The therapist expects to disagree as well as to agree, even though the patient hopes for complete agreement and supportive approval.

Another comment to indicate that a relationship must go beyond a purely supportive attitude: The therapist hopes that his attitude of having, on the one hand, a sincere tolerance toward certain aspects of the patient's life toward which the patient had been too self-critical and self-condemning and of having, on the other hand, a clear recognition of the need for a firm, realistic setting of limits about the acting-out of unacceptable behavior will be of value in helping the patient to become mature. He hopes that such a bilateral attitude will help the patient toward a more reliable and successful variety of inner control and social adjustment and hence to a greater independence.

Such a relationship, then, may lead to specific experiences and responses and modifications in the patient. Of these, two may be singled out for special comment: (*a*) the development of healthy identifications and (*b*) some corrective emotional experiences.

The therapist hopes that some of his own more mature attitudes, which become evident in the relationship, will be incorporated by the patient as part of his own attitudes, if they seem appropriate, just as a son may incorporate some of the attitudes of a good father. In other words, the therapist hopes that the patient will, through a process of identification, adopt some of the therapist's more successful defenses and adjustments. Such identifications may tend to counterbalance some of the patient's less healthy identifications with the unfavorable influences of his childhood and lead to a greater strength, to a diminution of anxiety and defenses, and more generally, to an increase in integrative capacity.

Further, the therapist hopes that some corrective emotional experiences will occur spontaneously, viz., that the patient will somehow be influenced by the fact that the therapist's attitudes and responses are different from the ones which his personality sickness has led him to expect from others. Such a contrast between expectation and actuality (e.g., between the expectation of being able to provoke the therapist to rejection and the actuality that it does not happen) can lead to distinct modification in patterns of interpersonal relations. (It is to be noted that in a relationship therapy there is merely the general expectation that a persistently good therapeutic attitude is likely to lead to some corrective emotional experiences. In an expressive psychotherapy, however, more specific corrective experiences are likely to occur, because specific patterns are being worked through and because there may be some planning for the occurrence of specific corrective experiences which the therapist regards as central for the treatment.)

To rephrase the processes just described, it may be said that, fundamentally, a relationship therapy provides the therapist with an opportunity to behave in a fashion different from the behavior of the patient's parents and, in a sense, to neutralize or to reverse the mistakes of the parents. If the patient had overly authoritarian parents, the therapist's friendly, nonauthoritarian attitude means that the patient has an opportunity to adjust to, to be led by, and to identify with a new type of parent-figure. And, in a similar fashion, patients who had overly indulgent, overly seductive, overly passive, or inconsistent parents can now have a new starting point, of being, in a sense, brought up again by a parent who is not making such mistakes or who may be responding in a way quite different from the patterns of the parents.

In many cases the mere fact that the therapist is responding fairly maturely provides enough of a contrast with the mistaken attitudes of the parents. In other instances, however, it may be wise for the therapist to emphasize the contrast, i.e., of being quite permissive if the parents were destructively restrictive or of being emphatically firm if the parents were destructively indulgent. Obviously, in many instances the patient cannot quickly adjust to, or be influenced by, such a contrasting attitude. Hence a relationship therapy is to be regarded as a slow process, which may take months or years.

Such a phrasing of the pattern of a relationship therapy may give the false impression that the therapist is placing the total responsibility for the patient's problems in the laps of the parents. Actually, serious problems may arise in childhood even when the parental attitudes are fundamentally sound. For example, a child, with little or no provocation from the parents, may develop hostile, destructive impulses toward the parents and then expect hostile, destructive retaliation from them. In such a setting he may develop severe anxiety, be provocative toward them, or be defensively resistant. And, at that point, believing his parents to be hostile people, he may identify with his "hostile parents" and consequently have a pattern which persists. And, of course, in such a situation, even mature parents may be bewildered and anxious and be provoked to hostility, which then can be a focus for conflict and identification in the child.

A relationship therapy can fit such a pattern as the one just described, as well as the patterns in which the primary responsibility is the parents'. In the pattern in which the child's destructive feelings initiated the interaction, a relationship therapy can be effective in this way: When the patient becomes hostile to the therapist and expects hostility in return, as an adult he is now better able to see the actual fact that he is not receiving a retaliatory hostility. (As a child, he was less able to distinguish fact from fancy.) He now can see that his hostility is not met with hostility; the effect is that of having him realize that his own hostile impulses are not so dangerous as they seemed, that parents or parent-figures are not so unfriendly as he thought, and that he no longer need identify with an image imbued with hostility. In addition, if the parents had, out of bewilderment, actually responded with hostility, the fact that the therapist does not, again offers a chance for a corrective experience.

At this point the comment should be made that one of the basic propositions of this chapter is that relationship therapy is a pervasive substrate of many of the forms of expressive psychotherapy discussed below. Further, one unsolved problem of psychotherapy, to be answered by further research, has to do with the possibility that some therapeutic results ordinarily credited to expressive therapy are in actuality to be credited to the concomitant therapeutic relationship.

A relationship therapy of itself is suitable for many varieties of psychogenic illness. It is especially to be chosen when the patient is too resistive to attempts at an expressive psychotherapy or is considered too ill for this type of treatment; and it is indicated when the skill and training of the therapist are not adequate for such psychotherapy or, on a more positive basis, when a gradual maturing process based on the elaboration of new foci for identification is regarded as the most promising line of modification.

Relationship therapy can form the backbone of the work of the psychiatrist whose training was not psychodynamically oriented; it is the vehicle for the success of many psychiatric social workers; and it can provide the best line of approach for the growing group of internists and other physicians whose psychosomatic interests call for the development of techniques of psychotherapy. Such a statement, of course, does not eliminate the possibility of the interweaving of a certain amount of expressive psychotherapy into relationship therapy, in the work of those whose training and skill are adequate.

(4) *Expressive psychotherapy.*—This is a broad and unsatisfactory term to include a variety of special techniques and procedures. Perhaps the essential characteristic of all of them is that they attempt to go beyond the goals of a supportive and of a relationship therapy. The goals of the various forms of expressive psychotherapy not only include the goals of the above-mentioned techniques, viz., a restoration of a disturbed equilibrium, the formation of new foci for identification, and the occurrence of spontaneous corrective emotional experiences; they also include the goals of a greater awareness of the determinants of the illness, an emotional reorientation and a more mature perspective with regard to these determinants, an increase in ego capacity and strength, and specific and central corrective experiences.

A variety of procedures may be called "expressive" or "exploratory" or "uncovering," and again there is a great deal of overlapping of techniques and terminology. The most superficial variety of expressive psychotherapy is a frank discussion of personal problems, of impulses, life-situations, and conflicts which are quite conscious to the patient but which he ordinarily would not discuss with others. This would include a sort of confession and ventilation of "worries," family problems, doubts, impulses, conscious anxieties, guilt feelings, etc., and a joint study of current conflicts and remembered past life-situations as they seem to relate to neurotic reactions or psychosomatic disorders. Such a series of discussions of conscious problems would include, of course, a good therapeutic attitude on the part of the psychiatrist, with the constructive effects hoped for in a relationship therapy. In addition, however, in this type of expressive psychotherapy, there is the added goal of some increase in understanding and insight. The therapist in such a program would not give interpretations of unconscious material but would limit himself to a clarification of conscious problems, to a linking of events and feelings with reactions and symptoms—a linkage which the patient had not noticed previously on his own. Even such superficial insight may lead to an increase in perspective and objectivity, to a lessening of anxiety, and to some undercutting of future automatic responses.

In addition, such a discussion of conscious issues may give the therapist a chance to correct the patient's misinformation on personal problems—a correction which may lead to some diminution of anxiety. Further, the verbalization of vague or unclear worries may have some therapeutic effect, since the process of verbalization itself may make the problem more specific and less vague. Vague dangers often seem greater than clear ones. Consequently, the process of verbalization may lead to a better perspective and objectivity.

This combination of superficial expressive psychotherapy with relationship therapy may then be deepened at times by the inclusion of a varying amount of dealing with unconscious material, via free association, understanding of the transference, some dream material, etc. Such psychotherapy goes by a number of labels, such as "brief psychotherapy," "therapeutic interviewing," or "psychoanalytically oriented psychotherapy." Intensively supervised training, with adequate emphasis on transference and countertransference problems, is a *sine qua non* for this type of therapy. (It is unnecessary to specify the details of this variety of psychotherapy, since it can be visualized quite simply as the deepening of relationship therapy and "conscious" expressive therapy described above, by the use of some of the facets of psychoanalysis, to be described in the following paragraphs.)

If, now, in other cases, the psychotherapy deals extensively and intensively with unconscious problems (with, however, as much attention to conscious problems and reality situations as the material calls for); if the therapeutic sessions are frequent enough to give extensive information about the complexities of the patient's patterns; if the emphasis is predominantly on dealing with transference and resistance and on the working-through of defenses to uncover and express preconscious and unconscious pathogenic material; if the patient can productively be given insight into the ways in which his patterns unconsciously have led to distorted attitudes to the therapist; and if both dynamic and genetic material play an important role in therapy, the technique is called a "psychoanalysis."

Since this is a textbook of dynamic psychiatry rather than of psychoanalysis per se, the technical aspects of psychoanalysis will not be considered in detail.

A psychoanalysis is built on the basis of a relationship therapy, with the above-mentioned effects of a persistent therapeutic attitude (nonjudgmental, etc.) and the possibility of new foci for identification and of corrective experiences. It deals also with the clarification of conscious anxieties and conflicts. Its additional and specific characteristics are the following: Its emphasis is on dealing with unconscious conflicts, with the goal of uncovering and verbalizing various unconscious drives and emotions and of alleviating unconscious anxieties. It places great emphasis on an understanding of unconscious problems as expressed in transference distortions. One of its major goals is the achievement by the patient of an increased insight into his unconscious trends, with a possibility of better integration, now that the impulse is to be dealt with by the adult ego rather than by the relatively weak ego of childhood. This process can be rephrased as the bringing into consciousness of unacceptable impulses so that they may be dealt with by conscious and adult acceptance or renunciation or modification rather than by repression, with its symptom-forming consequences. Another of the major goals of psychoanalysis is the corrective emotional experience of having previously unconscious and automatic attitudes, now directed toward the therapist, brought into consciousness and of seeing that they are reacted to by the therapist in a way far different from the patient's expectations.

As part of its emphasis on the exploration and expression of unconscious material, a psychoanalysis makes extensive use of dreams and the associations to them, of the various indications of hidden transference and defensive reactions, and of close observation of the sequence of ideas in free association, i.e., the type of expression of thoughts and feelings which occurs when one puts aside the usual attempt to censor one's talk or to present one's ideas or memories in a logical fashion.

In a sense a psychoanalysis deals with material on a "deeper level." This can be specified as meaning (*a*) that there is an extensive attempt to understand the unconscious dynamics, in addition to the conscious dynamics; (*b*) that interpretation of unconscious material plays a more important role than clarification of conscious material does; and (*c*) that the significance of the past in the formation of current problems is emphasized, as well as the significance of the current unconscious patterns and problems themselves.

Another variety of expressive psychotherapy is play therapy in children. In this, the child's play, when he is alone with the therapist, acts as a technical substitute for dreams and free association. The play may start with the spontaneous choice of one of a variety of toys and play situations, or the play situation may be planned by the therapist to facilitate the expression of anxiety-provoking impulses, e.g., the use of a family of dolls, on which the child may displace his interpersonal patterns. The goal of such therapy is either the development of a capacity for a greater expression of throttled emotions, in a safe and supervised therapeutic situation, or the use of the material so revealed for the development of insight and understanding or for the corrective living experience in the transference. Depending on the depth of the therapy, such work may be called "psychoanalytically oriented play therapy" or "child analysis."

Hypnotherapy is another variety of expressive psychotherapy, in which hypnosis is used in part to facilitate the expression of unconscious material, which then may be handled therapeutically.

Narcosynthesis is a comparable technique of facilitating the expression of suppressed or repressed material through the technique of the intravenous injection of sodium pentothal or sodium amytal to the point of thorough relaxation but not sleep. This technique seems to be effective chiefly when there have been recent severe traumatic experiences, which stirred impulses and anxiety to a degree that could not be handled without repression and symptom formation.

Certain varieties of group therapy (the open discussion, in a small group, of common or universal problems or of individual problems) not only have supportive value, as mentioned above, but also permit the expression of hidden anxieties and conflicts, and some insight and corrective experiences in relation to the leader and to the others of the group.

It is not possible to state in any brief fashion the indications and contraindications for the varieties of expressive psychotherapy. Essentially, they are more suitable for neurotic problems than for psychotic, since a relatively intact ego is essential for the integration of "expressed" material. Modifications of the techniques described, however, make them usable with some psychotic patients during their hospital stay. In general, the expressive psychotherapies are suitable for patients who are willing to cooperate in such a procedure, who in the diagnostic evaluation of the psychiatrist are capable of constructive modification through the expressive techniques, and who cannot be given adequate help through simpler procedures.

As a postscript to the above description of the varieties of psychotherapy, the following may be added: Except for certain previously repressed material which is uncovered in rather intensive expressive psychotherapy, the material brought by patients to psychotherapeutic sessions is approximately the same in all varieties of psychotherapy. The essential difference is what happens after the patient brings the material. Expressed with great oversimplification, the following contrast can be made. In any variety of psychotherapy the patient may tell the therapist of an anxiety dream or a nightmare of a small animal with big sorrowful eyes about to be devoured by an enormous spider. In a *suppressive* therapy the therapist would insist that the patient stop being concerned about dreams and stop being anxious over inconsequential nothings and would order him to forget his dreams and jump out of bed in the morning. In a *supportive* therapy the therapist might comment that dreams are disturbing at times to everyone, that this is a common enough type of dream, and that perhaps some mild sedative for sleep might temporarily be of value. In some cases he may try to get the patient to talk freely of his fears. In a *relationship* therapy the therapist would put to himself the question of whether in the dream he is the devouring spider or the endangered small animal or whether the patient is either. He is alerted to the probability that in the treatment the patient may be afraid or may soon be afraid either of being hurt or of hurting. He may make no direct comment to the patient about the dream other than a supportive comment, and then later help to steer the patient into some discussion of his conscious fears. Largely he uses the dream to put the question to himself as to whether he has done anything to frighten the patient or whether he has permitted the patient to frighten him, and so helps himself to continue in a good therapeutic attitude. In an *expressive* therapy that does not go deeply into unconscious material the therapist may use the dream material in the fashion just mentioned as part of relationship therapy but, in addition, may lead the discussion to some expression of the patient's fears, his thoughts about them, etc., and, noting the material touched on, be led to some clarification or interpretation of the patient's fear of women, etc. In an expressive therapy of a deeper variety, the therapist would have the patient associate freely to the elements of the dream and then or later give an interpretation of the unconscious problems revealed by the combination of the dream, the associations, and the patient's attitudes. In such a therapy, if the material justified it, the interpretation given (the latent meaning of the dream) may well be that the patient was deeply afraid of being devoured by women figures (and now by the therapist) because of his own desire to open his eyes wide to see what he felt he should not see. (Implicit in this is the attitude that the therapist knows of his impulses and will not punish him.) In other instances, the interpretation may be that the patient regards himself as the omnipotent devouring spider and expects the therapist to cower in fear. (And implicit in this is the fact that the therapist does not regard the patient as omnipotent or frightening, and that the therapist is not cowering in fear.)

2. THE TRAINING AND SKILL OF THE THERAPIST IN THE USE OF SPECIFIC TECHNIQUES

It is clear that special training must be called for in many of the techniques mentioned above. Only a neurosurgeon should remove a brain tumor. Only a psychiatrist trained in electro-convulsive therapy (as well as in general and dynamic psychiatry) should give that variety of shock therapy. Only an accredited psychoanalyst should do psychoanalysis.

Because of the overlapping of the fields of knowledge and of training, some varieties of therapy may be done by specialists in several fields. A psychiatric social worker, adequately trained (working either in a psychiatric clinic or in an agency which has close supervision by psychiatrists), may make use of some aspects of the techniques of supportive therapy, relationship therapy, and expressive therapy essentially limited to conscious material. Her work will largely be oriented to the patient's environmental and family problems, and her special experience in social pathology and family constellations can be specific assets in therapy. A clinical psychologist, if his training is adequate, may do the same varieties of psychotherapy while working as part of a psychiatric clinic team, although his primary responsibility is in the field of teaching, research, and the use of special diagnostic tests. The internist or general practitioner who has had no special training in psychotherapy should limit himself to supportive techniques, whereas, if he has had special training, his skills may include the use of relationship therapy and superficial expressive psychotherapy based on conscious material. The psychiatrist whose training was largely nondynamic should limit himself to supportive therapy, relationship therapy, expressive therapy dealing with conscious material, general care of psychotic patients, and shock therapy. The psychiatrist whose training included intensively supervised dynamic psychotherapy may, in addition, make "brief psychotherapy" the focus of his practice. The psychiatrist whose training included full training in psychoanalysis may use the method of psychoanalysis.

3. PRACTICAL ASPECTS OF TREATMENT

To recapitulate: The therapist must take into consideration the diagnostic formulations (clinical, dynamic, and genetic) and the transference and countertransference phenomena apparent during the exploratory period. He must consider the various types of acceptable therapy and their applicability in terms of the specific problem at hand. He must pay attention to the problem of the goals of treatment in the individual patient and fit the potentialities of the various treatment procedures to the needs and potentialities of the patient. Further, he must consider his own training and skill or those of the therapists to whom he might refer the patient.

In addition, his decisions about therapy must take into full consideration many practical issues. The age of the patient, his level of intelligence, the presence of serious physical defects, his cultural and educational background, his geographical location in respect to treatment—all are of importance in determining the feasibility of the therapy which may seem indicated.

The elements in the family constellation which foster improvement and those which block progress must be evaluated. The destructive aspects of the environment in which the patient must stay during treatment or to which he must return after treatment are often of crucial importance, particularly in childhood.

The resources of the community may have to be assessed as well. If private hospitalization is indicated, the availability of a vacancy in a good hospital, at a rate which the patient or the family can afford to pay, must be determined. If the patient should have ambulatory private care, the availability of an adequately trained therapist cannot be taken for granted. If the patient is unable to pay for private care, the existence of a good clinic in the community is crucial. (And if the patient's therapy would be benefited by his paying a small fee, the clinic should provide such a fee system as one of its therapeutic activities.)

The purpose of these final paragraphs, however, is not to give a full survey of practical considerations—rather it is to call attention to the danger that the therapist may become so fascinated by the discoveries of modern psychiatry and by the dynamic problems of the individual patient that he will minimize the need to consider the current realities. But when the therapist recognizes the urgent necessity of having his planning be realistic and appropriate, the practical issues in any individual situation become obvious and pertinent.

BIBLIOGRAPHY

1. AICHHORN, A. *Wayward Youth* (New York: Viking Press, 1945).
2. ALEXANDER, F. *Fundamentals of Psychoanalysis* (New York: W. W. Norton & Co., 1948), pp. 272–302.
3. ALEXANDER, F., and FRENCH, T. M. *Psychoanalytic Therapy* (New York: Ronald Press, 1946).
4. ALEXANDER, F., and HEALY, W. *Roots of Crime* (New York: Alfred A. Knopf, 1935).
5. BENNETT, A. E. "The Role of Psychotherapy in Electroshock Therapy," *Am. J. Psychiat.*, 105:392, 1948.
6. BINGER, C. *The Doctor's Job* (New York: W. W. Norton & Co., 1945).
7. BRENMAN, M., and GILL, M. M. *Hypnotherapy* (New York: International Universities Press, 1947).
8. COLEMAN, J. V. "Patient-Physician Relationship in Psychotherapy," *Am. J. Psychiat.*, 104:638, 1948.
9. DIETHELM, O. *Treatment in Psychiatry* (New York: Macmillan Co., 1951).
10. FEDERN, P. "Psychoanalysis of Psychoses," *Psychiat. Quart.*, 17:1, 246, 470, 1943.
11. FENICHEL, O. *Problems of Psychoanalytic Technique* (Albany, N.Y.: Psychoanalytic Quarterly, Inc., 1941).
12. FENICHEL, O. *The Psychoanalytic Theory of Neurosis* (New York: W. W. Norton & Co., 1945), pp. 547–89.
13. FINESINGER, J. E. "Psychiatric Interviewing. I. Some Principles and Procedures in Insight Therapy," *Am. J. Psychiat.*, 105:187, 1948.
14. FREUD, A. *Introduction to the Technic of Child Analysis* (London: George Allen & Unwin, 1931).
15. FREUD, S. *A General Introduction to Psychoanalysis* (New York: Boni & Liveright, 1935); or *Introductory Lectures on Psychoanalysis* (London: George Allen & Unwin, 1917).
16. FREUD, S. *New Introductory Lectures on Psycho-analysis* (New York: W. W. Norton & Co., 1933).
17. FREUD, S. Papers on Technique, in *Collected Papers*, Vol. 2 (London: Hogarth Press, 1924).
18. FROMM-REICHMANN, F. *Principles of Intensive Psychotherapy* (Chicago: University of Chicago Press, 1950).

19. GARRETT, A. *Interviewing: Its Principles and Methods* (New York: Family Welfare Association of America, 1942).

20. GRINKER, R. R., and SPIEGEL, J. P. *Men under Stress* (Philadelphia: Blakiston Co., 1945).

21. HENDRICK, I. *Facts and Theories of Psychoanalysis* (New York: Alfred A. Knopf, 1939).

22. HINSIE, L. E. *Concepts and Problems of Psychotherapy* (New York: Columbia University Press, 1937).

23. JESSNER, L., and RYAN, V. G. *Shock Treatment in Psychiatry* (New York: Grune & Stratton, 1941).

24. KALINOWSKI, L. B., and HOCH, P. H. *Shock Treatments and Other Somatic Procedures in Psychiatry* (New York: Grune & Stratton, 1946).

25. KLEIN, M. *The Psycho-analysis of Children* (London: Hogarth Press, 1932).

26. KNIGHT, R. P. "A Critique of the Present Status of the Psychotherapist," *Bull. New York Acad. Med.*, 25:100, 1949.

27. KNIGHT, R. P. "The Psychoanalytic Treatment in a Sanitarium of Chronic Addiction to Alcohol," *J.A.M.A.*, 111:1443, 1938.

28. KUBIE, L. S. *Practical Aspects of Psychoanalysis* (New York: W. W. Norton & Co., 1936).

29. KUBIE, L. S. "The Nature of Psychotherapy," *Bull. New York Acad. Med.*, 19:183, 1943.

30. LEVINE, M. "An Orientation Chart in the Teaching of Psychosomatic Medicine," *Psychosom. Med.*, 10:111, 1948.

31. LEVINE, M. *Psychotherapy in Medical Practice* (New York: Macmillan Co., 1942).

32. LEVY, D. M. "Attitude Therapy," *Am. J. Orthopsychiat.*, 7:103, 1937.

33. LEVY, D. M. "Trends in Therapy: Release Therapy," *Am. J. Orthopsychiat.*, 9:713, 1939.

34. LORAND, S. *Technique of Psychoanalytic Therapy* (New York: International Universities Press, 1946).

35. MENNINGER, K. *The Human Mind* (3d ed.; New York: Alfred A. Knopf, 1945), pp. 363-416.

36. NUNBERG, H. *Practice and Theory of Psychoanalysis* (New York: Nervous and Mental Disease Publishing Co., 1948), pp. 75, 105, 174.

37. POWDERMAKER, F. "The Techniques of the Initial Interview," *Am. J. Psychiat.*, 104:642, 1948.

38. *Proceedings of the Brief Psychotherapy Council* (Chicago: Institute for Psychoanalysis, 1942, 1944, 1946).

39. ROSEN, J. N. "The Treatment of Schizophrenic Psychoses by Direct Analytic Therapy," *Psychiat. Quart.*, 21:3, 1947.

40. SARGENT, W., and SLATER, E. *An Introduction to Physical Methods of Treatment in Psychiatry* (Baltimore: Williams & Wilkins Co., 1948).

41. SCHILDER, P. *Psychotherapy* (New York: W. W. Norton & Co., 1951).

42. SLAVSON, S. R. *The Practice of Group Therapy* (New York: International Universities Press, 1948).

43. SPOCK, B., and HUSCHKA, M. *Psychological Aspects of Pediatric Practice* (New York: New York State Committee on Mental Hygiene, 1938).

44. SZUREK, S. A. "Remarks on Training for Psychotherapy," *Am. J. Orthopsychiat.*, 19:36, 1949.

45. WITMER, H. L. (ed.). *Teaching Psychotherapeutic Medicine* (New York: Commonwealth Fund, 1947).

46. WHITEHORN, J. C. "Psychotherapy," in *Modern Medical Therapy in General Practice*, 1 (Baltimore: Williams & Wilkins Co., 1940), 3.

47. WHITEHORN, J. C. "Guide to Interviewing and Clinical Personality Study," *Arch. Neurol. & Psychiat.*, 52:197, 1944.

VIII

THE PSYCHOSOMATIC APPROACH IN MEDICINE

FRANZ ALEXANDER, M.D., AND THOMAS S. SZASZ, M.D.

WHAT IS PSYCHOSOMATIC MEDICINE?

THE psychosomatic approach in medical research and therapy consists in the co-ordinated application of somatic (i.e., anatomical, physiological, pharmacological, and surgical) methods and concepts, on the one hand, and psychological methods and concepts, on the other. Interest in the mutual influence of physiological and psychological processes is by no means new, as evidenced by such German expressions as were popular in the last century—*Psychophysiologie* (Wundt) or *Psychophysik* (Fechner). What is new in the modern psychosomatic approach is that both the physiological and the psychological processes are studied with the same scientific standards. This progress, like all fundamental scientific progress, became possible by improved methods. It is only since the advent of the psychoanalytic technique that psychological processes can be studied with precision. As a result, generalities, such as, for example, that the emotional state of a person may have a profound influence upon the course of any disease, can now be replaced by the precise study of these psychological influences.

Psychological processes are the functions of the central co-ordinator of the organism, i.e., of the highest integrative centers of the central nervous system. Essentially they are similar to other processes in the organism. The most important difference is that they are perceived subjectively. Accordingly, these processes can be studied by psychological techniques. Psychological methods, however, differ in many respects from all other methods used in medicine, such as physics, chemistry, anatomy, and physiology. Hence the co-ordination of these two types of approach meets with inherent difficulties, which are being overcome only gradually.

When psychoanalytic interest first turned to the problems of organic medicine, some pioneers, notably Georg Groddeck (51, 52, 53), attempted to understand somatic processes entirely *as if* they were the same as psychic processes and symptoms. He applied psychoanalytic concepts to physiologic processes, without due recognition of the fact that the latter require different conceptual tools for adequate description and understanding. The results thus arrived at were often bizarre, such as "interpreting" the fever of an infectious illness as "meaning" sexual excitement, or the increased blood flow to an organ, for whatever reason, as "meaning" a displaced erection.

Another example of such conceptual confusion may be seen in the approach of certain so-called "organicists." We are referring to the persistent attempts, both past and present, to find some histological or biochemical alteration in the central nervous system which would "explain" the neuroses or schizophrenia. Such findings, even if present, would no more explain the specific psychological pictures found in various psychiatric syndromes than the discovery of the syphilitic basis of paresis could explain the various psychic symptoms which occur in patients with this disorder.

The two examples cited are, of course, counterparts of each other. They illustrate the inappropriateness of simply transposing the concepts of psychology into physiology or vice versa. The creation of an *integrated conceptual system* which would combine the basic principles of these two diverse scientific approaches thus appears to be one of the most important goals of present-day research in psychosomatic medicine.

The current psychosomatic approach in medicine can be considered as a logical outcome of the basic orientation of Freud. From the beginning, Freud's approach to psychology was consistently biological. He considered psychological processes as functions of the living organism, which, like all other bodily functions, are in the service of survival and propagation. This, in his time, was in stark contrast to the traditional approach of psychology, which had its origin in philosophy. Since Descartes, emphasis has been placed upon the fact that all our knowledge about the surrounding world is based on such psychological processes as observing, knowing, and understanding (*cogito, ergo sum*). Hence the belief that psychological phenomena cannot be explained from external facts and that all other sciences are secondary to psychology. This epistemological emphasis gave psychology an extra-territorial status which was, in a sense, above and beyond all other sciences, and introspection was considered the only legitimate approach to psychic life.

Freud's biological orientation is best exemplified by his concept of the mental apparatus, the main function of which he considered to be the preservation of the equilibrium (stability) of the organism by satisfying its instinctual (biological) needs and protecting it from excessive external stimuli (45). This task it achieves by the perception of internal or instinctual needs, by the perception of existing conditions in the external environment upon which the satisfaction of instinctual needs depends, and, finally, by the confrontation of the data of internal and external perception with each other ("integrative function"). The ultimate function of the mental apparatus, however, is an executive one: the control of co-ordinated voluntary behavior, which is based on the integration of the data of internal and external perception by reasoning. According to Freud, all neurotic symptoms can be considered as failures of these functions; they are substitutes in fantasy for adequate, integrated acts. Whenever the relief of instinctual tensions by suitable co-ordinated behavior fails, these tensions seek other outlets. Neurotic symptoms are adaptations occurring in the face of such failures of adequate discharge of instinctual tensions; they are often inadequate, autoplastic substitutes for adequate, alloplastic action (44). Neurotic symptoms vary greatly in their effectiveness in relieving (draining) instinctual tensions; often they can relieve tensions only partially, and they may create secondary conflicts, leading to new tensions.

Often these chronic emotional tensions elicit chronic responses (dysfunctions) in the vegetative system, which have been called "functional" disorders, such as "nervous indigestion," diarrhea, cardiac neurosis, etc. The understanding of such conditions requires the co-ordinated use of psychological and physiological methods (9, 31, 88).

EARLY PSYCHOANALYTIC CONTRIBUTIONS

It is of interest to note that the first studies of Breuer and Freud (21) concerned themselves with hysterical conversion symptoms, i.e., with disorders in which certain isolated bodily changes occur in the field of the skeletomuscular and sensory systems (paralyses, contractures, and sensory disturbances). Such symptoms are motivated by unconscious thought-processes which cannot find outlet in motor behavior because of repression. Accordingly, they have a specific "meaning," which can be interpreted like any psychoneurotic symptom.

Otherwise, psychoanalytic research during the first two decades of this century was not primarily concerned with psychosomatic problems. This was the era during which the main interest of psychoanalysis was the exploration of unconscious processes. In addition to conversion hysteria, the chief syndromes studied were anxiety hysteria, obsessive-compulsive neurosis, depressions, and certain sexual and behavior disorders. In so far as the physiological processes or disorders were studied and interpreted, the pattern of thought was along the mechanism of hysterical conversions.

Among the early psychoanalysts, both Abraham and Ferenczi were interested in certain problems which today we would designate as psychosomatic, and both made important contributions to these problems. Abraham applied his concepts concerning the oral and anal stages of libido development to the explanation of certain disorders of the gastrointestinal tract. He described with great precision those emotional attitudes which in normal child development accompany the ingestion of food and the elimination of feces (1, 2, 3, 4).

He further pursued Freud's view that the infant's first attitude toward the contents of his bowels is a "coprophilic" one, i.e., the infant considers his feces at first a part of his own body and a valuable possession. In the course of toilet training he acquires the idea that he has to give up this possession in order to please his parents (mother), and subsequently he develops an attitude of disgust as a reaction formation against his earlier, repressed attitude toward bowel functions. Thus the excremental act becomes associated with hostile sadistic (soiling) impulses. Neurotic patients under emotional stress often regress to these emotional reactions. Such regressions may be important in many gastrointestinal disturbances in later life.

Ferenczi, too, was interested in many of the nonverbal (nonpsychological) means by which emotions may be expressed within the organism (36, 37, 39). Many of his thoughts concerning the psychological implications of fundamental physiological processes, such as growth and propagation, have influenced later psychosomatic research. In particular, his discrimination between the erotic and the utilitarian functions of different physiological processes has been further pursued by the theoretical formulations of Alexander and French.

Ferenczi also made extensive use of the concept of regression, the importance of which he demonstrated in all types of biological phenomena. In his concept of "patho-neurosis," he emphasized the fact that all injuries to the body may favor an autoerotic preoccupation with the affected organ (36). Although this term has not gained acceptance, Ferenczi's concepts concerning the narcissistic regression which occurs as a result of physical trauma or organic disease—including problems of war neurosis—have had a deep influence on subsequent psychoanalytic thinking (38). In a psychoanalytic study of patients with general paresis, made in collaboration with Hollos, Ferenczi for the first time used the concept of adaptation of the personality to its organic defects (57).

As has been emphasized before, most of the early psychosomatic contributions, particularly those of Jelliffe (59–63) and Groddeck (53), attempted to interpret physiological dysfunctions outside the neuromuscular and sensory systems with the same conceptual tools as had been used successfully in respect to hysterical conversion symptoms. In his early writings Felix Deutsch (27, 28, 29) also followed the same trend and tried to interpret many physiological disorders as hysterical conversions which express a definite unconscious psychic content.

One of the few early authors who did not fall into the foregoing methodological error is Paul Schilder. His book *The Image and Appearance of the Human Body* (78) contains a wealth of clinical observation and hypotheses. Schilder's concept of body image is closely connected with the psychoanalytic concept of the ego as a system of perception and perhaps also as an "entity." It has an important bearing on the problem of what constitutes a hysterical conversion.

THE PSYCHOSOMATIC ERA IN MEDICINE

In the last twenty years a new phase of psychosomatic research developed which was largely initiated by the conceptual clarification of the difference between hysterical conversion symptoms and vegetative responses to psychological stimuli (Alexander, 8). It was recognized that the similarity between a hysterical conversion symptom, such as the paralysis of a limb, on the one hand, and the vegetative responses to emotions, such as increased gastric secretion or increased blood pressure, on the other hand, consists merely in the fact that both conditions are "psychogenic," that is to say, they are caused by a chronically unrelieved emotional tension. The mechanisms involved, however, are fundamentally different, both physiologically and psychodynamically (8, 9). The hysterical conversion symptom is an attempt to relieve an emotional tension in a symbolic way; it is a symbolic (displaced) expression of a definite emotional content. This mechanism is restricted to the voluntary neuromuscular or perceptive systems whose functions are to express and relieve emotions. In contrast to this, a vegetative neurosis consists of a psychogenic dysfunction of a vegetative organ which is not under the control of the voluntary neuromuscular system and which therefore does not express any (primary) psychological meaning. The vegetative symptom is not a substitute expression of the emotion but its (normal) physiological concomitant. The pathologic nature of the condition consists primarily in the fact that, under continued emotional stimuli caused by unresolved conflicts, the vegetative responses become chronic. In time they may lead to irreversible tissue changes, resulting in clear-cut organic syndromes. This view introduced a new etiological concept into medicine: that organic illness may result, at least partially, from chronic neurotic conflicts.

This distinction between *two fundamentally different types of symptom formation* (conversion and vegetative neurosis) has become generally accepted, although it is frequently stated in somewhat different terms. It may be noted also that, according to Fenichel (35), the basic difference between what we today call "organ-neurotic"[1] symptoms on the one hand, and psychoneurotic symptoms, on the other, was recognized by Freud a long time ago. In a paper on psychogenic visual disturbances (43), Freud suggested the distinction between two types of psychogenic symptoms, differentiating the functions of an organ as it serves sexuality or utility. This distinction corresponds to Freud's views at that time (1910) concerning the duality of instincts (i.e., sexual and ego instincts). This idea was later taken up and elaborated by Ferenczi (36, 39).

1. The terms "organ neurosis" and "vegetative neurosis" are used synonymously.

The foregoing difference between two types of symptom formation was stated in still another way by Edward Glover, as follows:

Following this approach it is possible to draw two fundamental distinctions between the psychoneuroses and all psychosomatic disorders, first, that the *process of symptom-formation in the psychoneuroses follows a standardized psychic pattern*, and second, that *the psychoneuroses have psychic content and meaning. Psychosomatic disorders*, on the other hand, although influenced by psychic reactions at some point or another in their progress, *have in themselves no psychic content, and consequently do not represent stereotyped patterns of conflict*. Should they develop psychic meaning, it may be assumed that a psychoneurotic process has been superimposed on a psychosomatic foundation [48, pp. 170–71].

Thus both Alexander and Glover emphasize that organ-neurotic symptoms do not express any *primary* psychic meaning; in addition to this, Alexander connects hysterical symptoms with the voluntary neuromuscular and sensory perceptive systems, whereas Glover defines an additional difference in terms of the presence or absence of standardized or stereotyped patterns of conflict. Both these factors deserve further comment.

Glover's second distinction between psychoneuroses and psychosomatic disorders refers to the existence of a standardized pattern of conflict in the former and its absence in the latter. This point is of interest, since it has a bearing on the problem of specificity of somatic symptoms. In contrast to the specific pattern in which, for example, phobias or obsessions develop, the development of somatic symptoms in Glover's opinion is not governed by similar specific *psychological* patterns; he relates the nature of the choice of these symptoms to a number of determinants, such as constitutional factors, the depth of regression, the nature of the distribution of libido, etc.

Concerning the restriction of hysterical conversion symptoms to certain structures—defined on an anatomical and physiological basis—Szasz called attention to the fact that this rule applies only to motor (or discharge) symptoms. Thus, for example, in the case of hysterical pain the symptom does not depend upon any special type of peripheral innervation, such as the cerebrospinal conduction system. The mechanism in such a case does not rest on primarily physiological foundations but rather on the patient's own *body image*. That is to say, such a symptom may occur or, more precisely, may be referred to any part of the body which has a psychic representation. We may further note in this connection that when we think of "psychosomatic responses" we have in mind, as a rule, only motor or discharge phenomena. This follows inevitably from the fact that perception is, in the last analysis, a function of the ego or of the total psychological integration of the person at any particular time. Discussion of this interesting and important problem of perception in general and pain in particular, however, would lead us too far afield, and we cannot, therefore, pursue it any further at this time other than to state that here lies what appears to us a relatively unexplored area of psychosomatic research.

Gradually more and more systematic studies of emotional factors of different organic diseases were undertaken in different research centers. The fundamental theoretical concept underlying the psychosomatic studies conducted at the Chicago Institute for Psychoanalysis (10) was that emotional states do not express themselves in external behavior only but that the internal physiological processes also respond to every emotional state in an adaptive manner. This concept leaned heavily on Cannon's experimental studies of the physiological changes which regularly follow certain emotional states, such as anger and fear (22). These investigations, however, went further than studying the internal physiological responses to such basic emotional states as rage and fear. On the basis of their clinical studies, Alexander and his co-workers came to the conclusion that specific emotional states elicit specific physiological responses. They postulated, for example, that oral-incorporating cravings have a specific effect upon gastric secretion and motility; that rage, depending on its different psychological representations, may influence either the neuromuscular, the gastrointestinal, or the vascular system. In these studies the psychological processes observed were not brought into connection with the entire disease picture but rather with a specific physiological process, such as gastric secretion, vascular contraction, or muscular tension.

At the same time, Dunbar (30, 31, 32) and her collaborators paid more attention to the overt personality features which are commonly found in patients with certain organic disturbances. Stimulating though these studies were, they did not reveal any specific causal connection between psychological and organic processes. It is probable that what Dunbar observed were frequent and typical defense reactions against some basic conflicts which were present in certain organic diseases. In other words,

Dunbar observed rather distant end-results of the various psychological mechanisms which are more directly connected with disturbed organic functions.

At the present stage of development one of the central problems in psychosomatic medicine is that of the specific nature of the emotional stimuli involved in different organic disorders.

THE PROBLEM OF SPECIFICITY

There are three main schools of thought concerning this problem. According to the first view, mentioned above, the psychological factors which influence or disturb the functions of the vegetative organs are as specific as those which have been established in cases of conversion hysteria. They have an ideational content, a symbolic meaning, which can be interpreted in psychological terms: the affected visceral organ expresses the unconscious content, just as a hysterical conversion symptom is a symbolic expression of repressed psychological content. In psychoanalysis this view is the oldest one and at present is largely abandoned.

The second school of thought expresses a view which tends in the opposite direction. According to it, the nature of the active emotional factors may not determine the nature of the vegetative disturbance. Many different psychological stimuli may call forth the same vegetative responses. The nature of the vegetative disturbance depends largely on constitutional factors or on a previously acquired vulnerability of the affected organ. This view takes over only one component of the Freudian concept of hysterical conversion, namely, that of "bodily compliance." Under the influence of emotions, organic disturbances may develop according to the existing vulnerable spots within the organism. The person with a susceptible gastrointestinal system will react to emotional conflicts with stomach or bowel disorders. The person whose Achilles' heel is in the circulatory system will respond to emotional disturbances with cardiac or vascular symptoms. The vulnerability of the involved organ may be due to heredity, previous organic disease, or some other factors.

The third view which has been the working hypothesis of the investigative work at the Chicago Institute for Psychoanalysis takes an intermediary position between these two approaches. It does not discount the concept of the vulnerability of the affected organs, but it adds another factor, based primarily on

Cannon's original formulations (22, 23). According to this view, to every emotional state there corresponds a characteristic physiological response which in itself is not pathologic but is an integral part of the emotional state. Stimulation of the sympathoadrenal system, resulting in increased carbohydrate metabolism, faster heart action, and elevation of blood pressure, together with a relative inhibition of digestive functions, are all constituent parts of the state of rage. The physiological concomitants of anxiety are similar to, although probably not identical with, those of rage. Both states are common in emergency situations. Relaxation and emotional withdrawal from external affairs go with a physiological state which is the opposite of that found in emergency situations. The physiological concomitants of a relaxed state are characterized by increased anabolic and storing processes. The gastrointestinal functions are stimulated, while the functions of the skeletal muscles and of the circulatory and respiratory systems are inhibited. These changes—both in emergency and in the relaxed state—are adaptive reactions of the vegetative organs to the total situation in which the organism finds itself. They fulfil a physiological function. This theory gives full recognition to the local vulnerability of the affected organs but at the same time postulates a certain specific correlation between the emotional state and its physiological concomitants or sequelae: the nature of the emotional state determines the type of physiological response. The coexistence of both factors (the somatic local vulnerability of the affected organ and the specific emotional constellation) is responsible for the organic disturbance.

As has been mentioned before, Dunbar's point of view differs from the foregoing, inasmuch as it postulates certain overt personality features characteristic of different diseases. These features appear in overt behavior and can be described by personality profile studies, as proposed by Dunbar.

Alexander (9) emphasized that the specific correlation is not between overt personality features and vegetative response but between the latter and certain, mostly unconscious, emotional constellations which may be present in very different types of personalities and which may appear and disappear during the life of the same person. Accordingly, the specific relationship between disease and psychological factors is much less static than is postulated by Dunbar's concept.

PSYCHOSOMATIC MECHANISMS

In the present stage of psychosomatic medicine, there is a certain number of theoretical conceptions of a general nature which are utilized rather widely by workers currently active in this field. These conceptions rest on many well-established observations concerning psychophysiologic interrelations; they show the influence particularly of the views of Darwin, Cannon, and Freud.

VOLUNTARY BEHAVIOR

Psychologically, voluntary behavior can be described in terms of motives and goals. The physiological functions which are suited to achieve certain goals can thus be understood in terms of their utility, much as in the case of certain functions of a machine. These physiological functions are mediated by the voluntary nervous system, their end-organs being the striated musculature. From a nosological viewpoint, disturbances in these functions may give rise to hysterical conversion symptoms. (In a wider sense, there are many other types of failures in co-ordinated voluntary behavior, comprising essentially all disturbances in interpersonal relations. The mechanisms here described are not presented and cannot be used as a basis for a rigid classification of psychiatric syndromes.)

EXPRESSIVE INNERVATIONS

Expressive innervations are specific physiological processes, such as weeping, laughing, blushing, sighing, etc., which take place under the influence of specific emotional tensions (Darwin, 26). The physiological systems involved in these patterns of behavior include both the voluntary (cerebrospinal) and the autonomic nervous systems; moreover, in expressive innervations skeletal muscles may become activated through extra-pyramidal pathways, in contrast to the pyramidal conduction system which activates voluntary movements. Psychologically, expressive innervations cannot be understood in terms of utilitarian goals; they are discharge phenomena, and their only goal or "utility" is to secure relief from emotional tension. Thus weeping, for example, helps to discharge the painful feelings associated with grief. Disturbances of these functions are usually classified with hysterical conversion symptoms (e.g., hysterical laughter or weeping). However, it would be more nearly correct to regard such disturbances as bridging the gap between hysterical conversions and vegetative neuroses, since they combine features of both. In blushing or hysterical weeping, for example, the symptom may indeed be regarded as a hysterical conversion, since it expresses a specific unconscious psychological meaning in a bodily change; however, since the physiological pathways activated in this process include certain functions of the autonomic nervous system, a characteristic feature of a vegetative neurosis is also present.

PSYCHOSEXUAL PHENOMENA

Psychosexual phenomena are essentially similar to expressive innervations. Indeed, it is, par excellence, by means of sexual activity that the organism can rid itself of emotional tensions. Only in certain mature manifestations of sexuality is the aim of race preservation served also. The pregenital forms of sexuality discharge instinctual tensions which cannot be described in terms of utility, from the point of view either of self-preservation or of race preservation. The physiological mechanisms in sexual phenomena consist in complicated and not yet fully understood combinations of voluntary innervations, together with autonomic and hormonal changes (e.g., copulation, erection, ejaculation, orgasm, periodic changes in sexual receptivity, etc.) (15, 40). Because of this complex participation of cerebrospinal, autonomic, and endocrine responses, the disturbances of sexual functions cannot be rigidly classified as hysterical conversions or vegetative neuroses; different sexual disturbances may include features of both mechanisms, in varying proportions (e.g., frigidity and amenorrhea). The psychological aspects of these phenomena have been well explored by psychoanalytic studies of the last fifty years. Their physiology is still largely unknown.

VEGETATIVE RESPONSES

Vegetative responses consist of visceral reactions to emotional stimuli. Most of the current psychosomatic studies are concerned with these mechanisms.

1. *Adaptive responses, the "vegetative retreat," and "regressive innervations."*—As was postulated by Cannon (23), the main function of the sympathetic division of the autonomic nervous system is the regulation of internal vegetative functions in relation to external activities, particularly in emergency situations.

Thus adaptive responses in emergency situations consist of the stimulation of those functions which are needed for fight or flight; this is accomplished by the activation of the sympatho-adrenal system.

In the relaxed state, on the other hand, there is normally a withdrawal of interest from the environment, and the vegetative responses corresponding to this state are under the dominant influence of the parasympathetic branch of the autonomic nervous system; this results in stimulation of the digestive and storing (anabolic) functions and in a relative diminution in catabolic functions. While these responses are appropriate in the relaxed state, some patients react to effort, anxiety, and certain conflict situations with emotional withdrawal, and the corresponding vegetative responses ensue. In such cases these responses are paradoxical and can be interpreted as regressive solutions of the necessity to meet the emergency situation with adequate externally directed responses. This type of autoplastic response was designated by Alexander (9) as the "vegetative retreat."

Following upon this general schema, Szasz (87) found it possible to interpret certain autonomic dysfunctions more specifically as regressions to earlier, infantile modes of autonomic functioning. He also emphasized that, instead of speaking of a preponderance of one or the other branch of the autonomic nervous system or of an "autonomic imbalance" in psychosomatic disorders, what characterizes many of these syndromes is a localized *parasympathetic (cholinergic) hyperfunction* (e.g., peptic ulcer, diarrhea, asthma, neurodermatitis, etc.); *these autonomic dysfunctions represent regressions in specific physiological activities.* For example, the vagal hyperactivity of the patient with peptic ulcer was shown to be similar to the vagal preponderance which exists during the first two years of life, at a time when the sympathetic supply to the gastrointestinal tract is not yet fully developed (87). Similarly, some cases of diarrhea could be shown to be related to a reactivation of the gastrocolic reflex mechanism which is most active during infancy (85). On the basis of such examples, together with certain theoretical considerations, it was suggested that such patterns of autonomic response (localized parasympathetic hyperfunctions) be designated as "regressive innervations"; in contrast to this type of response, certain chronic sympathetic excitations of organs or organ-systems were designated as "concomitant innervations."

2. *Life-situations, emotions, and physiology.* — Harold G. Wolff, Stewart Wolf, and their associates studied a large number of physiological reactions under experimentally induced emotional states. Their study of the subject with gastric fistula, "Tom," now belongs among the medical classics (91). Their method in this case consisted of making careful observations of gastric activity, together with certain physiological measurements, under varying life-situations and in response to experimentally induced emotional conditions. They made similar studies on the eye (74), on the mucous membranes of the colon (50), bronchi (81, 82), nose (58), and on patients with essential hypertension (90) and diabetes mellitus (55, 56). Wolff interprets many of these reactions as serving the purpose of warding off or keeping out noxious stimuli. Illustrative of such an interpretation is the following:

Conspicuous among defensive protective reactions are those involving the nose and airways. It has been observed that in reaction to assaults and threats, certain individuals occlude their air passages and limit the ventilatory exchange by vasodilatation, turgescence, hypersecretion and contraction of smooth and skeletal muscle. The changes, especially in the upper respiratory airways, give rise to a variety of symptoms, notably pain and obstruction, the latter often leading to secondary infection, and the prolongation of morbid processes. Also the individual exhibits a behavior pattern and attitude of a non-participation in interpersonal relations [94, p. 1075].

Wolff's interpretation (92, 94) is essentially an extension of Cannon's basic philosophy concerning the mechanisms of "fight or flight" to a great many physiological reactions not considered or accounted for by Cannon. Yet Wolff's hypothesis contributes little toward the solution of the problem of specificity of symptoms, as it holds no clue to the question of why one particular organ-system should be affected in a particular case rather than in another. Moreover, although Wolff sometimes refers to the infantile prototypes of such reactions, he does not utilize the psychoanalytic concept of "regression." It is therefore implied that the reactions mentioned are considered *defensive in a temporally current sense* (that is, they are considered *currently useful*). It is readily seen that the psychoanalytic interpretation of such symptoms is similar, but with the difference that such symptoms are viewed as *regressions to earlier developmental patterns of reaction (defense), which are reactivated as a result of some current conflict.* The chief value of the work of Wolf and Wolff lies in their numerous and accurate observations concerning a wide variety of psychosomatic reactions. They do not differentiate, however, between conscious and unconscious psychological processes and make no reference to the psychoanalytically well-established phenomenon of regression, a conception without which the "defensive" nature of many physiological dysfunctions cannot be explained.

3. *Endocrinological responses in chronic stress.*—Physiological adaptations to stress occur in every part of the body. In addition to psychological adaptations, the most extensively studied and best-understood physiological changes which occur in response to stress are those mediated by the voluntary and autonomic nervous systems. That the endocrine system participates in the body's defenses in such situations has been known for some time, but it was only recently that a comprehensive theory concerning these endocrine reactions has been put forward. Hans Selye (79, 80) co-ordinated a vast number of observations under the name of the "general adaptation syndrome"; this term designates a complex chain of events, initiated by a variety of stressful situations ("stressors") and mediated by *hormonal* mechanisms. According to this theory, the first hormonal response to stress is the "alarm reaction." In the case of prolonged stress, chronic hormonal defensive reactions ensue ("the stage of resistance"); and it is these chronic and excessive hormonal changes, mediated primarily by the anterior pituitary and adrenal cortex, which lead to various pathologic changes in end-organs, designated as "diseases of adaptation" (e.g., arthritis, periarteritis nodosa, etc.). Understanding of the precise influence of psychological factors upon the endocrine system is still largely unexplored territory.

4. *Dissociation of physiologically co-ordinated functions.*—Sydney G. Margolin (68) and his associates recently reported that, in a patient under psychoanalytic observation, under certain circumstances various gastric functions may become dissociated; for example, there may occur changes in gastric motility and the secretion of hydrochloric acid and pepsin which do not run parallel to each other but vary in an independent and apparently random manner. Hitherto, most psychosomatic studies were concerned with hyperfunction or hypofunction. These observations point to dissociation of an organ's functions as another possible disease-producing mechanism. Szasz (83, 84) has raised a similar question in connection with the normally associated functions of the salivary and gastric glands. He noted that hypersalivation

occurs frequently in pregnant women, whereas the incidence of duodenal ulcers in such cases is extremely low. The question was raised whether the secretory activities of the salivary and gastric glands might become dissociated under such circumstances. The significance of these observations remains to be evaluated and depends on further studies of the phenomenon of dissociation of the functions of single organs or organ-systems.

PSYCHOLOGICAL FACTORS IN VEGETATIVE AND PSYCHOSEXUAL DISORDERS

During the last twenty years a great many psychosomatic studies concerned themselves with the detection of the role of specific emotional factors in different organic diseases. The essential features of the conceptual framework of these studies were described briefly in the previous section ("Psychosomatic Mechanisms"). It may be added now that each of the syndromes to be described will fall into one of two categories, depending on whether psychological factors lead to the physiological disturbance or vice versa. Examples of the first type of psychophysiologic interrelationship are found in cases of duodenal ulcer or asthma, and of the second type (i.e., physiological factors leading to psychological changes) in cases of diabetes mellitus and in the psychological changes accompanying the menstrual cycle in women.

In this chapter we cannot deal with the detailed result of the numerous psychosomatic studies reported in the literature. Only the most salient features of the best-established observations (largely based on psychoanalytic studies) will be summarized.

These studies consist primarily of the description of typical psychodynamic constellations which are found consistently in different organic diseases. Although these findings are largely empirical, in the conditions most extensively investigated the psychophysiological correlations are consistent with well-established physiological data. Thus, for example, the stimulation of gastric secretion by sustained and unrelieved receptive urges makes sense, so to speak, physiologically, since feeding activates gastric secretion and, at the same time, probably represents the earliest gratification of receptive urges. Similarly, the presence of chronic unrelieved aggressive impulses in hypertension is consistent with certain aspects of the physiology of rage; that is, elevation of the blood pressure is an integral part, on the physiological level, of the affect of rage.

On the other hand, the exact etiological significance, in specific individual syndromes, of many of the psychodynamic conflicts which will be described here is still far from being established. It is thus possible that some of the psychodynamic configurations which are now correlated with physiological changes may themselves represent derivatives of more basic conflicts. Further careful psychoanalytic studies of patients suffering from these diseases may thus necessitate modifications in current hypotheses.

Finally, it should be noted that the role of *quantitative* (psychic-economic) factors in the development of the various syndromes is not taken into account by formulations stressing psychodynamic factors only. This is a shortcoming of practically all current psychosomatic studies and is probably due, at least in part, to the methodological difficulties encountered in dealing with quantitative factors. There is, of course, no way of "measuring" the intensity of the various impulses which participate in a conflict. However, careful psychoanalytic observation makes it possible for the analyst to estimate the *relative* strength of various instinctual forces and of the defenses against them. Economic considerations appear indispensable for a complete understanding of physiological dysfunctions. The role of quantitative factors may also help in elucidating the connection between some so-called "psychosomatic" diseases and psychosis (13, 47). Cases have been reported in which the remission of psychotic symptoms is followed by the development of psychosomatic symptoms and vice versa. This relationship has been observed between ulcerative colitis and paranoid schizophrenia and between asthma and paranoid schizophrenia.

GASTROINTESTINAL DISTURBANCES

There are few vegetative functions which play such an important role in the emotional life as does the ingestion of food. From early life on, eating is associated with the feeling of security, of receiving love and care, and also with greed, possessiveness, and envy. The neurotic conflicts centering around these basic emotions may variously contribute to disturbances of the appetite (bulimia and anorexia) and of swallowing (nervous vomiting and cardiospasm) and also to dysfunctions of the digestive system (duodenal ulcer, constipation, diarrhea). What seems to be best established is that the accentuation and inhibition of the wish to receive love and protection, being deeply associated with feeding, may activate or inhibit almost any phase in the incorporation and digestion of food. Those functions which are under the control of autonomic innervations are activated or inhibited by emotional stimuli on the principle of the conditioned reflex. This is best demonstrated by the influence of the receptive cravings upon gastric secretion, which involves the following sequence of events: the wish to receive, to be taken care of, is associated on the psychological level with the wish to be fed and, physiologically, with increased gastric secretion (5, 11).

As was emphasized above, the recognition of these psychological components of illness does not constitute the full etiological theory of gastrointestinal disturbances. Similar emotional conflicts involving dependent receptive urges are found in individuals who do not suffer from any disorder of gastrointestinal functions. Still unknown coexisting local physiological or anatomical factors must be assumed to explain pathological developments as a result of this type of emotional conflict situation. In addition, quantitative (psychic-economic) factors may also play a role in determining the precise results of such conflict situations.

The excremental functions are also connected with distinct emotional attitudes from early life onward. These have been well described by the early psychoanalytic authors, particularly by Freud, Abraham, and Jones. Possessiveness, the sense of duty and obligation, the desire to give, the hostile impulses in the form of soiling, and early infantile sexual theories about pregnancy and birth (child = feces) have all been well established in fifty years of psychoanalytic studies. All these emotional attitudes influence the functions of the gastrointestinal tract and may contribute to their dysfunctions (different forms of diarrhea and constipation).

While the influence of this type of emotional attitude upon the excremental act itself, which is under voluntary control, does not raise particularly difficult theoretical questions, their influence upon peristalsis is more obscure. Recently, Szasz (85, 86) suggested the possibility that disturbances of peristalsis of the colon and rectum may result from variations in oral tendencies, through the mediation of the gastrocolic reflex. This theory rests upon what is considered as the basic rhythm of gastrointestinal activity, viz., the sequence of events in the nursing infant—hunger, feeding, defecation, and sleep. Activation of the upper portions of the gastrointestinal tract, by parasympathetic stimulation, is generally accompanied by inhibition of the colon and rectum, whereas a decrease in vagal tonus is accompanied by increased activation of the lower bowel. According to this theory, activation of oral cravings is thought to be paralleled by an increase in vagal activity, and this leads to a relative inhibition of colonic and rectal function and thus to constipation. It is postulated that satisfaction of the oral-intaking needs (either in reality or symbolically) or, more commonly, their inhibition by guilt on account of the sadistic nature of the impulses is paralleled by a decreased vagal activity; thus, through the chain of events indicated, there is increased stimulation of the sacral parasympathetics supplying the colon and rectum, and diarrhea ensues. The foregoing mechanisms may account for the effects of oral tendencies on lower gastrointestinal functions. While the role of such "oral mechanisms" appears to be considerable in many cases of constipation and diarrhea, it is likely that so-called "anal mechanisms" may also affect the functions of the colon and rectum. In other words, anal-erotic impulses may activate reflex mechanisms originating from the ano-rectal region (95).

BRONCHIAL ASTHMA

According to French, Alexander, *et al.* (41), the inhibition of the urge to cry seems to be the nuclear emotional factor in these cases. The function of crying in the infant is to call for maternal help and attention. Later the same effect is achieved by more complex physiological functions (speech), which, like crying, involve the expiratory phase of respiration. The inhibition to confess has been established by these studies as a superimposed factor upon the inhibition to cry. The fear of being separated from mother or the maternal figure brings about the urge to regain maternal love through confession of forbidden thoughts and impulses. If this urge is inhibited, the patient who has an allergic sensitivity may respond with a typical disturbance of the respiratory function known as "asthma."

As in the field of gastrointestinal disorders, here, too, the psychological factors appear usually in combination with specific somatic factors (allergic sensitivity). The coexistence of both factors explains why in many cases the symptoms may disappear by bringing about certain changes in either one of these two types of factors—the psychological or the allergic. In most cases, only the combination of both types of factors produces the illness.

RHEUMATOID ARTHRITIS

In this condition, as in essential hypertension, the central dynamic factor is thought to be the inhibition of hostile impulses. In these cases, however, a frequent finding is also an early propensity toward the muscular expressions of aggressive impulses. At the same time, there is a consistent history in early childhood of parental restriction of locomotory freedom. Often as a rebellion against this, there is, in arthritic women, a history of tomboyishness in pre-puberty, with great stress on physical exercise, indicating the presence of intensive muscle eroticism (Johnson, Shapiro, and Alexander, 64). In these studies correlations were attempted only between psychological factors and their possible relationship to chronic muscular tension. How chronic muscular tension may participate in the pathogenesis of the disease entity known as "rheumatoid arthritis" is not clear and requires further study (49).

ESSENTIAL HYPERTENSION

Among the great variety of cardiovascular disturbances, the most extensive studies have been made on essential hypertension. A continuous struggle against hostile impulses is the central issue described by most authors who have studied this condition (Binger *et al.*, 20; Alexander, 6, 7; Saul, 76). The inhibition of aggressive self-assertive impulses is frequently due to a conflict expressed by the overcompensation of an underlying repressed excessive dependence: for example, the fear of losing the affection of others through hostile behavior. Characteristic findings are temper tantrums in early childhood and the frequently sudden change, mostly during puberty, from openly aggressive behavior to excessive control.

SYNCOPE

As emphasized by Engel (33), the term "syncope," or fainting, denotes only a symptom which may be due to a variety of causes. He also suggested that the underlying pathological processes which lead to syncope may be most conveniently classified according to three basic mechanisms: "1. Altered cerebral metabolism due to circulatory disturbances; 2. Altered cerebral metabolism due to metabolic factors; 3. Psychological mechanisms not involving any known disturbance in cerebral metabolism or circulation" (33, p. 5).

The two most common types of fainting in young adults are vasodepressor and hysterical. The physiological mechanism underlying vasodepressor syncope is that of a sudden fall in blood pressure; although the fainting reaction may be initiated in any position, extreme hypotension and unconsciousness are much more likely to occur in the erect than in the recumbent position, because of the hydrostatic effect of gravity. Psychologically, fainting of this type tends to occur in situations of fear and danger, particularly when the overt expression of fear must be suppressed. Both the physiological and the psychodynamic aspects of this syndrome were studied and described with great care by Engel and Romano (33, 34, 75). Vasodepressor syncope is thus a typical example of a vegetative neurosis. In hysterical fainting, on the other hand, there are no physiological disturbances of the cardiovascular system, and the symptom represents the substitutive or symbolic expression of a repressed instinctual impulse.

MIGRAINE

The physiological mechanisms involved in migraine have been studied by many workers, and there is general agreement concerning the role of vasomotor disturbances of the cranial arteries (93). There is disagreement, however, as to whether vasoconstriction is the primary disturbance and vasodilatation is a compensatory reaction or whether vasodilatation has an independent origin. There is also extensive literature concerning the emotional factors which may induce or contribute to these local changes in cranial blood flow. Most authors have noted the significance of repressed destructive impulses (Fromm-Reichmann, 46; Wolberg, 89; Wolff, 93). As has been stated above, the same emotional factors appear as the outstanding psychological feature in essential hypertension and in arthritis. Whether specific psychological (dynamic and economic) factors are responsible for the fact that one patient develops hypertension, another arthritis, and a third migraine headaches is still an open question. The hypothesis that the nature of the hostile impulses is important in determining the resulting physiological disturbance still needs further validation. According to Alexander (9), fully consummated aggressive behavior has three phases: (1) The conceptual phase: the preparation of the attack in fantasy, its planning and mental visualization. (2) The vegetative preparation of the body for concentrated activity. This consists in changes in metabolism and circulation. (3) The neuromuscular phase: the consummation of the aggressive act itself through co-ordinated muscular activity. The nature of the physical symptoms may depend upon the phase which is accentuated or in which the complete psychosomatic process of hostile attack becomes arrested or inhibited. If the process is arrested after the first phase, migraine headache may develop. If it progresses to the vegetative stage, hypertension may result. And if the hostile behavior is inhibited only in its last phase, namely, the actual hostile attack, arthritic symptoms will be favored. The somatic compliance resulting from vulnerability of the involved system must also be considered as a determining factor.

HYPERTHYROIDISM

The significance of emotional factors in thyrotoxicosis has long been known through numerous clinical observations. On the basis of the studies of a number of investigators (Lidz and Whitehorn, 66, 67; Conrad, 24; Mittelmann, 73; Ham et al., 54), the following features appear characteristic of this syndrome. In some cases hyperthyroidism develops suddenly following exposure to a traumatic situation; this syndrome was accordingly designated as "shock-Basedow." Usually, however, the disease develops less precipitately, and one often finds a lifelong urge toward accelerated maturation; this is thought to be a more or less specific defense against anxiety on the part of these patients (Ham et al., 55). It was accordingly suggested that this continuous urge for self-sufficiency, so dominant in these patients from early childhood onward, may constitute a chronic stimulus for thyroid function, finally leading to hyperthyroidism. The fact that the primary physiological function of the thyroid gland is closely related to growth and metabolic rate is consistent with this hypothesis. The physiological details of the mechanism—of how such continual stress may stimulate thyroid hyperfunction —remain to be explained.

DIABETES MELLITUS

Interesting psychoanalytic studies of patients with diabetes have been reported by Daniels (25) and Meyer et al. (70). It is difficult to ascertain the etiological significance of the psychological observations described in these cases. One of the chief difficulties in elucidating the psychosomatic aspects of this syndrome is the fact that the physiological mechanisms responsible for the development of diabetes are not fully understood. Present studies (Benedek, Mirsky *et al.*, 18) indicate that in this disease the typical psychological phenomenon—which appears as an insatiable oral need, similar to that seen in bulimia—may be an adaptation on the part of the organism to a probably hereditary metabolic insufficiency. Much of the psychological material observed in these cases can thus be interpreted as various defenses of the ego against the perception and demands of this excessive oral need.

FATIGUE STATES

Certain recurrent or chronic fatigue states connected with disturbances of the carbohydrate-regulating mechanisms offer in many respects an opposite picture from that found in arthritis, hypertension, and migraine. This picture consists in emotional withdrawal from activity and rebellion against the necessity for continued effort, particularly against routine work undertaken without zest. According to McCulloch, Carlson, Alexander, and Portis (69, 12), continued zest and interest, much like rage, have a stimulating effect upon carbohydrate metabolism. If the organism has to perform effort-requiring accomplishments over a prolonged period of time without interest in the performance, it appears that the promptness of the carbohydrate regulation necessary for effort suffers. This may explain why extreme fatigue attacks frequently develop in persons who have to engage in such effort-requiring activities under external or internal compulsion without having interest in their task. Attacks of fatigue are particularly likely to occur when the patient has given up hope of achieving some cherished aim.

SKIN DISEASES

Although the influence of emotional factors on diseases of the skin has been known, in one way or another, ever since biblical times (Job), precise data concerning psychophysiological interrelations in this organ-system are still relatively meager. The most extensively studied conditions are neurodermatitis, eczema, and urticaria. On the basis of psychoanalytic observations in patients with neurodermatitis, Miller (71, 72) emphasized the importance of sado-masochistic and exhibitionistic trends. Scratching, which is of paramount importance in most skin disorders, once they have developed—and may even be of some etiological importance in neurodermatitis—often expresses specific psychological conflicts; the role of both hostile and erotic (masturbatory) impulses in this activity is well established (14). In urticaria a specific correlation of the symptom with inhibited weeping has been described by Saul and Bernstein (77). Kepecs *et al.* (65) have recently described some experimental studies concerning the relationship between weeping and exudation into the skin. They found that weeping is accompanied by increased fluid secretion into the skin (using an experimentally produced blister), whereas inhibition of weeping results, first, in a drop in exudation rate, followed by a rise if the inhibition is sustained.

Itching and scratching, leading to skin changes as a result of chronic traumata to the skin, are closely related to erotization of different parts of the body (such as the anus); in such cases, scratching often provides a conscious erotic pleasure and is clearly a masturbatory equivalent.

DISTURBANCES OF SEXUAL FUNCTIONS

The existence of an intimate interrelation between emotions and sexual functions is a matter of common knowledge. Indeed, what we now consider a relatively new approach to medicine, namely, the psychosomatic approach, had already characterized the earliest psychoanalytic studies concerned with the problem of sexuality. In his essay *Three Contributions to the Theory of Sex* (42), Freud described certain behavioral manifestations of infants and children which he considered the developmental precursors of adult sexual activities. Indeed, a precise description of the "psychosexual development" of human beings was one of the first discoveries of psychoanalysis.[2] The course of the psychosexual development of the individual forms the core of the development of the entire personality (17).

For a proper understanding of disturbances of the sexual functions, precise knowledge of the normal functions of these organ-systems—as in the case of all other organ-systems—is essential. We shall not undertake a detailed presentation of this information here but will merely indicate briefly the interrelations between

2. It is of interest to note that the term "psychosexual" attempted to bridge the gap between the psychological and the somatic aspects of behavior, to which later the much-criticized term "psychosomatic" was applied.

certain endocrine functions and sexual behavior. In the male the full development of mature sexual function is dependent on the normal development of testicular function, which takes place during puberty under the influence of pituitary stimulation. The secondary sex characteristics of the male develop in response to androgenic stimulation. Similarly, in the female the development of mature sexual function depends on the activation of the ovaries by the pituitary; but, whereas in the male the testes produce but a single type of hormone, in the female there is a cyclical production of two different types of hormones—estrogens and progesterone, the hormones which control menstruation.[3]

Some disturbance of sexual function occurs in every neurosis and psychosis. A classification of such dysfunctions is, however, extremely difficult. The various terms in common usage designating sexual disturbances do not refer to syndromes or disease entities but are rather *descriptions of symptoms*.

The term "impotence" actually refers to a number of symptoms which are all characterized by some disturbance in performing the act of intercourse with orgasm. It may include such varied manifestations as lack of interest in the sexual act, inability to have or maintain an erection, premature or retarded ejaculation, or intercourse and ejaculation without orgasm, etc. From the psychological point of view, the most important conflict in all these symptoms is usually related to *castration anxiety*, that is to say, to unconscious fears connected with injury to the penis; on an even deeper unconscious level this may be equated in some cases with fears of complete annihilation and death. In addition to this basic factor—which may be regarded as a common denominator among all symptoms of sexual dysfunction—a number of other psychological factors may be of varying importance. Foremost among these is the nature of the *pregenital organization of the libido* in the particular person; in other words, the relative importance of oral, anal, urethral, skin, and other bodily areas in the childhood sexual history of the individual. In connection with this we may also mention the importance of *infantile sexual theories*, which often have the profoundest influence on the later development and manifestations of the sexual drive.

Parallel with the foregoing psychological phenomena, there occur physiological changes in the genitals which lead to the

3. For a more detailed consideration of this subject, as well as of the various psychosexual dysfunctions, see Benedek (16).

actual somatic manifestations of the disorder. The precise physiological changes responsible for many of these symptoms are still poorly understood, as, indeed, are the exact hormonal and neurophysiological control of erection and ejaculation (40). There is an intimate connection between anal, urethral, and genital functions (39).

The psychosexual dysfunctions of women may be divided into two large groups: (1) disturbances connected with the act of intercourse and (2) disturbances connected with the process of menstruation and childbearing. *Frigidity* is probably the commonest dysfunction. The psychological motivations of this symptom are analogous to those of impotence in men; they usually relate to fears of being damaged by the penis and of fears of pregnancy and childbirth. The term "frigidity," like "impotence," does not refer to any single condition but denotes a rather wide variety of phenomena, ranging from severe phobic abhorrence of intercourse and vaginismus to cases where the sexual act may be pleasurable in varying degrees but is without orgasm.

Disturbances of menstruation and childbearing are numerous and complex. The interplay between the various hormonal stimulations and emotions, as seen during the menstrual cycle, has been discussed elsewhere (17). Severe disturbances of menstruation, including complete amenorrhea, may be the physiological manifestation of severe conflicts over sexuality with profound inhibition of sexual functions.

Conflicts related to childbearing may find expression in such diverse symptoms as pseudocyesis, sterility (which may consist of an inability to conceive as well as an inability to carry a pregnancy to term), or hyperemesis gravidarum and may lead to postpartum psychosis.

One of the most significant psychosomatic studies belonging to this field is that of Benedek and Rubenstein (19). These authors attempted to correlate the psychological attitudes in women with changes in the estrogen and progesterone level occurring during the ovarian cycle. They found that increased estrogen production goes with an increased turning of libidinal interest toward heterosexual contacts. To the increased progesterone production following ovulation, on the other hand, there corresponds a turning of the libidinal charge toward the self (narcissistic regression).

It was emphasized that psychosomatic medicine, as a method of investigation, consists essentially in the combination of the investigative techniques of medicine and psychoanalysis. It follows that there is no such thing as a specific technique of psychosomatic therapy. The psychosomatic approach must rather be considered as a universal principle of medicine (one could say a medical "Weltanschauung") which should be applied to every patient, for every patient, in addition to being the carrier of a diseased organ, is also an individual human being whose emotional reactions are involved in the specific disease process. The nature of the psychophysiological interaction may vary from case to case; in some, psychological (interpersonal) stress may be etiologically related to the ensuing disease, while in others the person's emotional reactions are of an essentially reactive nature to a primarily somatic (e.g., genetic, traumatic) disease process.

Knowledge of personality development and psychodynamics is increasingly considered one of the basic sciences of medicine, to be taught to every physician. Psychopathology, at the same time, is seeking its place as a counterpart of somatic pathology. And, accordingly, psychiatric diagnosis and management are becoming indispensable in an integrated therapeutic approach to all chronic diseases. Although every physician must be able to make at least a rough psychological diagnosis, decisions concerning psychotherapy—as in the case of other specialized treatments—must rest with the psychiatric specialist. It is important to emphasize that whenever the psychological approach consists in more than providing emotional support, that is to say, whenever it attempts to penetrate behind the ego's defenses and uncover etiological factors, it is likely to activate emotional tension and cause an exacerbation of somatic symptoms. Indeed, we are only now beginning to understand the functional value of somatic illness for the total personality. Also in patients with organic disease psychological treatment may have to be supplemented by, or intelligently co-ordinated with, somatic measures, whenever the latter type of treatment is indicated. Finally, it should be noted that attempts to treat patients with certain organic diseases through psychoanalysis are of relatively recent origin and that the analysis of such patients often presents special problems, not unlike the problems encountered in the analysis of psychotic patients.

BIBLIOGRAPHY

1. ABRAHAM, KARL. "The First Pregenital Stage of the Libido," in *Selected Papers* (London: Hogarth Press, 1927), chap. xii.
2. ABRAHAM, KARL. "The Narcissistic Evaluation of Excretory Processes in Dreams and Neurosis," in *Selected Papers* (London: Hogarth Press, 1927), chap. xvii.
3. ABRAHAM, KARL. "Contributions to the Theory of the Anal Character," in *Selected Papers* (London: Hogarth Press, 1927), chap. xxiii.
4. ABRAHAM, KARL. "The Influence of Oral Erotism on Character-Formation," in *Selected Papers* (London: Hogarth Press, 1927), chap. xxiv.
5. ALEXANDER, FRANZ. *The Medical Value of Psychoanalysis* (New York: W. W. Norton & Co., 1936).
6. ALEXANDER, FRANZ. "Psychoanalytic Study of a Case of Essential Hypertension," *Psychosom. Med.*, 1:139, 1939.
7. ALEXANDER, FRANZ. "Emotional Factors in Essential Hypertension," *Psychosom. Med.*, 1:173, 1939.
8. ALEXANDER, FRANZ. "Fundamental Concepts of Psychosomatic Research: Psychogenesis, Conversion, Specificity," *Psychosom. Med.*, 5:205, 1943.
9. ALEXANDER, FRANZ. *Psychosomatic Medicine: Its Principles and Applications* (New York: W. W. Norton & Co., 1950).
10. ALEXANDER, FRANZ; FRENCH, T. M.; *et al. Studies in Psychosomatic Medicine: An Approach to the Cause and Treatment of Vegetative Disturbances* (New York: Ronald Press, 1948).
11. ALEXANDER, FRANZ, *et al.* "The Influence of Psychologic Factors upon Gastrointestinal Disturbances: A Symposium," *Psychoanalyt. Quart.*, 3:501, 1934.
12. ALEXANDER, FRANZ, and PORTIS, S. A. "A Psychosomatic Study of Hypoglycaemic Fatigue," *Psychosom. Med.*, 6:191, 1944.
13. APPEL, JESSE, and ROSEN, S. R. "Psychotic Factors in Psychosomatic Illness," *Psychosom. Med.*, 12:236, 1950.
14. BARTEMEIER, L. H. "A Psychoanalytic Study of a Case of Chronic Exudative Dermatitis," *Psychoanalyt. Quart.*, 7:216, 1938.
15. BEACH, F. A. *Hormones and Behavior: A Survey of Interrelationships between Endocrine Secretions and Patterns of Overt Response* (New York: Paul B. Hoeber, 1948).
16. BENEDEK, THERESE. "The Functions of the Sexual Apparatus and Their Disturbances," in FRANZ ALEXANDER, *Psychosomatic Medicine* (New York: W. W. Norton & Co., 1950), chap. xv.
17. BENEDEK, THERESE. "Development of the Personality," *this volume*, chap. iv.
18. BENEDEK, THERESE; MIRSKY, I. A.; *et al.* Unpublished observations.
19. BENEDEK, THERESE, and RUBENSTEIN, B. B. *The Sexual Cycle in Women: The Relation between Ovarian Function and Psychodynamic Processes* ("Psychosomatic Medicine Monographs," Vol. 3, Nos. 1 and 2 [1942]).

20. BINGER, C. A. L.; ACKERMAN, N. W.; COHN, A. E.; SCHROEDER, H. A.; and STEELE, J. H. *Personality in Arterial Hypertension* (New York: American Society for Research in Psychosomatic Problems, 1945).

21. BREUER, JOSEPH, and FREUD, SIGMUND. *Studies in Hysteria* (New York: Nervous and Mental Disease Publishing Co., 1936).

22. CANNON, W. B. *Bodily Changes in Pain, Hunger, Fear, and Rage: An Account of Recent Researches into the Function of Emotional Excitement* (New York: D. Appleton & Co., 1929).

23. CANNON, W. B. *The Wisdom of the Body* (New York: W. W. Norton & Co., 1939).

24. CONRAD, AGNES. "The Psychiatric Study of Hyperthyroid Patients," *J. Nerv. & Ment. Dis.*, 79:505, 1934.

25. DANIELS, G. E. "Analysis of a Case of Neurosis with Diabetes Mellitus," *Psychoanalyt. Quart.*, 5:513, 1936.

26. DARWIN, C. R. *The Expression of the Emotions in Man and Animals* (London: J. Murray, 1872).

27. DEUTSCH, FELIX. "Psychoanalyse und Organkrankheiten," *Internat. Ztschr. f. Psychoanal.*, 8:290, 1922.

28. DEUTSCH, FELIX. "Zur Bildung des Konversionssymptoms," *Internat. Ztschr. f. Psychoanal.*, 10:380, 1924.

29. DEUTSCH, FELIX. "Der gesunde und der kranke Körper in psychoanalytischer Betrachtung," *Internat. Ztschr. f. Psychoanal.*, 12:493, 1926.

30. DUNBAR, FLANDERS. *Psychosomatic Diagnosis* (New York: Paul B. Hoeber, 1943).

31. DUNBAR, FLANDERS. "Psychosomatic Medicine," in SANDOR LORAND (ed.), PSYCHOANALYSIS TODAY (New York: International Universities Press, 1944), pp. 23–41.

32. DUNBAR, FLANDERS. *Mind and Body: Psychosomatic Medicine* (New York: Random House, 1947).

33. ENGEL, G. L. *Fainting: Physiological and Psychological Considerations* (Springfield, Ill.: Charles C. Thomas, 1950).

34. ENGEL, G. L., and ROMANO, JOHN. "Studies of Syncope. IV. Biologic Interpretation of Vasodepressor Syncope," *Psychosom. Med.*, 9:288, 1947.

35. FENICHEL, OTTO. *The Psychoanalytic Theory of Neurosis* (New York: W. W. Norton & Co., 1945).

36. FERENCZI, SANDOR. "Disease- or Patho-neuroses," in *Further Contributions to the Theory and Technique of Psycho-analysis* (London: Hogarth Press, 1926), Paper No. 5.

37. FERENCZI, SANDOR. "The Phenomena of Hysterical Materialization," in *Further Contributions to the Theory and Technique of Psycho-analysis* (London: Hogarth Press, 1926), Paper No. 6.

38. FERENCZI, SANDOR. "Two Types of War Neuroses," in *Further Contributions to the Theory and Technique of Psycho-analysis* (London: Hogarth Press, 1926), Paper No. 11.

39. FERENCZI, SANDOR. *Thalassa: A Theory of Genitality* (New York: Psychoanalytic Quarterly, Inc., 1938).

40. FORD, C. S., and BEACH, F. A. *Patterns of Sexual Behavior* (New York: Harper & Bros., 1951).

41. FRENCH, T. M.; ALEXANDER, FRANZ; *et al. Psychogenic Factors in Bronchial Asthma*, Parts I and II (Psychosomatic Medicine Monographs, Vol. 1, No. 4; Vol. 2, Nos. 1 and 2 [1941]).

42. FREUD, SIGMUND. *Three Contributions to the Theory of Sex* (4th ed.; New York: Nervous and Mental Disease Publishing Co., 1930).

43. FREUD, SIGMUND. "Psychogenic Visual Disturbance According to Psychoanalytical Conceptions," in *Collected Papers* (London: Hogarth Press, 1925), Vol. 2, Paper No. 9.

44. FREUD, SIGMUND. *Inhibitions, Symptoms and Anxiety* (London: Hogarth Press, 1936).

45. FREUD, SIGMUND. *An Outline of Psychoanalysis* (New York: W. W. Norton & Co., 1949).

46. FROMM-REICHMANN, FRIEDA. "Contribution to the Psychogenesis of Migraine," *Psychoanalyt. Rev.*, 24:26, 1937.

47. FUNKENSTEIN, D. H. "Psychophysiologic Relationship of Asthma and Urticaria to Mental Illness," *Psychosom. Med.*, 12:377, 1950.

48. GLOVER, EDWARD. *Psycho-analysis: A Handbook for Medical Practitioners and Students of Comparative Psychology* (2d ed.; New York: Staples Press, 1949).

49. GOTTSCHALK, L. A.; SEROTA, H. M.; and SHAPIRO, L. B. "Psychologic Conflict and Neuromuscular Tension. I. Preliminary Report on a Method, as Applied to Rheumatoid Arthritis," *Psychosom. Med.*, 12:315, 1950.

50. GRACE, W. J.; WOLF, STEWART; and WOLFF, H. G. *The Human Colon* (New York: Paul B. Hoeber, 1951).

51. GRODDECK, GEORG. "Ueber die Psychoanalyse des Organischen im Menschen," *Internat. Ztschr. f. Psychoanal.*, 7:252, 1921.

52. GRODDECK, GEORG. "Traumarbeit und Arbeit des organischen Symptoms," *Internat. Ztschr. f. Psychoanal.*, 12:504, 1926.

53. GRODDECK, GEORG. *The Book of the It: Psychoanalytic Letters to a Friend* (New York: Nervous and Mental Disease Publishing Co., 1928).

54. HAM, G. C.; ALEXANDER, FRANZ; and CARMICHAEL, H. T. "A Psychosomatic Theory of Thyrotoxicosis," *Psychosom. Med.*, 13:18, 1951.

55. HINKLE, L. E., and WOLF, STEWART. "Experimental Study of Life Situations, Emotions, and the Occurrence of Acidosis in a Juvenile Diabetic," *Am. J. M. Sc.*, 217:130, 1949.

56. HINKLE, L. E.; WOLF, STEWART; *et al.* "Studies in Diabetes Mellitus: Changes in Glucose, Ketone, and Water Metabolism during Stress," in *Life Stress and Bodily Disease* (Baltimore: Williams & Wilkins Co., 1950), chap. xxii.

57. HOLLOS, STEFAN, and FERENCZI, SANDOR. *Psychoanalysis and the Psychic Disorder of General Paresis* (New York: Nervous and Mental Disease Publishing Co., 1925).

58. HOLMES, T. H.; GOODELL, HELEN; WOLF, STEWART; and WOLFF, H. G. *The Nose: An Experimental Study of Reactions within the*

Nose in Human Subjects during Varying Life Experiences (Springfield, Ill.: Charles C. Thomas, 1950).

59. JELLIFFE, S. E. "Dupuytren's Contracture and the Unconscious: A Preliminary Statement of a Problem," *Internat. Clin.*, 3:41st ser., 184, 1931.

60. JELLIFFE, S. E. "Psychoanalysis and Internal Medicine," in SANDOR LORAND (ed.), *Psychoanalysis Today* (New York: International Universities Press, 1944), pp. 12–22.

61. JELLIFFE, S. E. "Psychopathology and Organic Disease," *Arch. Neurol. & Psychiat.*, 8:639, 1922.

62. JELLIFFE, S. E. "Somatic Pathology and Psychopathology at the Encephalitis Crossroad: A Fragment," *J. Nerv. & Ment. Dis.*, 61:561, 1925.

63. JELLIFFE, S. E., and EVANS, E. "Psoriasis as an Hysterical Conversion Symbolization," *New York State J. Med.*, 104:1077, 1916.

64. JOHNSON, A. M.; SHAPIRO, L. B.; and ALEXANDER, FRANZ. "A Preliminary Report on a Psychosomatic Study of Rheumatoid Arthritis," *Psychosom. Med.*, 9:295, 1947.

65. KEPECS, J. G.; ROBIN, MILTON; and BRUNNER, M. J. "Relationship between Certain Emotional States and Exudation into the Skin," *Psychosom. Med.*, 13:10, 1951.

66. LIDZ, THEODORE. "Emotional Factors in the Etiology of Hyperthyroidism: The Report of a Preliminary Survey," *Psychosom. Med.*, 11:2, 1949.

67. LIDZ, THEODORE, and WHITEHORN, J. C. "Life Situations, Emotions, and Graves' Disease," *Psychosom. Med.*, 12:184, 1950.

68. MARGOLIN, S. G.; ORRINGER, DAVID; KAUFMAN, M. R.; *et al.* "Variations of Gastric Functions during Conscious and Unconscious Conflict States," in *Life Stress and Bodily Disease* (Baltimore: Williams & Wilkins Co., 1950), chap. xliv.

69. McCULLOCH, W. S.; CARLSON, H. B.; and ALEXANDER, FRANZ. "Zest and Carbohydrate Metabolism," in *Life Stress and Bodily Disease* (Baltimore: Williams & Wilkins Co., 1950), chap. xxiv.

70. MEYER, ALBRECHT; BOLLMEIER, L. N.; and ALEXANDER, FRANZ. "Correlation between Emotions and Carbohydrate Metabolism in Two Cases of Diabetes Mellitus," *Psychosom. Med.*, 7:335, 1945.

71. MILLER, M. L. "Psychodynamic Mechanisms in a Case of Neurodermatitis," *Psychosom. Med.*, 10:309, 1948.

72. MILLER, M. L. "A Psychological Study of a Case of Eczema and a Case of Neurodermatitis," *Psychosom. Med.*, 4:82, 1942.

73. MITTELMANN, BELA. "Psychogenic Factors and Psychotherapy in Hyperthyreosis and Rapid Heart Imbalance," *J. Nerv. & Ment. Dis.*, 77:465, 1933.

74. RIPLEY, H. S., and WOLFF, H. G. "Life Situations, Emotions, and Glaucoma," *Psychosom. Med.*, 12:215, 1950.

75. ROMANO, JOHN, and ENGEL, G. L. "Studies of Syncope. III. The Differentiation between Vasodepressor Syncope and Hysterical Fainting," *Psychosom. Med.*, 7:3, 1945.

76. Saul, L. J. "Hostility in Cases of Essential Hypertension," *Psychosom. Med.*, 1:153, 1939.

77. Saul, L. J., and Bernstein, Clarence, Jr. "The Emotional Settings of Some Attacks of Urticaria," *Psychosom. Med.*, 3:349, 1941.

78. Schilder, Paul. *The Image and Appearance of the Human Body: Studies in the Constructive Energies of the Psyche* (London: K. Paul, Trench, Trubner & Co., 1935).

79. Selye, Hans. "The General Adaptation Syndrome and the Diseases of Adaptation," *J. Clin. Endocrinol.*, 6:117, 1946.

80. Selye, Hans. *The Physiology and Pathology of Exposure to Stress: A Treatise Based on the Concepts of the General-Adaptation-Syndrome and the Diseases of Adaptation* (Montreal: Acta, Inc., 1950).

81. Stevenson, Ian. "Variations in the Secretion of Bronchial Mucus during Periods of Life Stress," in *Life Stress and Bodily Disease* (Baltimore: Williams & Wilkins Co., 1950), chap. xxxviii.

82. Stevenson, Ian, and Wolff, H. G. "Life Situations, Emotions, and Bronchial Mucus," *Psychosom. Med.*, 11:223, 1949.

83. Szasz, T. S. "Psychosomatic Aspects of Salivary Activity. I. Hypersalivation in Patients with Peptic Ulcer," in *Life Stress and Bodily Disease* (Baltimore: Williams & Wilkins Co., 1950), chap. xliii.

84. Szasz, T. S. "Psychosomatic Aspects of Salivary Activity. II. Psychoanalytic Observations concerning Hypersalivation," *Psychosom. Med.*, 12:320, 1950.

85. Szasz, T. S. "Physiologic and Psychodynamic Mechanisms in Constipation and Diarrhea," *Psychosom. Med.*, 13:112, 1951.

86. Szasz, T. S. "Oral Mechanisms in Constipation and Diarrhea," *Internat. J. Psycho-Analysis*, 32:196, 1951.

87. Szasz, T. S. "Psychoanalysis and the Autonomic Nervous System," to be published in *Psychoanalyt. Rev.*

88. Weiss, Edward, and English, O. S. *Psychosomatic Medicine* (2d ed.; Philadelphia: W. B. Saunders Co., 1949).

89. Wolberg, L. R. "Psychosomatic Correlations in Migraine: Report of a Case," *Psychiat. Quart.*, 19:60, 1945.

90. Wolf, Stewart; Pfeiffer, J. B.; Ripley, H. S.; Winter, O. S.; and Wolff, H. G. "Hypertension as a Reaction Pattern to Stress: Summary of Experimental Data on Variations in Blood Pressure and Renal Blood Flow," *Ann. Int. Med.*, 29:1056, 1948.

91. Wolf, Stewart, and Wolff, H. G. *Human Gastric Function: An Experimental Study of a Man and His Stomach* (2d ed.; New York: Oxford University Press, 1947).

92. Wolff, H. G. "Protective Reaction Patterns and Disease," *Ann. Int. Med.*, 27:944, 1947.

93. Wolff, H. G. *Headache and Other Head Pain* (New York: Oxford University Press, 1948).

94. Wolff, H. G. "Life Stress and Bodily Disease—a Formulation," in *Life Stress and Bodily Disease* (Baltimore: Williams & Wilkins Co., 1950), chap. lxix.

95. Youmans, W. B. *Nervous and Neurohumoral Regulation of Intestinal Motility* (New York: Inter-Science Publishers, 1949), chap. xvi.

INDEX OF NAMES

293

INDEX OF SUBJECTS